Evaluation and Clinical Management of Alzheimer's Disease

Evaluation and Clinical Management of Alzheimer's Disease

Editor: Blake Finn

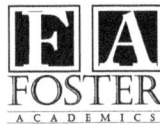

FA
FOSTER
A C A D E M I C S

www.fosteracademics.com

www.fosteracademics.com

FA
FOSTER
ACADEMICS

Cataloging-in-Publication Data

Evaluation and clinical management of Alzheimer's disease / edited by Blake Finn.
    p. cm.
Includes bibliographical references and index.
ISBN 978-1-63242-788-5
1. Alzheimer's disease. 2. Alzheimer's disease--Diagnosis. 3. Alzheimer's disease--Treatment.
4. Alzheimer's disease--Patients--Care. I. Finn, Blake.
RC523 .E83 2019
616.831--dc23

Foster Academics,
118-35 Queens Blvd., Suite 400,
Forest Hills, NY 11375, USA

ISBN 978-1-63242-788-5 (Hardback)

Contents

Preface IX

Chapter 1   What is the impact of regulatory guidance and expiry of drug patents on
            dementia drug prescriptions in England? A trend analysis in the Clinical
            Practice Research Datalink 1
            Venexia M. Walker, Neil M. Davies, Patrick G. Kehoe and Richard M. Martin

Chapter 2   Cardiorespiratory fitness attenuates age-associated aggregation of white
            matter hyperintensities in an at-risk cohort 12
            Clayton J. Vesperman, Vincent Pozorski, Ryan J. Dougherty, Lena L. Law,
            Elizabeth Boots, Jennifer M. Oh, Catherine L. Gallagher, Cynthia M. Carlsson,
            Howard A. Rowley, Yue Ma, Barbara B. Bendlin, Sanjay Asthana,
            Mark A. Sager, Bruce P. Hermann, Sterling C. Johnson, Dane B. Cook and
            Ozioma C. Okonkwo

Chapter 3   In vivo quantification of neurofibrillary tangles with [¹⁸F]MK-6240 19
            Tharick A. Pascoal, Monica Shin, Min Su Kang, Mira Chamoun,
            Daniel Chartrand, Sulantha Mathotaarachchi, Idriss Bennacef, Joseph Therriault,
            Kok Pin Ng, Robert Hopewell, Reda Bouhachi, Hung-Hsin Hsiao,
            Andrea L. Benedet, Jean-Paul Soucy, Gassan Massarweh, Serge Gauthier and
            Pedro Rosa-Neto

Chapter 4   Clinical dementia severity associated with ventricular size is differentially
            moderated by cognitive reserve in men and women 33
            Shraddha Sapkota, Joel Ramirez, Donald T. Stuss, Mario Masellis and
            Sandra E. Black

Chapter 5   Non-beta-amyloid/tau cerebrospinal fluid markers inform staging and
            progression in Alzheimer's disease 46
            Umesh Gangishetti, J. Christina Howell, Richard J. Perrin, Natalia Louneva,
            Kelly D. Watts, Alexander Kollhoff, Murray Grossman, David A. Wolk,
            Leslie M. Shaw, John C. Morris, John Q. Trojanowski, Anne M. Fagan,
            Steven E. Arnold and William T. Hu

Chapter 6   Modifiable dementia risk score to study heterogeneity in treatment effect
            of a dementia prevention trial: a post hoc analysis in the preDIVA trial using
            the LIBRA index 56
            Tessa van Middelaar, Marieke P. Hoevenaar-Blom, Willem A. van Gool,
            Eric P. Moll van Charante, Jan-Willem van Dalen, Kay Deckers,
            Sebastian Köhler and Edo Richard

Chapter 7   Does taking statins affect the pathological burden in autopsy-confirmed
            Alzheimer's dementia? 66
            Jana Crum, Jeffrey Wilson and Marwan Sabbagh

Chapter 8   Patterns of cognitive function in middle-aged and elderly Chinese
            adults—findings from the EMCOA study 72
            Yu An, Lingli Feng, Xiaona Zhang, Ying Wang, Yushan Wang, Lingwei Tao,
            Yanhui Lu, Zhongsheng Qin and Rong Xiao

Chapter 9   **Functional connectivity in cognitive control networks mitigates the impact of white matter lesions in the elderly** 89
Gloria Benson, Andrea Hildebrandt, Catharina Lange, Claudia Schwarz,
Theresa Köbe, Werner Sommer, Agnes Flöel and Miranka Wirth

Chapter 10   **The EMIF-AD PreclinAD study: study design and baseline cohort overview** 101
Elles Konijnenberg, Stephen F. Carter, Mara ten Kate, Anouk den Braber,
Jori Tomassen, Chinenye Amadi, Linda Wesselman, Hoang-Ton Nguyen,
Jacoba A. van de Kreeke, Maqsood Yaqub, Matteo Demuru, Sandra D. Mulder,
Arjan Hillebrand, Femke H. Bouwman, Charlotte E. Teunissen, Erik H. Serné,
Annette C. Moll, Frank D. Verbraak, Rainer Hinz, Neil Pendleton,
Adriaan A. Lammertsma, Bart N. M. van Berckel, Frederik Barkhof,
Dorret I. Boomsma, Philip Scheltens, Karl Herholz and Pieter Jelle Visser

Chapter 11   **Vascular Endothelial Growth Factor remains unchanged in cerebrospinal fluid of patients with Alzheimer's disease and vascular dementia** 113
Ananya Chakraborty, Madhurima Chatterjee, Harry Twaalfhoven,
Marta Del Campo Milan, Charlotte E. Teunissen, Philip Scheltens,
Ruud D. Fontijn, Wiesje M. van Der Flier and Helga E. de Vries

Chapter 12   **Exome sequencing in an Italian family with Alzheimer's disease points to a role for seizure-related gene 6 (SEZ6) rare variant R615H** 119
Lara Paracchini, Luca Beltrame, Lucia Boeri, Federica Fusco, Paolo Caffarra,
Sergio Marchini, Diego Albani and Gianluigi Forloni

Chapter 13   **Synergistic interaction between APOE and family history of Alzheimer's disease on cerebral amyloid deposition and glucose metabolism** 139
Dahyun Yi, Younghwa Lee, Min Soo Byun, Jun Ho Lee, Kang Ko,
Bo Kyung Sohn, Young Min Choe, Hyo Jung Choi, Hyewon Baek,
Chul-Ho Sohn, Yu Kyeong Kim, Dong Young Lee

Chapter 14   **Discovery and validation of autosomal dominant Alzheimer's disease mutations** 150
Simon Hsu, Brian A. Gordon, Russ Hornbeck, Joanne B. Norton, Denise Levitch,
Adia Louden, Ellen Ziegemeier, Robert Laforce Jr., Jasmeer Chhatwal,
Gregory S. Day, Eric McDade, John C. Morris, Anne M. Fagan,
Tammie L. S. Benzinger, Alison M. Goate, Carlos Cruchaga, Randall J. Bateman,
Dominantly Inherited Alzheimer Network (DIAN) and Celeste M. Karch

Chapter 15   **MRI predictors of amyloid pathology: results from the EMIF-AD Multimodal Biomarker Discovery study** 158
Mara ten Kate, Alberto Redol i, Enrico Peira, Isabelle Bos,
Stephanie J. Vos, Rik Vandenberghe, Silvy Gabel, Jolien Schaeverbeke,
Philip Scheltens, Olivier Blin, Jill C. Richardson, Regis Bordet, Anders Wallin,
Carl Eckerstrom, José Luis Molinuevo, Sebastiaan Engelborghs,
Christine Van Broeckhoven, Pablo Martinez-Lage, Julius Popp,
Magdalini Tsolaki, Frans R. J. Verhey, Alison L. Baird, Cristina Legido-Quigley,
Lars Bertram, Valerija Dobricic, Henrik Zetterberg, Simon Lovestone,
Johannes Streffer, Silvia Bianchetti, Gerald P. Novak, Jerome Revillard,
Mark F. Gordon, Zhiyong Xie, Viktor Wottschel, Giovanni Frisoni,
Pieter Jelle Visser and Frederik Barkhof

Chapter 16   **Single-word comprehension deficits in the nonfluent variant of primary progressive aphasia** 170
Jolien Schaeverbeke, Silvy Gabel, Karen Meersmans, Rose Bruffaerts,
Antonietta Gabriella Liuzzi, Charlotte Evenepoel, Eva Dries, Karen Van Bouwel,
Anne Sieben, Yolande Pijnenburg, Ronald Peeters, Guy Bormans,
Koen Van Laere, Michel Koole, Patrick Dupont and Rik Vandenberghe

Chapter 17   **Alzheimer disease pathology and the cerebrospinal fluid proteome**...........................190
Loïc Dayon, Antonio Núñez Galindo, Jérôme Wojcik, Ornella Cominetti,
John Corthésy, Aikaterini Oikonomidi, Hugues Henry, Martin Kussmann,
Eugenia Migliavacca, India Severin, Gene L. Bowman and Julius Popp

Permissions

List of Contributors

Index

Preface

Alzheimer's disease is a chronic neurodegenerative disease. Usually it begins slowly, but worsens with the passage of time. In most of the cases, it is the cause of dementia, i.e., a decrease in the ability to think and remember. Symptoms of Alzheimer's disease include short-term memory loss, mood swings, disorientation, problems with language and inability to manage self. The causes of Alzheimer's disease are found to be genetic in most of the cases. Cognitive testing with medical imaging and blood tests is often used for the purpose of diagnosis. There is no known cure for Alzheimer's disease. It is managed with pharmaceutical and psychosocial therapies. Some medications used to treat the cognitive issues linked with the disease are acetylhocholinesterase inhibitors and mematine. Psychological interventions encompass emotion-, behavior-, cognition-, and stimulation- oriented approaches. These are used along with pharmaceutical treatment. The topics included in this book on Alzheimer's disease are of utmost significance and bound to provide incredible insights to readers. It aims to shed light on some of the unexplored aspects of evaluation and management of this disease. This book will serve as a reference to a broad spectrum of readers.

The information shared in this book is based on empirical researches made by veterans in this field of study. The elaborative information provided in this book will help the readers further their scope of knowledge leading to advancements in this field.

Finally, I would like to thank my fellow researchers who gave constructive feedback and my family members who supported me at every step of my research.

Editor

What is the impact of regulatory guidance and expiry of drug patents on dementia drug prescriptions in England? A trend analysis in the Clinical Practice Research Datalink

Venexia M. Walker[1,2]*, Neil M. Davies[1,2], Patrick G. Kehoe[3,4] and Richard M. Martin[1,2]

Abstract

Background: Drugs for dementia have been available in England since 1997. Since their launch, there have been several changes to national guidelines and initiatives that may have influenced prescribing. These include changes in National Institute for Health and Care Excellence (NICE) guidance, several government dementia strategies, the addition of dementia to the Quality and Outcomes Framework (QOF), and the expiry of drug patents. Despite this, there has been little research into the effect of these events on prescribing. This paper examines prescribing trends in England using data from the U.K. Clinical Practice Research Datalink since the launch of drugs for dementia up to 1st January 2016.

Methods: We considered the monthly proportion of patients eligible for treatment, with a diagnosis of probable Alzheimer's disease, receiving their first prescription for each drug class—namely, acetylcholinesterase (AChE) inhibitors (donepezil, rivastigmine, galantamine) and N-methyl-D-aspartate (NMDA) receptor antagonists (memantine). Trend analysis using joinpoint models was then applied to identify up to two trend changes per treatment of interest.

Results: The overall trend was for increasing prescriptions in each drug class over the period in which they were studied. This was indicated by the average monthly percentage change, which was 6.0% (95% CI, − 6.4 to 19.9; June 1997 to December 2015) for AChE inhibitors and 15.4% (95% CI, − 77.1 to 480.9; January 2003 to December 2015) for NMDA receptor antagonists. Prescriptions of AChE inhibitors increased at the end of 2012, probably in response to the patent expiry of these drugs earlier that year. The Prime Minister's Dementia Challenge launched in May 2012 may also have contributed to the observed increase. However, neither this strategy nor patent expiry appeared to influence prescriptions of NMDA receptor antagonists. Instead trend changes in this drug class were driven by NICE guidance released in 2011 that allowed access to these drugs outside of clinical trials.

Conclusions: Dementia drug prescribing does not always respond to factors such as regulatory guidance, recommendations, or patent expiry, and when it does, not necessarily in a predictable way. This suggests that communication with clinicians may need to be improved to use drugs for dementia more cost-effectively.

Keywords: Alzheimer disease, Dementia, Donepezil, Rivastigmine, Galantamine, Memantine, Clinical Practice Research Datalink, National Institute for Health and Care Excellence, Quality and Outcomes Framework, England

---

* Correspondence: venexia.walker@bristol.ac.uk
[1]Bristol Medical School: Population Health Sciences, University of Bristol, Bristol, UK
[2]MRC Integrative Epidemiology Unit, University of Bristol, Bristol, UK
Full list of author information is available at the end of the article

Background

There are currently four licensed treatments that provide symptomatic relief for patients with Alzheimer's disease in England—three acetylcholinesterase (AChE) inhibitors (donepezil, rivastigmine, galantamine) and one N-methyl-D-aspartate (NMDA) receptor antagonist (memantine). These drugs are collectively referred to as *drugs for dementia* in the British National Formulary, despite their licensing for Alzheimer's disease only [1]. Since the first of these drugs became available in 1997, there have been several changes in national guidelines for the treatment of Alzheimer's disease, as well as several initiatives to encourage better diagnosis and treatment of the disease. Despite this, there has been little research into whether such changes to guidelines and initiatives have directly influenced clinical practice [2, 3]. We examined how prescription rates in England have changed since the launch of these drugs up to 1st January 2016, using data from the U.K. Clinical Practice Research Datalink (CPRD). We investigated how prescribing was affected by changes in National Institute for Health and Care Excellence (NICE) guidance (including the 2006 guidance that was subject to legal challenges), the addition of dementia to the Quality and Outcomes Framework (QOF), the introduction of ambitious government dementia strategies, and the expiry of drug patents. The timing of each of these changes, which may have influenced aspects of drug prescribing and clinical practice, is discussed further below and summarized in Table 1.

NICE guidance on the prescribing of drugs for dementia

In the past NICE guidance has used scores from the Mini Mental State Examination (MMSE), in combination with other measures, to guide whether a patient should be prescribed a drug for dementia. The test, proposed in 1975 by Folstein et al., assesses a patient's cognition out of a total possible score of 30, where normal cognition is considered as a score of 24 or more [4]. The original NICE guidance, issued in 2001, on the use of drugs to treat Alzheimer's disease recommended that the three AChE inhibitors should be used for all patients scoring 12 or above on the MMSE until the drugs were deemed no longer effective [5, 6]. In November 2006, NICE revised their guidance so that the use of AChE inhibitors was restricted to patients with moderate Alzheimer's disease; this was defined as patients scoring between 10 and 20 points on the MMSE. The 2006 guidance was also the first to consider the use of the NMDA receptor antagonist memantine, which was recommended for use only in clinical trials for patients with moderate to severe disease [7]. This revision of the guidance was controversial because of the way in which it assessed cost-effectiveness, which was expected to

Table 1 Events prior to 1st January 2016 that potentially affected prescription rates

Event date	Event
May 1997	Donepezil first recorded in CPRD
September 1998	Rivastigmine first recorded in CPRD
January 2001	Galantamine first recorded in CPRD and first NICE guidance released
December 2002	Memantine first recorded in CPRD
November 2006	NICE recommended restricting drug access
September 2007	QOF revised to include dementia
February 2009	First National Dementia Strategy launched
March 2011	NICE removed recommendation restricting drug access
January 2012	Galantamine patent expired
February 2012	Donepezil patent expired
May 2012	Prime Minister's Dementia Challenge launched
July 2012	Rivastigmine patent expired
April 2014	Memantine patent expired
February 2015	Prime Minister's Challenge on Dementia 2020 launched

CPRD Clinical Practice Research Datalink, *NICE* National Institute for Health and Care Excellence, *QOF* Quality and Outcomes Framework

restrict access to these drugs, and was ultimately the subject of a high court challenge by the Alzheimer's Society and two drug manufacturers, Eisai and Pfizer [8–10]. This led to a further revision being made to the NICE guidance at the end of March 2011, which recommended AChE inhibitors for patients with mild to moderate Alzheimer's disease and memantine for patients with moderate to severe Alzheimer's disease or who could not tolerate AChE inhibitors [11]. For the duration of our present study, treatment had to be initiated by a specialist and deemed effective as long as there has been 'an improvement or no deterioration in MMSE score, together with evidence of global improvement on the basis of behavioral and/or functional assessment' [6].

Inclusion of dementia on the QOF

QOF is a voluntary incentive program, introduced in 2004, to improve services in primary care [12]. Dementia first appeared in QOF as an 'indicator' in September 2007 [13]. There are currently three indicators for dementia included in the framework. The first requires that the practice establish and maintain a register of patients diagnosed with dementia, and the other two indicators refer to the ongoing management of the disease [14]. The inclusion of dementia on the QOF could therefore have encouraged a greater focus on the diagnosis and pharmacological management of the disease in participating practices.

Government dementia strategies

The first National Dementia Strategy was launched by the Department of Health in February 2009. The aim of that strategy was 'to ensure that significant improvements are made to dementia services across three key areas: improved awareness, earlier diagnosis and intervention, and a higher quality of care' [15]. This strategy was followed in 2012 by the Prime Minister's Dementia Challenge, which looked to improve care and research by 2015, and more recently by the Prime Minister's Challenge on Dementia 2020 [16, 17]. The most recent strategy aims to build on the work of its predecessors to make England the best place for both dementia care and research. In general such strategies may help to increase the awareness of dementia for both the public and health services [18, 19].

Drug patents

The King's Fund charity found that the prescription of generic drugs over their patented alternatives has 'saved the NHS around £7.1 billion and allowed more than 490 million more items to be prescribed to patients' between 1976 and 2013 [20]. AChE inhibitors for the treatment of Alzheimer's disease became available generically from 2012, whereas NMDA receptor antagonists became available generically from 2014 (Table 2) [21]. Therefore, in recent years the cost of drugs for dementia has decreased significantly from previous years. This serves as a potential factor in rates of prescribing, particularly in publicly funded health care services such as the NHS in England.

Methods

Aim

The aim of the study was to examine prescribing trends in England from the launch of the drugs for dementia up to 1st January 2016, using data from the CPRD.

Design

This study was a joinpoint analysis of the proportion of patients eligible for treatment, with a diagnosis of 'probable Alzheimer's disease', receiving their first prescription

for the treatment of interest in each month. We defined patients as eligible for their first prescription if they had the diagnosis of interest with no previous prescription for the treatment of interest. The time period was measured in units of 1 month because this was the smallest clinically meaningful measure we could realistically define. We investigated treatment rates as a proportion of eligible patients because the underlying rate of diagnosis of Alzheimer's disease, as well as non-Alzheimer's disease and mixed dementias, has changed over time in the CPRD (Fig. 1). The joinpoint analysis used in this study has been developed for incidence rates, so prevalent drug use, which requires consideration of both incidence and continued drug use, was not studied.

The four drugs for dementia were separated according to drug class (i.e., AChE inhibitors and NMDA receptor antagonists). Exposure date was taken to be the date on which the first prescription requesting the drug(s) being considered was recorded. This allowed patients who had previously been prescribed AChE inhibitors to be included in the NMDA receptor antagonist analysis. This is necessary because NMDA receptor antagonists may be prescribed alongside AChE inhibitors and are often given to patients later in the course of their disease, potentially following exposure to AChE inhibitors.

Setting

In this study we used data from the CPRD, an ongoing U.K.-based primary care database established in 1987. The data used in this study were obtained as part of a larger project investigating whether commonly prescribed drugs can be repurposed for the prevention or treatment of Alzheimer's and other neurodegenerative diseases [22]. For this project, we sampled patients older than 40 years of age with at least 12 consecutive months of records classified as 'acceptable' by the CPRD from an 'up to standard' practice. The data were taken from the March 2016 CPRD GOLD database snapshot, which covered the period from 1st January 1987 to 29th February 2016, inclusive.

Sample

For this study, we considered the data available from 1st January 1987 to 31st December 2015, inclusive, from practices with a last data collection date in 2016; this

Table 2 Patent information for the drugs used for dementia [21]

Generic name	Patent name (manufacturer)	Drug class	Patent expiry
Donepezil	Aricept (Eisai / Pfizer)	AChE inhibitor	January 2012
Rivastigmine	Exelon (Novartis)	AChE inhibitor	February 2012
Galantamine	Reminyl (Shire)	AChE inhibitor	July 2012
Memantine	Ebixa (Lundbeck)	NMDA receptor antagonist	April 2014

AChE Acetylcholinesterase, NMDA N-methyl-D-aspartate

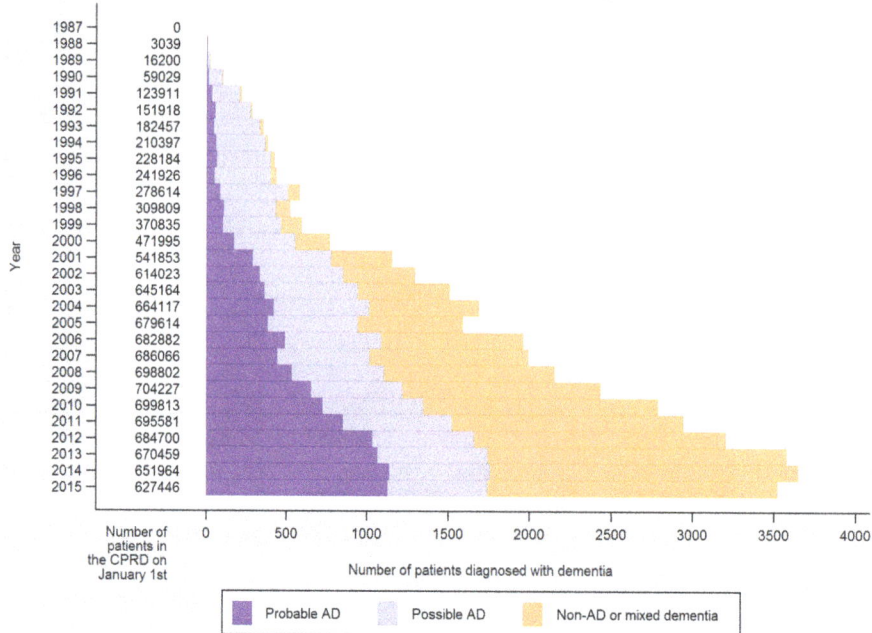

Fig. 1 Bar graph illustrating the number of patients diagnosed with dementia, by diagnosis type. The data presented are restricted to patients who received a diagnosis prior to 1st January 2016 and are from an English practice with a last data collection date in 2016 to reflect the main analysis. Definitions for each of the diagnoses are presented in Table 3.

ensured that all data were complete for the time frame being considered. We also restricted the data to English practices. This is because guidelines and initiatives can differ by nation in the United Kingdom; for example, all nations are subject to patent expiry, but the National Dementia Strategy is applicable only to England, with other nations having their own strategies. Additional file 1 presents a sensitivity analysis investigating the effect of limiting the study to practices in England. The analysis concludes that because the majority of the CPRD data is obtained from English practices and the proportion of people included in the study is similar for England and the CPRD as whole, the representativeness of the CPRD is likely to have been preserved. To be included in the study, a patient had to have a diagnosis of dementia as determined by a read or product code (see reference [23] for code lists). Read and product codes uniquely identify clinical terms and prescriptions, respectively, in the CPRD and are recorded by the general practitioner at the time of the consultation with the date [24]. The validity of codes for dementia diagnoses in the CPRD has previously been studied and was found to be in concordance with depersonalized written records relating to the diagnosis [25]. The diagnoses and their definitions as used in the present study are provided in Table 3. We used treatment to define diagnosis under the assumption that treatment implies diagnosis. Diagnosis date was taken to be the first date on which a code from any of

the lists was recorded. We performed a sensitivity analysis to test the diagnosis definitions, which is presented in full in Additional file 2. The analysis considered the sensitivity and specificity of the diagnoses in the CPRD dataset using linked data from the Office of National Statistics (ONS) death registry and the Hospital Episode Statistics (HES) inpatient dataset. We found there to be high specificity (HES, 62.9–79.1%; ONS, 57.5–75.1%) and variable sensitivity (HES, 37.3–71.6%; ONS, 36.0–80.4%). The high specificity demonstrated in this analysis reflects our conservative approach when constructing the code lists. Consequently, we expected a lower sensitivity, and this is in line with what we observed.

Analysis

The analysis of each treatment of interest started on the first day of the month following the first recorded prescription for that treatment. For example, the first prescription for NMDA receptor antagonists occurred on 16th December 2002, so the analysis of this drug class started on 1st January 2003. For each patient, we used the month and year of diagnosis (Table 3) and first prescription. For each month, we calculated the following: (A) the number of patients receiving their first prescription in that month and (B) the number of patients with a diagnosis who had not received treatment before the first of the month. Dividing A by B provided the proportion of patients with diagnoses who received their first

Table 3 Diagnosis definitions used in the study, presented with the number of patients

Diagnosis	Definition	Patients
Probable AD	Patients with one or more codes on the list 'probable AD'. Patients may also have codes on the lists 'possible AD', 'donepezil', 'rivastigmine', 'galantamine' and 'memantine'.	10,651
Possible AD	Patients with one or more codes on the list 'possible AD'. Patients may also have codes on the lists 'donepezil', 'rivastigmine', 'galantamine' and 'memantine'.	12,167
Non-AD and mixed dementias	Patients with one or more codes on any of the following lists: 'probable AD', 'possible AD', 'other dementia', 'vascular dementia', 'non-specific dementia', 'donepezil', 'rivastigmine', 'galantamine' and 'memantine', who do not meet the above criteria.	17,384

AD Alzheimer's disease

The data presented are restricted to patients who received a diagnosis prior to 1st January 2016 and are from an English practice with a last data collection date in 2016 to reflect the main analysis. The total number of patients with 'any dementia' is 40,202

prescription for the treatment of interest each month. We also calculated the SE of this proportion [26]. Trend analysis using joinpoint models was then conducted. The optimal number of joinpoints, as determined by the software and up to a maximum number of 2, was used to select the model. We refer to the period between two joinpoints as a 'segment' and number them chronologically. Our model assumes that the rate of prescription 'changes at a constant percentage of the rate of the previous year' [27] and so is determined by the following equation: $\ln y = xb$. This allows us to consider the monthly percent change. The trend over the entire study period is summarized using the average monthly percent change. This is calculated as the average of the monthly percent changes, weighted by segment length [28]. All analysis was conducted using Joinpoint Regression Program (version 4.3.1.0; National Cancer Institute, Bethesda, MD, USA) and Stata (version 14.1; Stata-Corp, College Station, TX, USA) software [29, 30]. The model specifications for the joinpoint analyses are the software's default with dependent variable type set to 'proportion' and the maximum number of join points set to 2. The Stata code used in this analysis is available from GitHub (https://github.com/venexia/DementiaDrugsCPRD) [31].

News search

Several of the national guidelines and initiatives considered in this study may have increased awareness of dementia, including Alzheimer's disease. To investigate this, we downloaded the Google Trends (https://trends.google.com/trends/) data for news searches in England for the disease term 'Alzheimer's disease' from 1st January 2008 up to 1st January 2016 [32]. Unfortunately, data were not recorded prior to 2008, so we cannot comment on the effect media coverage may have had on trend changes identified before this point in time. As with the main analysis, data were processed and plotted using Stata (version 14.1; StataCorp, College Station, TX, USA), and the code is available from GitHub (https://github.com/venexia/DementiaDrugsCPRD) [29, 30].

Results

Trend analysis for AChE inhibitors

The proportion of patients with probable Alzheimer's disease receiving their first prescription for an AChE inhibitor increased throughout the study period (Fig. 2). This is reflected in the average monthly percent change, which was 6.0 (95% CI, – 6.4 to 19.9) for the period from June 1997 to December 2015. For much of the study period, the trend was for an increasing proportion of patients to receive their first prescription for an AChE inhibitor with a monthly percent change of 5.4 (95% CI, 4.2 to 6.7). In October 2012 (95% CI; September 2011 to April 2013; $p = 0.816$), the prescription rate surged with a monthly percent change of 67.2 (95% CI, – 96.6 to 8179.8). Less than 1 year later, in May 2013 (95% CI; November 2012 to April 2014; $p = 0.789$), the trend reversed so that prescription rates were falling. In the months that followed, the monthly percent change had a value of – 1.6 (95% CI, – 10.4 to 8.1), falling below zero for the first time since the launch of these drugs.

Trend analysis for NMDA receptor antagonists

Figure 3 presents the equivalent analysis for the NMDA receptor antagonist memantine. Memantine became available in January 2003 and was prescribed much less often than the other drugs, despite similar numbers of eligible patients. This is partly related to the indication of these drugs. Memantine is generally recommended for more advanced disease than the AChE inhibitors and is often added to a prescription of AChE inhibitors following progression of the disease. Despite this, as observed for the AChE inhibitors, the proportion of patients with probable Alzheimer's disease receiving their first prescription for an NMDA receptor antagonist increased on average throughout the study period. The average monthly percent change for the period from January 2003 to December 2015 was 15.4 (95% CI, – 77.1 to 480.9), though the 95% CI around this estimate is large. The initial trend for prescribing of this drug showed a reduced number of prescriptions in the time that followed the launch with a monthly percent change of – 5.3 (95% CI, – 12.6 to 2.6). This changed around

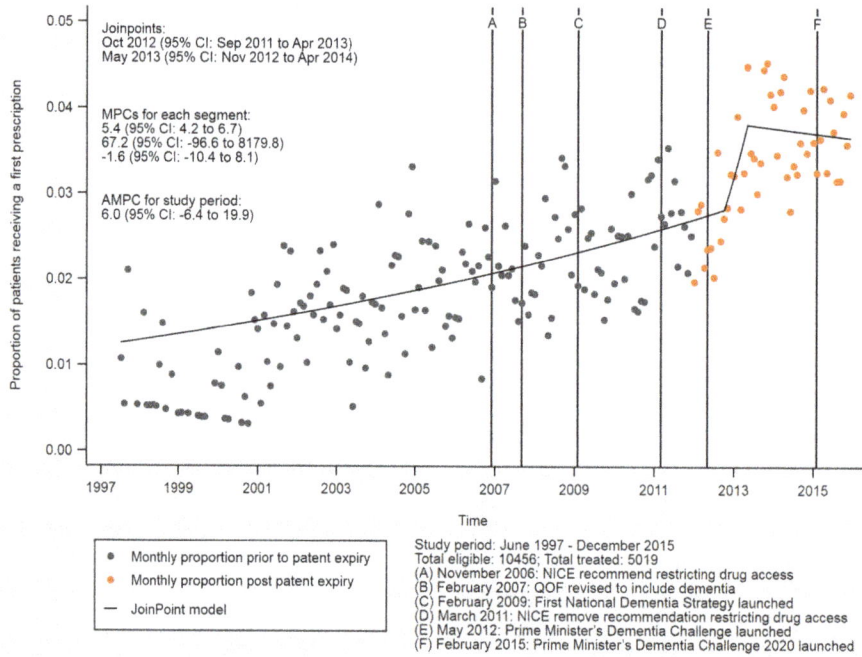

Fig. 2 Indicative graph of acetylcholinesterase (AChE) inhibitor prescriptions in patients with probable Alzheimer's disease. This graph shows the proportion of patients with probable Alzheimer's disease receiving their first prescription for an AChE inhibitor each month from June 1997 to December 2015. The fixed lines indicate events with the potential to affect prescription rates during the study period. The joinpoints, monthly percent change (MPC) for each segment, and the average monthly percent change (AMPC) for the entire study period are also presented

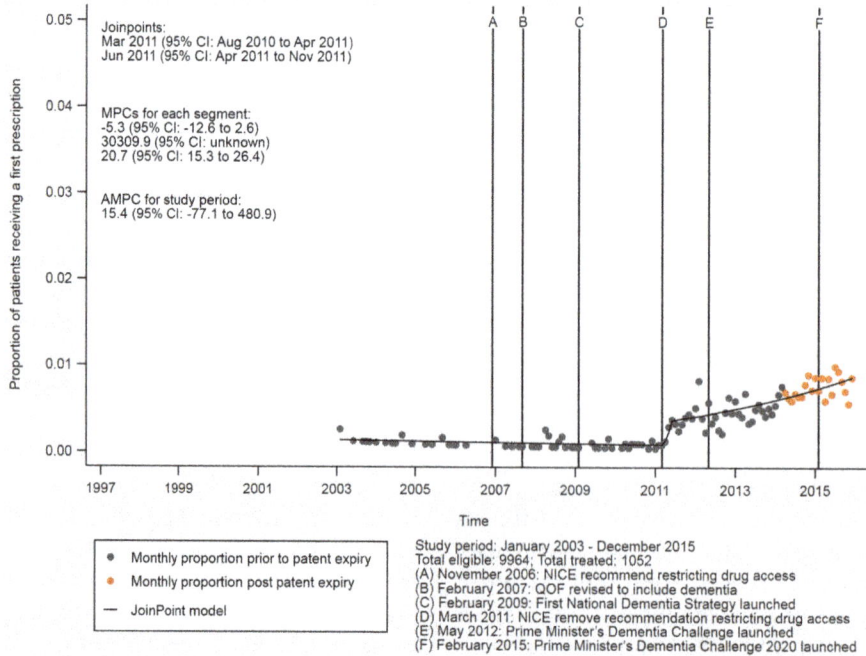

Fig. 3 Indicative graph of N-methyl-D-aspartate (NMDA) receptor antagonist prescriptions in patients with probable Alzheimer's disease. This graph shows the proportion of patients with probable Alzheimer's disease receiving their first prescription for an NMDA receptor antagonist each month from January 2003 to December 2015. The fixed lines indicate events with the potential to affect prescription rates during the study period. The joinpoints, the monthly percent change (MPC) for each segment, and the average monthly percent change (AMPC) for the study period are also presented

March 2011 (95% CI, August 2010 to April 2011, $p = 0.892$) to a very strong trend for increased prescribing. From the second trend change in June 2011 (95% CI, April 2011 to November 2011, $p = 0.896$) until the end of the study in December 2015, this trend reduced to a monthly percent change of 20.7 (95% CI, 15.3 to 26.4). This indicates a continuing increase in the prescriptions for NMDA receptor antagonists in recent years, albeit substantially reduced from the rise observed between March and June 2011. The complete output for both this analysis and that relating to AChE inhibitors is provided in Additional file 3.

Sensitivity analyses

We repeated the main analysis, which considers the diagnosis 'probable Alzheimer's disease', with relaxed diagnosis definitions to test the sensitivity of our results. We did this in two ways: (1) introducing codes that represented what may be lesser degrees of confidence in the accuracy of Alzheimer's disease diagnosis (termed *any Alzheimer's disease*) and (2) introducing codes capturing other types of dementia (termed *any dementia*). The results of these further analyses are provided in Additional file 3, and a summary of all results can be found in Table 4. For NMDA receptor antagonists, the joinpoint analysis is consistent regardless of the diagnosis definition used. However, for AChE inhibitors, the joinpoint analysis varies according to the diagnosis definition used, though the two sensitivity analyses are reasonably consistent with each other.

News search

Figure 4 presents the Google Trends data for news searches in England for the disease term 'Alzheimer's disease' each month from January 2008 to December 2015, inclusive. There were no strong trends in the interest for the search term, with values indicating both low and high interest occurring throughout the period studied. Months with insufficient data, indicating little interest in the search term, became less common over the period studied, with the most recent occurring in August 2015. Interest peaked in September 2012 and was also high in January 2011 (88%), January 2010 (82%) and April 2008 (81%).

Discussion

The first trend change for the proportion of patients with probable Alzheimer's disease receiving their first prescription for an AChE inhibitor occurred in October 2012 (95% CI, September 2011 to April 2013, $p = 0.816$). At this time, a long-term steadily increasing trend became a very strong increasing trend. This surge could be related to two factors. Firstly, the patents expired on the three drugs in this class in 2012—galantamine in January 2012, donepezil in February 2012 and rivastigmine in July 2012. Secondly, the Prime Minister's Dementia Challenge launched in May 2012. It is likely that the reduction in cost of these drugs, which resulted from their patents expiring, in combination with increased awareness of dementia due to the Prime Minister's Dementia Challenge, led to this substantial change in prescription rates we observed. In addition to these factors, a large amount of literature concerning AChE inhibitors had been published ahead of the revisions to the NICE guidance in 2011. Although this is unlikely to have caused the sharp surge that we observed, it could have contributed to the long-term steadily increasing trend observed prior to this change. A systematic review which covers the literature through November 2014 (i.e., after all join points identified in our analysis but 13 months before the end of our study) summarizes the literature available at that time [33]. It shows that several studies published

Table 4 Comparison of the sample sizes and joinpoint estimates, presented with 95% confidence intervals, for all analyses

	Probable AD	Any AD	Any dementia
Source	Main analysis	Additional file 3	Additional file 3
Diagnoses	Probable AD	Probable AD Possible AD	Probable AD Possible AD Non-AD and mixed dementias
AChE inhibitors	Eligible: 10,456 Treated: 5019 Joinpoint 1: Oct 2012 (Sep 2011–Apr 2013) Joinpoint 2: May 2013 (Nov 2012–Apr 2014)	Eligible: 21,342 Treated: 6449 Joinpoint 1: Jun 1999 (Apr 1998–Dec 2000) Joinpoint 2: Jun 2001 (Sep 2000–Mar 2002)	Eligible: 38,650 Treated: 9896 Joinpoint 1: Aug 2000 (Jun 1998–Nov 2000) Joinpoint 2: Jan 2001 (Sep 2000–Nov 2001)
NMDA receptor antagonists	Eligible: 9964 Treated: 1052 Joinpoint 1: Mar 2011 (Aug 2010–Apr 2011) Joinpoint 2: Jun 2011 (Apr 2011–Nov 2011)	Eligible: 18,930 Treated: 1309 Joinpoint 1: Sep 2010 (Dec 2009–Apr 2011) Joinpoint 2: Nov 2011 (Apr 2011–Mar 2012)	Eligible: 35,625 Treated: 1961 Joinpoint 1: Aug 2010 (Nov 2009–Dec 2010) Joinpoint 2: Nov 2011 (Aug 2011–Mar 2012)

AChE Acetylcholinesterase, *AD* Alzheimer's disease, *NMDA* N-methyl-ᴅ-aspartate

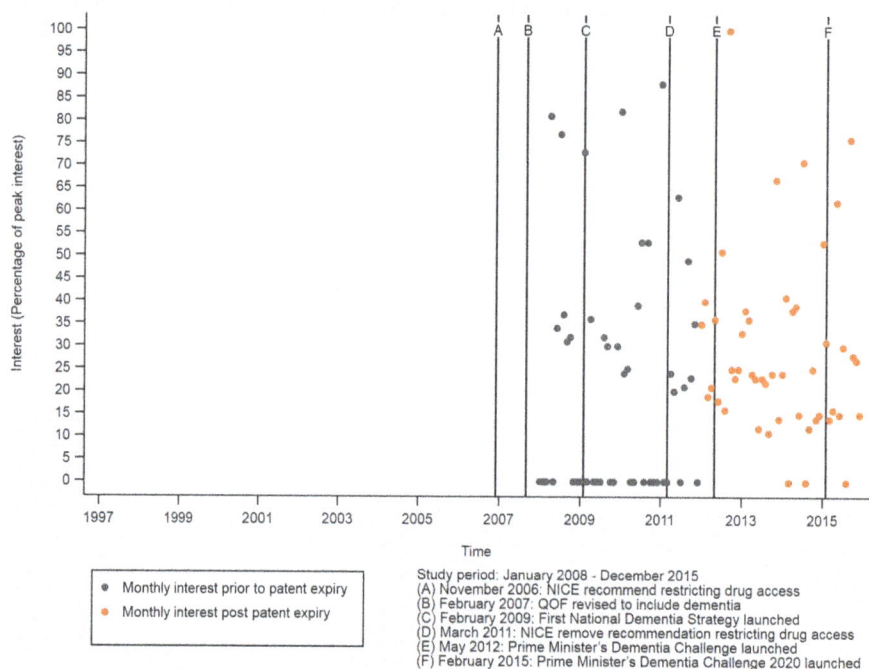

Fig. 4 Google Trends data for news searches in England for the disease term 'Alzheimer's disease'. This graph shows the interest in the disease term 'Alzheimer's disease' each month from January 2008 to December 2015, inclusive. Interest is given as a percentage scaled against peak popularity, which is represented as a value of 100% and occurred for the downloaded data in September 2012. Values of zero indicate insufficient data for that month

between 2003 and 2008 suggested that patients with mild to moderate Alzheimer's disease could benefit from AChE inhibitors with estimated 'improvements on the order of 1.5 MMSE (30-point scale)'. We therefore cannot rule out a potential effect of the literature on prescribing, even though the authors of the review questioned whether such an improvement was clinically meaningful when all the evidence was presented together. Further to the support from the literature, the Google Trends data for news searches in England also suggested increased awareness around the time of this trend change. The interest for the search term 'Alzheimer's disease' was at its maximum in September 2012 (based on the data available from January 2008 to December 2015, inclusive), which could indicate interest among the public.

The second trend change in the AChE inhibitor analysis occurred in May 2013 (95% CI, November 2012 to April 2014, $p = 0.789$), less than 1 year after the initial change for this drug class and with overlapping 95% CIs. This change signals the end of the surge in prescribing and the start of a decreasing trend in prescriptions. This is not unexpected, because patent expiry may have led to a form of 'catch-up prescribing' whereby people who were previously denied access to the drug were granted access at this time owing to its newly reduced cost. This would result in the apparent decreasing trend once

'catch-up prescribing' was complete, which is suggested by the trend analysis but is not as clear when considering the raw data points. These results differ from the sensitivity analyses that considered relaxed diagnosis definitions, though the 'any Alzheimer's disease' and 'any dementia' analyses were in line with each other. This suggests that prescribing for patients with probable Alzheimer's disease was more consistent, as one might expect, across the study than for other groups. This could indicate that patients with dementias other than probable Alzheimer's disease (i.e., with unlicensed indications) were receiving these drugs and that their prescriptions were subject to change over the period studied. Further to this, large increases in prescriptions are observed as the diagnosis definition is relaxed. This could provide further evidence for the possible unlicensed use of this drug class. The literature at that time also reflects ongoing discussion concerning the benefit of these drugs for indications other than Alzheimer's disease. For example, a 2012 review by Rodda and Carter discusses their use in vascular dementia, dementia with Lewy bodies and Parkinson's disease dementia [34]. Alternatively, it could be attributed to the fluctuating course of symptoms that some people with dementia experience or increased recognition of mixed diagnoses where there is evidence of Alzheimer's disease in addition to other forms of dementia, both of which might lead to treatment changes.

The trend changes in the NMDA receptor antagonist analysis occurred in March 2011 (95% CI, August 2010 to April 2011, $p = 0.891$) and June 2011 (95% CI, April 2011 to November 2011, $p = 0.896$). Notably, the 95% CI for the first trend change ends in April 2011, which is when the 95% CI for the second trend change begins. This suggests that the trend changes may be related. The first of these trend changes marks the start of a strong increasing trend that changes to a steadily increasing trend following the second trend change. In March 2011 NICE introduced guidelines that recommended the prescription of memantine for patients with moderate to severe Alzheimer's disease or for those people who could not tolerate AChE inhibitors. This replaced existing guidelines that restricted access to memantine to patients participating in clinical trials. It would therefore seem that these trend changes relate to the transition between the existing guidelines and those introduced in March 2011. In addition, we observed the second highest peak in interest (88% of maximum interest) for the disease term 'Alzheimer's disease' in the Google Trends data for news searches in England in January 2011. In this month, the 'Final Appraisal Determination on Donepezil, galantamine, rivastigmine and memantine for the treatment of Alzheimer's disease' was released. NICE defined this document as 'the appraisal committee's final draft guidance about using a treatment or group of treatments in the NHS', which becomes guidance if not appealed [35]. The increase in news searches around this time, and its alignment with the release of the final draft guidance, supports the idea of a transition in prescribing practice due to the NICE guidance. Finally, the evidence concerning the use of memantine is summarized in a technology appraisal conducted by NICE in 2011 to support their guidance [11]. We cannot disentangle the role that this information from several studies published prior to the trend change might have played in changes to prescribing.

Interestingly, neither of the trend changes in the NMDA receptor antagonist analysis aligns with those observed for the AChE inhibitors. This suggests that the NICE guidelines, which were implemented at the same time for both drug classes, may not have been as effective for AChE inhibitors. This is likely due to the fact that these drugs were available outside of clinical trials prior to the restrictive guidelines recommended in 2006. The sensitivity analyses conducted for the NMDA receptor antagonists were consistent with these results, regardless of the diagnosis definition used. The first of the joinpoints for all NMDA receptor antagonist analyses occurred in the 7-month period between August 2010 and March 2011, and the second occurred in the 6-month period between June 2011 and November 2011. This high level of consistency across diagnosis definitions

indicates a clear pattern in prescribing, suggestive of a distinct change in practice. This provides additional support for our inferences concerning the impact of the 2011 NICE guidance on the NMDA receptor antagonist drug class.

Strengths and limitations

The key strength of this study is the large sample of primary care data with prescribing information, provided by the CPRD. The CPRD is 'broadly representative of the UK general population' and was generally comparable to the last census in 2011 for age, sex and ethnicity despite young people and smaller practices tending to be slightly underrepresented [36, 37]. Our data extract contains 40,202 patients diagnosed with dementia in England up to 1st January 2016 (note that data are restricted to practices with a last data collection date in 2016), including 10,651 with probable Alzheimer's disease and a further 12,167 with possible Alzheimer's disease. A further strength of our study is the long follow-up of patients that allowed us to consider patients who did not receive immediate treatment. This is important because pharmacological interventions for Alzheimer's disease have historically considered severity as part of the prescribing decision, so there is likely to be a treatment delay after initial diagnosis for those presenting with mild disease.

The main limitation of our study is the likelihood of missed diagnoses. This is demonstrated within our dataset, because there were 1231 patients receiving one of the treatments of interest who did not have any form of recorded dementia diagnosis. Missed diagnoses are likely to be due to (1) outdated or non-specific diagnoses (i.e., type of dementia is not updated once established), (2) diagnoses received outside of primary care (i.e., from a specialist service) and (3) unrecorded diagnoses in primary care (i.e., a diagnosis is given but not added to a record). Missed diagnoses have been explored in sensitivity analyses by testing the sensitivity and specificity of our diagnosis definitions (Additional file 2) and by relaxing the diagnosis definition from 'probable Alzheimer's disease' to include other less certain codes for the disease and other types of dementia (Additional file 3). Neither of these sensitivity analyses provided any cause for concern. A final limitation of this study is the difficulty in determining the lag time between an event and a trend change to assess the impact of the event. To allow for this, we have focused on events that are considered to be of greatest impact—for example, changes at a national level—and so we expect any effect associated with them to be evident if present. However, this prevents us from covering all the factors that may influence prescriptions for drugs for dementia during the study period; for example, we cannot comment on all papers concerning these drugs published during this time.

Conclusions

Analysis of both drug classes indicates that inclusion of dementia in QOF had no effect on prescribing trends and the other factors had mixed effects. NICE guidance on the prescribing of drugs for dementia aligned with trend changes for NMDA receptor antagonists but not AChE inhibitors. The guidance that had the noticeable effect was released in March 2011 and allowed the NMDA receptor antagonist memantine to be used outside of clinical trials. All other guidance for both this drug and AChE inhibitors, including that which recommended restricting access, did not align with trend changes. Government dementia strategies also appear to have had mixed results, with the Prime Minister's Dementia Challenge (launched May 2012) being the only strategy to align with a trend change. Although this strategy is likely to have increased awareness of dementia around the time of the October 2012 trend change for AChE inhibitors, we believe that the more likely cause of this change is the patent expiry of the drugs in this class. This will have reduced the cost of these drugs and potentially led to a surge in prescribing, such as that observed in our trend analysis. The events considered here highlight the many factors that may have influenced prescribing rates and the challenges in assessing the impact of a given event. Overall it would seem that the proportion of patients receiving prescriptions increased over the period studied, regardless of changing guidelines and other initiatives. Furthermore, given the increase in diagnoses of dementia and, more specifically, Alzheimer's disease reported in the CPRD (Fig. 1), the absolute number of prescriptions has increased considerably over the period studied.

To our knowledge, there are two other studies that have considered prescribing trends, and these were focused mainly on the impact of the National Dementia Strategy [2, 3]. Our study extends the findings of these previous studies because it considers trends since the launch of these drugs and implements a joinpoint model as a hypothesis-free approach for the factors affecting prescribing. We have observed that prescription rates in England do not always respond to factors such as regulatory guidance, recommendations or patent expiry, and when they do, not necessarily in a predictable way. This suggests that communication with clinicians may need to be improved to use drugs for dementia more cost-effectively. In addition to this, the present study provides insight into the factors that may have influenced prescription rates of drugs for dementia in England since their launch in 1997. This is essential for accurate assessment of the effectiveness of these treatments and to adjust for them in other forms of analyses, particularly as factors that may modify the rates of disease progression. This study may also help to inform the handling of regulatory guidance and recommendations concerning drugs for dementia in the future.

Abbreviations

AChE: Acetylcholinesterase; AD: Alzheimer's disease; AMPC: Average monthly percent change; CPRD: Clinical Practice Research Datalink; HES: Hospital Episode Statistics; MMSE: Mini Mental State Examination; MPC: Monthly percent change; NICE: National Institute for Health and Care Excellence; NMDA: N-methyl-D-aspartate; ONS: Office of National Statistics; QOF: Quality and Outcomes Framework

Acknowledgements

We acknowledge Dr. Elizabeth Coulthard (University of Bristol) for input during the initial stages of this study.

Funding

This work was supported by the Perros Trust and the Integrative Epidemiology Unit. The Integrative Epidemiology Unit is supported by the Medical Research Council and the University of Bristol (grant number MC_UU_12013/9). PGK has a professorship supported by the Sigmund Gestetner Foundation.

Authors' contributions

All authors contributed to planning the analysis. VMW conducted the analysis and drafted the manuscript. All other authors edited and revised the manuscript. PGK and RMM were responsible for securing the funding. All authors read and approved the final manuscript.

Competing interests

The authors declare that they have no competing interests.

Author details

[1]Bristol Medical School: Population Health Sciences, University of Bristol, Bristol, UK. [2]MRC Integrative Epidemiology Unit, University of Bristol, Bristol, UK. [3]Dementia Research Group, University of Bristol, Bristol, UK. [4]Bristol Medical School: Translational Health Sciences, University of Bristol, Bristol, UK.

References

1. British National Formulary (BNF). Section 4.11: drugs for dementia. London: BNF; 2015. https://www.medicinescomplete.com/mc/bnflegacy/current/PHP3236-dementia.htm. Accessed 11 Jan 2016

2. Donegan K, Fox N, Black N, Livingston G, Banerjee S, Burns A. Trends in diagnosis and treatment for people with dementia in the UK from 2005 to 2015: a longitudinal retrospective cohort study. Lancet Public Health. 2017;2:e149–56.

3. Mukadam N, Livingston G, Rantell K, Rickman S. Diagnostic rates and treatment of dementia before and after launch of a national dementia policy: an observational study using English national databases. BMJ Open. 2014;4:e004119.

4. Folstein MF, Folstein SE, McHugh PR. "Mini-mental state": a practical method for grading the cognitive state of patients for the clinician. J Psychiatr Res. 1975;12:189–98.

5. National Institute for Health and Care Excellence (NICE). NICE consults on revised first draft guidance on the use of drugs to treat Alzheimer's disease (including a review of existing guidance no. 19) [press release]. https://www.nice.org.uk/guidance/TA111/documents/2006001-nice-consults-on-revised-first-draft-guidance-on-the-use-of-drugs-to-treat-alzheimers-disease2. Accessed 24 Nov 2016.

6. National Institute for Health and Care Excellence (NICE). Alzheimer's disease (mild to moderate) - donepezil, galantamine, rivastigmine and memantine (part review): final scope. London: NICE; 2009. https://www.nice.org.uk/guidance/TA217/documents/alzheimers-disease-mild-to-moderate-donepezil-galantamine-rivastigmine-and-memantine-part-review-final-scope2. Accessed 6 Feb 2017

7. National Institute for Health and Care Excellence (NICE). Dementia: supporting people with dementia and their carers in health and social care. London: NICE; 2006. http://www.nice.org.uk/guidance/cg42/resources/dementia-supporting-people-with-dementia-and-their-carers-in-health-and-social-care-975443665093. Accessed 6 Feb 2017.

8. Dyer C. NICE's decision on dementia drugs was "irrational," High Court is told. BMJ. 2007;334:1337.

9. Kmietowicz Z. NICE hears appeals over dementia drugs. BMJ. 2006;333:165.

10. Iliffe S. The National Institute for Health and Clinical Excellence (NICE) and drug treatment for Alzheimer's disease. CNS Drugs. 2007;21:177–84.

11. National Institute for Health and Care Excellence (NICE). Donepezil, galantamine, rivastigmine and memantine for the treatment of Alzheimer's disease. NICE technology appraisal guidance 217. London: NICE; 2011. https://www.nice.org.uk/guidance/ta217/resources/donepezil-galantamine-rivastigmine-and-memantine-for-the-treatment-of-alzheimers-disease-pdf-82600254699973. Accessed 20 Nov 2017.

12. NHS Digital. Quality and Outcome Framework. 2015. http://content.digital.nhs.uk/qof. Accessed 18 Jan 2017.

13. Information Centre, Government Statistical Service. National Quality and Outcomes Framework statistics for England 2006/07. 2007. http://content.digital.nhs.uk/catalogue/PUB05997/qof-eng-06-07-bull-rep.pdf. Accessed 11 Jan 2017.

14. NHS Digital. Summary of QOF indicators. https://assets.publishing.service.gov.uk/government/uploads/system/uploads/attachment_data/file/213226/Summary-of-QOF-indicators.pdf. Accessed 18 Jan 2017.

15. Department of Health. Living well with dementia: a national dementia strategy. 2009. https://assets.publishing.service.gov.uk/government/uploads/system/uploads/attachment_data/file/168220/dh_094051.pdf. Accessed 14 Sept 2016.

16. Department of Health. Prime minister's challenge on dementia - delivering major improvements in dementia care and research by 2015. 2012. https://assets.publishing.service.gov.uk/government/uploads/system/uploads/attachment_data/file/215101/dh_133176.pdf. Accessed 16 Dec 2016.

17. Department of Health. Prime minister's challenge on dementia 2020. 2015. https://assets.publishing.service.gov.uk/government/uploads/system/uploads/attachment_data/file/414344/pm-dementia2020.pdf. Accessed 16 Dec 2016.

18. Abdi Z, Burns A. Championing of dementia in England. Alzheimers Res Ther. 2012;4:36.

19. Wortmann M. Importance of national plans for Alzheimer's disease and dementia. Alzheimers Res Ther. 2013;5:40.

20. Alderwick H, Robertson R, Appleby J, Dunn P, Maguire D. Better value in the NHS: the role of changes in clinical practice. https://www.kingsfund.org.uk/sites/default/files/field/field_publication_file/better-value-nhs-Kings-Fund-July%202015.pdf. Accessed 13 Dec 2016.

21. Boarer C, Solomons K. Acetylcholinesterase inhibitors: maximising benefits to the Surrey healthcare economy from the loss of exclusivity of donepezil, galantamine and rivastigmine in 2012–13. 2012. http://pad.res360.net/Content/Documents/Loss%20of%20patent%20exclusivity%20of%20acetylcholinesterase%20inhibitors.pdf. Accessed 16 Dec 2016.

22. Walker VM, Davies NM, Jones T, Kehoe PG, Martin RM. Can commonly prescribed drugs be repurposed for the prevention or treatment of Alzheimer's and other neurodegenerative diseases? Protocol for an observational cohort study in the UK Clinical Practice Research Datalink. BMJ Open. 2016;6:e012044.

23. Walker V, Davies N, Kehoe PG, Martin R. CPRD codes: neurodegenerative diseases and commonly prescribed drugs. 2017. https://doi.org/10.5523/bris.1plm8il42rmlo2a2fqwslwckm2. Accessed 16 Oct 2017.

24. Health & Social Care Information Centre. Read codes. http://webarchive.nationalarchives.gov.uk/20160921135209/http://systems.digital.nhs.uk/data/uktc/readcodes. Accessed 16 Dec 2016

25. Seshadri S, Zornberg GL, Derby LE, Myers MW, Jick H, Drachman DA. Postmenopausal estrogen replacement therapy and the risk of Alzheimer disease. Arch Neurol. 2001;58:435–40.

26. Statistical Methodology and Applications Branch, Surveillance Research Program, National Cancer Institute. Dependent variable—Joinpoint help system 4.5.0.1. https://surveillance.cancer.gov/help/joinpoint/setting-parameters/input-file-tab/dependent-variable. Accessed 20 Nov 2017.

27. Statistical Methodology and Applications Branch, Surveillance Research Program, National Cancer Institute. APC Definition - Joinpoint Help System 4.6.0.0. https://surveillance.cancer.gov/help/joinpoint/tech-help/frequently-asked-questions/apc-definition. Accessed 18 May 2018.

28. Kim HJ, Fay MP, Feuer EJ, Midthune DN. Permutation tests for joinpoint regression with applications to cancer rates. Stat Med. 2000;19:335–51.

29. Statistical Methodology and Applications Branch, Surveillance Research Program, National Cancer Institute. Joinpoint regression program. Bethesda, MD: National Institutes of Health; 2016.

30. StataCorp. Stata statistical software. College Station, TX: StataCorp LP; 2015.

31. Walker V. DementiaDrugsCPRD. GitHub. 2017. https://github.com/venexia/DementiaDrugsCPRD. Accessed 7 Sep 2017.

32. Google. Interest over time on Google Trends for Alzheimer's disease - England, 1/1/08–12/1/15. https://g.co/trends/TTrq9. Accessed 4 Apr 2018.

33. Buckley JS, Salpeter SR. A risk-benefit assessment of dementia medications: systematic review of the evidence. Drugs Aging. 2015;32:453–67.

34. Rodda J, Carter J. Cholinesterase inhibitors and memantine for symptomatic treatment of dementia. BMJ. 2012;344:e2986.

35. National Institute for Health and Care Excellence (NICE). Glossary. https://www.nice.org.uk/glossary?letter=f. Accessed 4 Apr 2018.

36. Herrett E, Gallagher AM, Bhaskaran K, Forbes H, Mathur R, van Staa T, et al. Data resource profile: Clinical Practice Research Datalink (CPRD). Int J Epidemiol. 2015;44:827–36.

37. Mathur R, Bhaskaran K, Chaturvedi N, Leon DA, vanStaa T, Grundy E, et al. Completeness and usability of ethnicity data in UK-based primary care and hospital databases. J Public Health (Oxf). 2014;36:684–92.

Cardiorespiratory fitness attenuates age-associated aggregation of white matter hyperintensities in an at-risk cohort

Clayton J. Vesperman[1,2] (iD), Vincent Pozorski[1,5], Ryan J. Dougherty[2,4], Lena L. Law[1,2], Elizabeth Boots[8,9], Jennifer M. Oh[1,2], Catherine L. Gallagher[1,2,5], Cynthia M. Carlsson[1,2,3], Howard A. Rowley[2,7], Yue Ma[2], Barbara B. Bendlin[1,2,3], Sanjay Asthana[1,2], Mark A. Sager[2,3], Bruce P. Hermann[2,3,5], Sterling C. Johnson[1,2,3], Dane B. Cook[4,6] and Ozioma C. Okonkwo[1,2,3,10]*

Abstract

Background: Age is the cardinal risk factor for Alzheimer's disease (AD), and white matter hyperintensities (WMH), which are more prevalent with increasing age, may contribute to AD. Higher cardiorespiratory fitness (CRF) has been shown to be associated with cognitive health and decreased burden of AD-related brain alterations in older adults. Accordingly, the aim of this study was to determine whether CRF attenuates age-related accumulation of WMH in middle-aged adults at risk for AD.

Methods: One hundred and seven cognitively unimpaired, late-middle-aged adults from the Wisconsin Registry for Alzheimer's Prevention underwent 3 T magnetic resonance imaging and performed graded maximal treadmill exercise testing from which we calculated the oxygen uptake efficiency slope (OUES) as our measure of CRF. Total WMH were quantified using the Lesion Segmentation Tool and scaled to intracranial volume. Linear regression adjusted for APOE4 carriage, family history, body mass index, systolic blood pressure, and sex was used to examine relationships between age, WMH, and CRF.

Results: As expected, there was a significant association between age and WMH ($p < .001$). Importantly, there was a significant interaction between age and OUES on WMH ($p = .015$). Simple main effects analyses revealed that the effect of age on WMH remained significant in the Low OUES group ($p < .001$) but not in the High OUES group ($p = .540$), indicating that higher CRF attenuates the deleterious age association with WMH.

Conclusions: Higher CRF tempers the adverse effect of age on WMH. This suggests a potential pathway through which increased aerobic fitness facilitates healthy brain aging, especially among individuals at risk for AD.

Keywords: Alzheimer's disease, White matter hyperintensities, Cardiorespiratory fitness

Background

With the aging population, the number of people with Alzheimer's disease (AD) in the United States is projected to reach 13.8 million people by 2050, in the absence of preventative or curative therapies [1]. White matter hyperintensities (WMH), commonly observed in older adults, are characterized by bright areas on magnetic resonance imaging (MRI) using T2-weighted or T2 fluid-attenuated inversion recovery (FLAIR) sequences [16, 47]. WMH have been shown to predict AD earlier in life, and may be the "second hit" required to progress a person to clinical AD [8, 16, 33, 40]. Indeed, WMH are now considered by some to be a core component of AD pathophysiology, and/or caused by chronic ischemia associated with cerebral small vessel disease [9, 33]. The factors that most contribute to the development of WMH are aging and cardiovascular disease [34, 39, 49].

* Correspondence: ozioma@medicine.wisc.edu
[1]Geriatric Research Education and Clinical Center, William S. Middleton Memorial Veterans Hospital, Madison, WI 53705, USA
[2]Wisconsin Alzheimer's Disease Research Center, University of Wisconsin School of Medicine and Public Health, Madison, WI 53792, USA
Full list of author information is available at the end of the article

Cardiorespiratory fitness (CRF), an index of habitual physical activity, has been associated with preserved cognitive function and brain structure in older adults [10, 20, 21, 25, 27, 38]. It has also been associated with a lower risk of dementia in the elderly [14, 18, 46]. Interestingly, individuals with higher CRF have also been shown to have lower WMH [7, 13, 37]. This association may indicate that by leading a physically active lifestyle, an individual might slow their accumulation of WMH as they age, and thus enjoy healthier brain aging.

Although peak oxygen consumption ($VO_{2\,peak}$) is traditionally regarded as the gold standard measure for CRF [2], older adults as a whole are known to struggle with meeting the criteria for peak effort during maximal graded exercise testing (GXT). The oxygen uptake efficiency slope (OUES) was developed as an effort-independent measure of CRF that is nonetheless highly correlated with $VO_{2\,peak}$ [3, 24]. Accordingly, the OUES served as our index of CRF in this study, which examined associations between CRF, age, and WMH [19]. We hypothesized that older age would be associated with more WMH, but that higher CRF would attenuate this deleterious effect of aging on WMH.

Methods

Participants
We utilized data provided by 107 participants enrolled in an ancillary study—Fitness, Aging, and the Brain—of the Wisconsin Registry for Alzheimer's Prevention (WRAP). WRAP is a longitudinal study consisting of approximately 1500, late-middle-aged adults who were free of dementia and were between the ages of 40 and 65 years at study entry [28]. The cohort is enriched with risk factors for AD including positive family history for AD (FH) and/or apolipoprotein E ε4 allele (APOE4) carriage [28, 32, 42]. Participants were enrolled in the ancillary study if they were determined to have no MRI contraindications and could perform a GXT safely. The mean amount of time between the MRI and GXT was 1.04 ± 1.04 years. All study procedures were approved by the University of Wisconsin Institutional Review Board and each participant provided informed consent prior to participation.

Graded exercise testing
GXT was performed using a modified Balke protocol [4]. A comfortable, yet quick, walking speed was determined for each participant before testing, as a safety measure. For those able to, a walking speed of 3.5 miles per hour was used throughout the test. Every 2 min, the incline of the treadmill was increased by 2.5% until the participant reached volitional exhaustion. Oxygen uptake (VO_2), carbon dioxide production, minute ventilation (VE), heart rate, and work rate were measured continuously using a metabolic cart and two-way nonrebreathing valve (TrueOne® 2400; Parvomedics, Sandy, UT, USA). The

OUES was determined for each participant by calculating the regression slope from the linear relationship of absolute VsO_2 ($ml\cdot min^{-1}$) plotted as a function of $\log_{10}$ VE ($ml\cdot min^{-1}$) (i.e., $VO_2 = a\log_{10}VE + b$) [3]. The OUES values were then adjusted for body surface area (BSA) to account for individual differences [24]. BSA was calculated using the Mosteller formula (BSA = $0.016667 \times W^{0.5} \times H^{0.5}$). A higher OUES value (i.e., a steeper VO_2 / VE slope) indicates more efficient oxygen extraction from the cardiopulmonary system by the working skeletal muscles [3]. Because the OUES value is calculated as a regression slope, the unit is arbitrary. The OUES computation only included metabolic data collected during the GXT and excluded the warm up and recovery stages due to irregular ventilation that is often observed during those stages. We have previously shown excellent reliability (ICC = .995, $p < .001$) between OUES values calculated at 75%, 90%, and 100% of the exercise duration [19]. Therefore, we used the OUES values that sampled the entire exercise duration (100%) as the primary CRF variable for the current study.

Brain imaging acquisition
MRI scanning was performed on a GE × 750 3 T scanner (General Electric, Waukesha, WI, USA) with an eight-channel head coil and parallel imaging with the Array Spatial Sensitivity Encoding Technique. A T1-weighted volume scan was acquired in the axial plane with a 3D fast spoiled gradient-echo sequence using the following parameters: inversion time (TI) = 450 ms; repetition time (TR) = 8.2 ms; echo time (TE) = 3.2 ms; flip angle = 12°; acquisition matrix = 256 mm × 256 mm, field of view (FOV) = 256 mm; slice thickness = 1.0 mm, no gap, yielding a voxel resolution of 1 mm isometric. A 3D T2 FLAIR sequence was acquired in the sagittal plane using the following parameters: TI = 1868 ms; TR = 6000 ms; TE = 123 ms; flip angle = 90°; acquisition matrix = 256 mm × 256 mm, FOV = 256 mm; slice thickness = 2.0 mm, no gap, yielding a voxel resolution of 1 mm × 1 mm × 2 mm. Additional details have been previously described [6, 7].

White matter hyperintensities segmentation
The Lesion Segmentation Tool (LST) version 1.2.3 in SPM12 was used to calculate the total volume of WMH [43]. This toolbox is open source and uses automated segmentation with high reliability. For lesion segmentation, LST seeds lesions based on spatial and intensity probabilities from T1 images and hyperintense outliers on T2 FLAIR images. The intracranial volume (ICV) was calculated using the "reverse brain masking" method [30]. Total WMH was then divided by ICV and multiplied by 100 to obtain a measure of lesion-to-cranial

volume in percent units [6, 7, 43]. This measure served as the dependent variable in all analyses and was log-transformed to normalize its distribution, as required by the assumptions for ordinary least squares regression [45].

Statistical analysis

Multiple linear regression was used to examine relationships between CRF, age, and WMH. We first fitted a model that investigated the relationship between age and WMH while controlling for APOE4, FH, body mass index, systolic blood pressure, and sex (Model 1). These covariates were applied to account for their contributions to interindividual variations in brain size, WMH, and/or risk for AD [1, 22, 41, 48].

Next, we refitted the original model while additionally including the OUES and age × OUES terms (Model 2). The OUES and age were centered at the mean of each variable. Where significant, the age × OUES term would indicate that the effect of age on WMH differs by CRF. A significant age × OUES interaction was further interrogated using simple main effects analyses. All analyses were conducted using IBM SPSS version 24. Statistical tests were considered significant at $p < .05$.

Results

Similar to the larger WRAP cohort, many participants in this sample had a positive FH (71%) and were APOE4 positive (43%). The sample studied was 65.4% female. Other sample characteristics are presented in Table 1.

The results of Model 1 (see Table 2) revealed a strong positive association between age and WMH (β(SE) = .01 (.003); $t = 3.89$; $p < .001$). Sex was also a significant predictor of WMH (β(SE) = −.082 (.03); $t = −2.71$, $p = .008$), with men harboring less WMH burden compared to women. Of note, APOE4 was not a significant predictor of WMH (β(SE) = −.015 (.031); $t = −0.50$, $p = .620$). Similarly, FH was not a significant predictor of WMH (β(SE) = .029 (.034); $t = 0.85$, $p = .396$).

Model 2 (see Table 3) showed a significant interaction between age and CRF on WMH (β(SE) = −.000024 (.0000096); $t = −2.47$; $p = .015$). Per standard practice [12], we followed up on this interaction by conducting simple main effects analyses of the effect of age on WMH for Low OUES vs High OUES. To accomplish this, we set anchor points for Young vs Old and for Low OUES vs High OUES at one standard deviation below vs above the mean of each variable (see Table 1 for the respective values). As depicted in Fig. 1, these simple main effects analyses revealed that the effect of age on WMH accumulation remained significant in the Low OUES group (β(SE) = .19 (.043); $t = 4.41$; $p < .001$) but not in the High OUES group (β(SE) = .029 (.047); $t = 0.62$; $p = .540$).

Table 1 Background characteristics

Characteristic	Value
Age (years)	64.19 (5.85) (49.58–74.96)
Female (%)	65.40
Education (years)	16.30 (2.35) (12–22)
FH (%)	71
APOE4 (%)	43
MMSE	29.37 (1.01) (24–30)
Hypertension (%)	14.0
Diabetes (%)	1.8
Smoker (%)	34.6
Beta blocker usage (%)	6.5
BMI (kg/m^2)	27.84 (5.31) (17.65–48.03)
Systolic blood pressure (mmHg)	123.72 (15.66) (94–162)
Diastolic blood pressure (mmHg)	70.41 (9.62) (44–90)
OUES	1153.52 (290.72) (460–2290)
WMH (ml)	2.90 (5.23) (0.011–28.03)
ICV (ml)	1466.46 (140.65) (1175–1927)
Interval between MRI and GXT (years)	1.04 (1.04) (0–4.42)

All values presented as mean (standard deviation) (range) unless noted otherwise

FH family history of Alzheimer's disease, APOE4 apolipoprotein E ε4 allele carriage, MMSE Mini-Mental State Examination, BMI body mass index, OUES oxygen uptake efficiency slope, WMH white matter hyperintensities, ICV intracranial volume, MRI magnetic resonance imaging, GXT graded exercise testing

As noted earlier, our set of covariates (i.e., APOE4, FH, body mass index, systolic blood pressure) were selected based on prior evidence that they influence WMH and/or AD risk. However, in this study, none of these covariates were significantly associated with WMH at the .05 threshold (all $p \geq .124$). Therefore, we repeated our analyses after excluding these covariates. Our original findings remained essentially unchanged. That is, there remained a positive association between age and WMH (β(SE) = .01 (.002); $t = 4.3223$; $p < .001$) and there remained a significant interaction between CRF and age on WMH (β(SE) = −.000025 (.000009); $t = −2.62$;

Table 2 Association between age and WMH

Variable	β (SE)	t	p
Age	.01(.003)	3.89	<.001
Sex	−.082 (.03)	−2.71	.008
SBP	.001 (.001)	0.35	.728
FH	.029 (.034)	0.85	.396
BMI	−.001 (.003)	−0.34	.731
APOE4	−.015 (.031)	−0.50	.620

WMH white matter hyperintensities, SE standard error, SBP systolic blood pressure, FH family history of Alzheimer's disease, BMI body mass index, APOE4 apolipoprotein E ε4 allele carriage

Table 3 CRF attenuates the effect of age on WMH

Variable	β (SE)	t	p
Age	.009 (.003)	3.48	.001
Sex	−.073 (.035)	−2.07	.041
SBP	.000088 (.001)	0.091	.928
FH	.027 (.033)	0.81	.419
BMI	−.001 (.003)	−0.50	.619
APOE4	−.011 (.031)	−0.34	.732
OUES	−.000043 (.000063)	−0.68	.495
Age × OUES	−.000024 (.0000096)	−2.47	.015

CRF cardiorespiratory fitness, WMH white matter hyperintensities, SE standard error, SBP systolic blood pressure, FH family history of Alzheimer's disease, BMI body mass index, APOE4 apolipoprotein E ε4 allele carriage, OUES oxygen uptake efficiency slope

$p = .01$). For completeness sake, we opted to retain the original model that included the covariates.

Furthermore, we ran additional analyses to investigate whether our primary findings were influenced by potential confounders such as vascular risk factors (e.g., hypertension, smoking, and diabetes), beta blocker usage, and physical activity (as measured by caloric expenditure on the CHAMPS questionnaire [44]). The relationship between age and WMH remained significant when further adjusted for these covariates (β(SE) = .01 (.003); $t = 3.23$; $p = .002$). Similarly, the interaction between age and CRF on WMH also remained significant (β(SE) = −.000022 (.00001); $t = -2.22$; $p = .029$). Accordingly, we opted to retain our original findings.

Discussion

In this study, we found that older age was associated with greater accumulation of WMH. Importantly, our results showed that aerobic fitness attenuates the relationship between age and WMH. For those with low aerobic fitness, there was a significant difference in white matter lesion volume between younger and older participants. However, for those with high CRF, a similar deleterious effect of age on the prevalence of white matter lesions was not observed.

A prior study from our group reported that advancing age predisposes individuals to an aggregation of WMH, and that an increase in WMH is associated with decreased cognitive function [6]. Other groups have also found that WMH track with older age in the general population [15, 17, 31, 49]. Our results mirror these past findings despite the fact that our cohort is relatively younger. Of interest, we present novel results showing that CRF moderates the relationship between age and WMH. Given that WMH contributes to the clinical manifestation of AD [8, 16, 33, 40], CRF's curtailment of WMH accumulation raises the possibility that CRF may, thereby, slow progression toward the clinical syndrome of AD.

Previous reports have found significant relationships between CRF and WMH using $VO_{2\ peak}$ as the index of CRF [11, 23, 50]. As discussed earlier, although deemed the gold standard for measuring CRF, true $VO_{2\ peak}$ is often unattainable by older adults. Hence, various alternatives have been considered in the literature such as

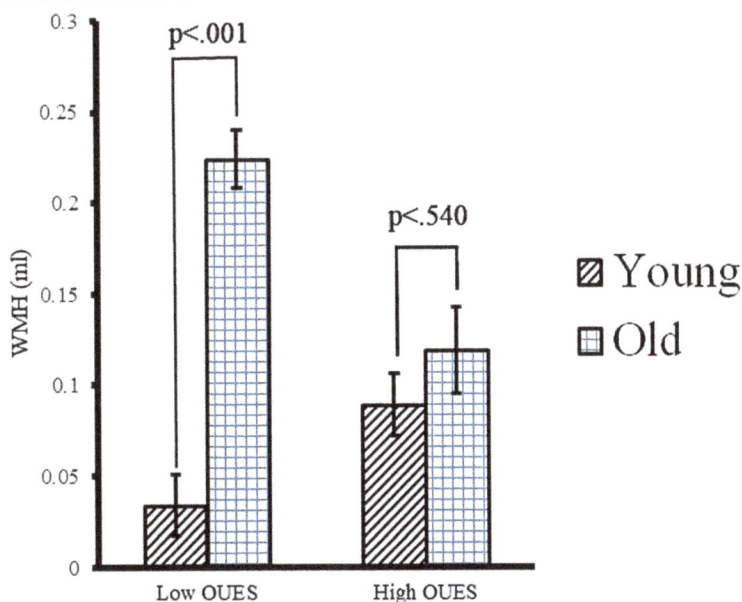

Fig. 1 Estimated WMH as a function of age and OUES. Although age and OUES were modeled as continuous variables in our analyses, to depict these simple main effects, Low OUES vs High OUES were set to one standard deviation below vs above mean OUES. Similarly, Young vs Old were set to one standard deviation below vs above mean age WMH white matter hyperintensities, OUES oxygen uptake efficiency slope

non-GXT-based measures of CRF [7, 29] and OUES [3, 24]. Consistent with our recent publication [19], our present findings support the utility of the OUES as a viable metric for CRF in older adults, and highlight its sensitivity to important health outcomes such as cerebrovascular disease, brain aging, and risk for AD.

One possible mechanism for the results found in this study relates to cerebral perfusion. Previous studies in cognitively normal individuals have shown that an increase in WMH is associated with lower cerebral blood flow [9, 36]. Also, higher cardiorespiratory fitness is associated with increased cerebral blood flow and better cognition in older adults [9, 26]. Therefore, it is possible that higher cardiorespiratory fitness may protect against reductions in cerebral blood flow with advancing age, which then translates to a reduction in WMH. A formal test of this hypothesis will be the focus of future studies from our group.

This study is not without limitations. Neither APOE4 nor FH was significantly associated with WMH in our sample, even though other studies have previously reported such associations [5, 35]. Similarly, we did not assess relationships between WMH and β-amyloid or tau, the core pathological characteristics of AD, as such an investigation was not the objective of this study. Accordingly, we cannot definitively say that interindividual variations in WMH in this sample are AD specific. Our design is cross-sectional in nature, which limits our ability to draw causal inferences. Future studies incorporating longitudinal observations would provide clearer insights into the evolution of WMH over time and how CRF affects that trajectory. Also, because the WRAP cohort is largely composed of highly educated, non-Hispanic white individuals harboring specific risk factors for AD, there is a potential restriction of the generalizability of our results to the larger population. Relatedly, WRAP participants who volunteer for additional ancillary studies might differ in unmeasured ways from those who do not (e.g., our study sample was slightly older (mean age 64.19 years) than the larger WRAP cohort (mean age 62.89 years)). Lastly, we did not have information about the physical fitness of the participants earlier in their life, so we cannot determine how that may affect their current physical fitness or our outcomes of interest.

Conclusion

We found that in a small sample at risk for AD, advancing age was associated with an accumulation of WMH. However, higher CRF attenuated this adverse impact of age on WMH. These findings contribute to the larger body of evidence highlighting the potential benefits of a physically active lifestyle, specifically as relates to improved cerebrovascular health and healthier brain aging.

Acknowledgements
Special thanks to the researchers and staff at the Waisman Center, University of Wisconsin–Madison, where the brain scans took place, and to participants in the Wisconsin Registry for Alzheimer's Prevention for their continued dedication.

Funding
This work was supported by National Institute on Aging grants K23 AG045957 (OCO), R21 AG051858 (OCO), R01 AG037639 (BBB), R01 AG027161 (SCJ), R01 AG021155 (SCJ), and P50 AG033514 (SA); and by a Clinical and Translational Science Award (UL1RR025011) to the University of Wisconsin, Madison. Portions of this research were supported by the Extendicare Foundation, Alzheimer's Association, Wisconsin Alumni Research Foundation, the Helen Bader Foundation, Northwestern Mutual Foundation, and from the Veterans Administration including facilities and resources at the Geriatric Research Education and Clinical Center of the William S. Middleton Memorial Veterans Hospital, Madison, WI, USA.

Authors' contributions
Study design, drafting of manuscript, and statistical analysis were done by CJV and OCO. Acquisition, analysis, and interpretation of data and critical revision of the manuscript was done by CJV, VP, RJD, LLL, EB, JMO, CLG, CMC, HAR, YM, BBB, SA, MAS, BPH, SCJ, DBC, and OCO. Funding was obtained by BBB, SCJ, SA, and OCO. All authors read and approved the final manuscript.

Consent for publication
Not applicable.

Competing interests
The data described in this manuscript have not been published in any prior reports and are not presently under consideration for possible publication by another journal. The authors do not have any conflicts of interest to report pertaining to this manuscript.

Author details
[1]Geriatric Research Education and Clinical Center, William S. Middleton Memorial Veterans Hospital, Madison, WI 53705, USA. [2]Wisconsin Alzheimer's Disease Research Center, University of Wisconsin School of Medicine and Public Health, Madison, WI 53705, USA. [3]Wisconsin Alzheimer's Institute, University of Wisconsin School of Medicine and Public Health, Madison, WI 53705, USA. [4]Department of Kinesiology, University of Wisconsin School of Education, Madison, WI 53792, USA. [5]Department of Neurology, University of Wisconsin School of Medicine and Public Health, Madison, WI 53705, USA. [6]Research Service, William S. Middleton Memorial Veterans Hospital, Madison, WI 53705, USA. [7]Department of Radiology, University of Wisconsin School of Medicine and Public Health, Madison, WI 53705, USA. [8]Department of Psychology, University of Illinois-Chicago, Chicago, IL 60607, USA. [9]Rush Alzheimer's Disease Center, Rush University Medical Center, Chicago, IL 60612, USA. [10]Department of Medicine and Alzheimer's Disease Research Center, University of Wisconsin School of Medicine and Public Health, Madison, WI 53792, USA.

References
1. Alzheimer's Association. 2016 Alzheimer's Disease Facts and Figures. 2016 Retrieved from http://www.alz.org/facts/

2. American College of Sports Medicine, Pescatello LS. ACSM's guidelines for exercise testing and prescription. 9th ed. Philadelphia: Wolters Kluwer/Lippincott Williams & Wilkins Health; 2014.

3. Baba R, Nagashima M, Goto M, Nagano Y, Yokota M, Tauchi N, Nishibata K. Oxygen uptake efficiency slope: a new index of cardiorespiratory functional reserve derived from the relation between oxygen uptake and minute ventilation during incremental exercise. J Am Coll Cardiol. 1996;28(6):1567–72.

4. Balke B, Ware RW. An experimental study of physical fitness of Air Force personnel. U S Armed Forces Med J. 1959;10(6):675–88.

5. Bendlin BB, Ries ML, Canu E, Sodhi A, Lazar M, Alexander AL, et al. White matter is altered with parental family history of Alzheimer's disease. Alzheimers Dement. 2010;6(5):394–403. https://doi.org/10.1016/j.jalz.2009.11.003.

6. Birdsill AC, Koscik RL, Jonaitis EM, Johnson SC, Okonkwo OC, Hermann BP, et al. Regional white matter hyperintensities: aging, Alzheimer's disease risk, and cognitive function. Neurobiol Aging. 2014;35(4):769–76. https://doi.org/10.1016/j.neurobiolaging.2013.10.072.

7. Boots EA, Schultz SA, Oh JM, Larson J, Edwards D, Cook D, et al. Cardiorespiratory fitness is associated with brain structure, cognition, and mood in a middle-aged cohort at risk for Alzheimer's disease. Brain Imaging Behav. 2015;9(3):639–49. https://doi.org/10.1007/s11682-014-9325-9.

8. Brickman AM, Provenzano FA, Muraskin J, Manly JJ, Blum S, Apa Z, et al. Regional white matter hyperintensity volume, not hippocampal atrophy, predicts incident Alzheimer disease in the community. Arch Neurol. 2012; 69(12):1621–7. https://doi.org/10.1001/archneurol.2012.1527.

9. Brickman AM, Zahra A, Muraskin J, Steffener J, Holland CM, Habeck C, et al. Reduction in cerebral blood flow in areas appearing as white matter hyperintensities on magnetic resonance imaging. Psychiatry Res. 2009; 172(2):117–20. https://doi.org/10.1016/j.pscychresns.2008.11.006.

10. Brown AD, McMorris CA, Longman RS, Leigh R, Hill MD, Friedenreich CM, Poulin MJ. Effects of cardiorespiratory fitness and cerebral blood flow on cognitive outcomes in older women. Neurobiol Aging. 2010;31(12):2047–57. https://doi.org/10.1016/j.neurobiolaging.2008.11.002.

11. Burzynska AZ, Chaddock-Heyman L, Voss MW, Wong CN, Gothe NP, Olson EA, et al. Physical activity and cardiorespiratory fitness are beneficial for white matter in low-fit older adults. PLoS One. 2014;9(9):e107413. https://doi.org/10.1371/journal.pone.0107413.

12. Cohen J, Cohen P, West SG, Aiken LS. Applied multiple regression/correlation analysis for behavioral sciences. 3rd ed. Mahwah: Lawrence Erlbaum Associates Publishers; 2003.

13. Colcombe SJ, Erickson KI, Raz N, Webb AG, Cohen NJ, McAuley E, Kramer AF. Aerobic fitness reduces brain tissue loss in aging humans. J Gerontol A Biol Sci Med Sci. 2003;58(2):176–80.

14. de Bruijn RF, Schrijvers EM, de Groot KA, Witteman JC, Hofman A, Franco OH, et al. The association between physical activity and dementia in an elderly population: the Rotterdam Study. Eur J Epidemiol. 2013;28(3):277–83. https://doi.org/10.1007/s10654-013-9773-3.

15. de Leeuw FE, de Groot JC, Achten E, Oudkerk M, Ramos LM, Heijboer R, et al. Prevalence of cerebral white matter lesions in elderly people: a population based magnetic resonance imaging study. The Rotterdam Scan Study. J Neurol Neurosurg Psychiatry. 2001;70(1):9–14.

16. Debette S, Markus HS. The clinical importance of white matter hyperintensities on brain magnetic resonance imaging: systematic review and meta-analysis. BMJ. 2010;341:c3666. https://doi.org/10.1136/bmj.c3666.

17. DeCarli C, Massaro J, Harvey D, Hald J, Tullberg M, Au R, et al. Measures of brain morphology and infarction in the framingham heart study: establishing what is normal. Neurobiol Aging. 2005;26(4):491–510. https://doi.org/10.1016/j.neurobiolaging.2004.05.004.

18. Defina LF, Willis BL, Radford NB, Gao A, Leonard D, Haskell WL, et al. The association between midlife cardiorespiratory fitness levels and later-life dementia: a cohort study. Ann Intern Med. 2013;158(3):162–8. https://doi.org/10.7326/0003-4819-158-3-201302050-00005.

19. Dougherty RJ, Lindheimer JB, Stegner AJ, Van Riper S, Okonkwo OC, Cook DB. An objective method to accurately measure cardiorespiratory fitness in older adults who cannot satisfy widely used oxygen consumption criteria. J Alzheimers Dis. 2018;61(2):601–11.

20. Dougherty RJ, Schultz SA, Boots EA, Ellingson LD, Meyer JD, Van Riper S, et al. Relationships between cardiorespiratory fitness, hippocampal volume, and episodic memory in a population at risk for Alzheimer's disease. Brain Behav. 2017;7(3):e00625. https://doi.org/10.1002/brb3.625.

21. Gordon BA, Rykhlevskaia EI, Brumback CR, Lee Y, Elavsky S, Konopack JF, et al. Neuroanatomical correlates of aging, cardiopulmonary fitness level,

22. Gottesman RF, Coresh J, Catellier DJ, Sharrett AR, Rose KM, Coker LH, et al. Blood pressure and white-matter disease progression in a biethnic cohort: Atherosclerosis Risk in Communities (ARIC) study. Stroke. 2010;41(1):3–8. https://doi.org/10.1161/STROKEAHA.109.566992.

23. Hayes SM, Salat DH, Forman DE, Sperling RA, Verfaellie M. Cardiorespiratory fitness is associated with white matter integrity in aging. Ann Clin Transl Neurol. 2015;2(6):688–98. https://doi.org/10.1002/acn3.204.

24. Hollenberg M, Tager IB. Oxygen uptake efficiency slope: an index of exercise performance and cardiopulmonary reserve requiring only submaximal exercise. J Am Coll Cardiol. 2000;36(1):194–201.

25. Honea RA, Thomas GP, Harsha A, Anderson HS, Donnelly JE, Brooks WM, Burns JM. Cardiorespiratory fitness and preserved medial temporal lobe volume in Alzheimer disease. Alzheimer Dis Assoc Disord. 2009;23(3):188–97. https://doi.org/10.1097/WAD.0b013e31819cb8a2.

26. Johnson NF, Gold BT, Bailey AL, Clasey JL, Hakun JG, White M, et al. Cardiorespiratory fitness modifies the relationship between myocardial function and cerebral blood flow in older adults. Neuroimage. 2016;131: 126–32. https://doi.org/10.1016/j.neuroimage.2015.05.063.

27. Johnson NF, Kim C, Clasey JL, Bailey A, Gold BT. Cardiorespiratory fitness is positively correlated with cerebral white matter integrity in healthy seniors. Neuroimage. 2012;59(2):1514–23. https://doi.org/10.1016/j.neuroimage.2011.08.032.

28. Johnson SC, Koscik RL, Jonaitis EM, Clark LR, Mueller KD, Berman SE, et al. The Wisconsin Registry for Alzheimer's Prevention: a review of findings and current directions. Alzheimers Dement (Amst). 2018;10:130–42. https://doi.org/10.1016/j.dadm.2017.11.007.

29. Jurca R, Jackson AS, LaMonte MJ, Morrow JR Jr, Blair SN, Wareham NJ, et al. Assessing cardiorespiratory fitness without performing exercise testing. Am J Prev Med. 2005;29(3):185–93. https://doi.org/10.1016/j.amepre.2005.06.004.

30. Keihaninejad S, Heckemann RA, Fagiolo G, Symms MR, Hajnal JV, Hammers A, Alzheimer's Disease Neuroimaging, I. A robust method to estimate the intracranial volume across MRI field strengths (1.5T and 3T). Neuroimage. 2010;50(4):1427–37. https://doi.org/10.1016/j.neuroimage.2010.01.064.

31. King KS, Peshock RM, Rossetti HC, McColl RW, Ayers CR, Hulsey KM, Das SR. Effect of normal aging versus hypertension, abnormal body mass index, and diabetes mellitus on white matter hyperintensity volume. Stroke. 2014;45(1): 255–7. https://doi.org/10.1161/STROKEAHA.113.003602.

32. Koscik RL, La Rue A, Jonaitis EM, Okonkwo OC, Johnson SC, Bendlin BB, et al. Emergence of mild cognitive impairment in late middle-aged adults in the wisconsin registry for Alzheimer's prevention. Dement Geriatr Cogn Disord. 2014;38(1–2):16–30. https://doi.org/10.1159/000355682.

33. Lee, S., Viqar, F., Zimmerman, M. E., Narkhede, A., Tosto, G., Benzinger, T. L., … Dominantly Inherited Alzheimer, N. White matter hyperintensities are a core feature of Alzheimer's disease: evidence from the dominantly inherited Alzheimer network. Ann Neurol, 2016 79(6), 929–939. doi:https://doi.org/10.1002/ana.24647.

34. Liao D, Cooper L, Cai J, Toole JF, Bryan NR, Hutchinson RG, Tyroler HA. Presence and severity of cerebral white matter lesions and hypertension, its treatment, and its control. The ARIC Study. Atherosclerosis Risk in Communities Study. Stroke. 1996;27(12):2262–70.

35. Lunetta, K. L., Erlich, P. M., Cuenco, K. T., Cupples, L. A., Green, R. C., Farrer, L. A., … Group, M. S. Heritability of magnetic resonance imaging (MRI) traits in Alzheimer disease cases and their siblings in the MIRAGE study. Alzheimer Dis Assoc Disord, 2007 21(2), 85–91. doi:https://doi.org/10.1097/WAD.0b013e3180653bf7.

36. Marstrand JR, Garde E, Rostrup E, Ring P, Rosenbaum S, Mortensen EL, Larsson HB. Cerebral perfusion and cerebrovascular reactivity are reduced in white matter hyperintensities. Stroke. 2002;33(4):972–6.

37. Perea RD, Vidoni ED, Morris JK, Graves RS, Burns JM, Honea RA. Cardiorespiratory fitness and white matter integrity in Alzheimer's disease. Brain Imaging Behav. 2016;10(3):660–8. https://doi.org/10.1007/s11682-015-9431-3.

38. Prakash RS, Voss MW, Erickson KI, Lewis JM, Chaddock L, Malkowski E, et al. Cardiorespiratory fitness and attentional control in the aging brain. Front Hum Neurosci. 2011;4:229. https://doi.org/10.3389/fnhum.2010.00229.

39. Prins ND, Scheltens P. White matter hyperintensities, cognitive impairment and dementia: an update. Nat Rev Neurol. 2015;11(3):157–65. https://doi.org/10.1038/nrneurol.2015.10.

40. Provenzano, F. A., Muraskin, J., Tosto, G., Narkhede, A., Wasserman, B. T., Griffith, E. Y., … Alzheimer's Disease Neuroimaging, I. White matter

hyperintensities and cerebral amyloidosis: necessary and sufficient for clinical expression of Alzheimer disease? JAMA Neurol,2013 70(4), 455–461. doi:https://doi.org/10.1001/jamaneurol.2013.1321.

41. Ruigrok AN, Salimi-Khorshidi G, Lai MC, Baron-Cohen S, Lombardo MV, Tait RJ, Suckling J. A meta-analysis of sex differences in human brain structure. Neurosci Biobehav Rev. 2014;39:34–50. https://doi.org/10.1016/j.neubiorev. 2013.12.004.

42. Sager MA, Hermann B, La Rue A. Middle-aged children of persons with Alzheimer's disease: APOE genotypes and cognitive function in the Wisconsin Registry for Alzheimer's Prevention. J Geriatr Psychiatry Neurol. 2005;18(4):245–9. https://doi.org/10.1177/0891988705281882.

43. Schmidt P, Gaser C, Arsic M, Buck D, Forschler A, Berthele A, et al. An automated tool for detection of FLAIR-hyperintense white-matter lesions in multiple sclerosis. Neuroimage. 2012;59(4):3774–83. https://doi.org/10.1016/j. neuroimage.2011.11.032.

44. Stewart AL, Mills KM, King AC, Haskell WL, Gillis D, Ritter PL. CHAMPS physical activity questionnaire for older adults: outcomes for interventions. Med Sci Sports Exerc. 2001;33(7):1126–41.

45. Tabachnick BG, Fidell LS. Using multivariate statistics. 5th ed. Boston: Pearson/Allyn & Bacon; 2007.

46. Vidoni ED, Honea RA, Billinger SA, Swerdlow RH, Burns JM. Cardiorespiratory fitness is associated with atrophy in Alzheimer's and aging over 2 years. Neurobiol Aging. 2012;33(8):1624–32. https://doi.org/10.1016/j. neurobiolaging.2011.03.016.

47. Wardlaw, J. M., Smith, E. E., Biessels, G. J., Cordonnier, C., Fazekas, F., Frayne, R., … nEuroimaging, S. T. f. R. V. c. o. Neuroimaging standards for research into small vessel disease and its contribution to ageing and neurodegeneration Lancet Neurol, 2013 12(8), 822–838. doi:https://doi.org/ 10.1016/S1474-4422(13)70124-8.

48. Windham BG, Lirette ST, Fornage M, Benjamin EJ, Parker KG, Turner ST, et al. Associations of brain structure with adiposity and changes in adiposity in a middle-aged and older biracial population. J Gerontol A Biol Sci Med Sci. 2017;72(6):825–31. https://doi.org/10.1093/gerona/glw239.

49. Yoshita M, Fletcher E, Harvey D, Ortega M, Martinez O, Mungas DM, et al. Extent and distribution of white matter hyperintensities in normal aging, MCI, and AD. Neurology. 2006;67(12):2192–8. https://doi.org/10.1212/01.wnl. 0000249119.95747.1f.

50. Zhu N, Jacobs DR Jr, Schreiner PJ, Launer LJ, Whitmer RA, Sidney S, et al. Cardiorespiratory fitness and brain volume and white matter integrity: The CARDIA Study. Neurology. 2015;84(23):2347–53. https://doi.org/10.1212/ WNL.0000000000001658.

In vivo quantification of neurofibrillary tangles with [18F]MK-6240

Tharick A. Pascoal[1,2], Monica Shin[1], Min Su Kang[1,2], Mira Chamoun[2], Daniel Chartrand[2], Sulantha Mathotaarachchi[1,2], Idriss Bennacef[3], Joseph Therriault[1], Kok Pin Ng[1], Robert Hopewell[2], Reda Bouhachi[2], Hung-Hsin Hsiao[2], Andrea L. Benedet[1], Jean-Paul Soucy[2], Gassan Massarweh[2], Serge Gauthier[1] and Pedro Rosa-Neto[1,2,4*]

Abstract

Background: Imaging agents capable of quantifying the brain's tau aggregates will allow a more precise staging of Alzheimer's disease (AD). The aim of the present study was to examine the in vitro properties as well as the in vivo kinetics, using gold standard methods, of the novel positron emission tomography (PET) tau imaging agent [18F]MK-6240.

Methods: In vitro properties of [18F]MK-6240 were estimated with autoradiography in postmortem brain tissues of 14 subjects (seven AD patients and seven age-matched controls). In vivo quantification of [18F]MK-6240 binding was performed in 16 subjects (four AD patients, three mild cognitive impairment patients, six healthy elderly individuals, and three healthy young individuals) who underwent 180-min dynamic scans; six subjects had arterial sampling for metabolite correction. Simplified approaches for [18F]MK-6240 quantification were validated using full kinetic modeling with metabolite-corrected arterial input function. All participants also underwent amyloid-PET and structural magnetic resonance imaging.

Results: In vitro [18F]MK-6240 uptake was higher in AD patients than in age-matched controls in brain regions expected to contain tangles such as the hippocampus, whereas no difference was found in the cerebellar gray matter. In vivo, [18F]MK-6240 displayed favorable kinetics with rapid brain delivery and washout. The cerebellar gray matter had low binding across individuals, showing potential for use as a reference region. A reversible two-tissue compartment model well described the time–activity curves across individuals and brain regions. Distribution volume ratios using the plasma input and standardized uptake value ratios (SUVRs) calculated after the binding approached equilibrium (90 min) were correlated and higher in mild cognitive impairment or AD dementia patients than in controls. Reliability analysis revealed robust SUVRs calculated from 90 to 110 min, while earlier time points provided inaccurate estimates.

Conclusions: This evaluation shows an [18F]MK-6240 distribution in concordance with postmortem studies and that simplified quantitative approaches such as the SUVR offer valid estimates of neurofibrillary tangle load 90 min post injection. [18F]MK-6240 is a promising tau tracer with the potential to be applied in the disease diagnosis and assessment of therapeutic interventions.

Keywords: Tau positron emission tomography, Neurofibrillary tangles, Alzheimer's disease

* Correspondence: pedro.rosa@mcgill.ca
[1]Translational Neuroimaging Laboratory, The McGill University Research Centre for Studies in Aging, 6825 LaSalle Boulevard, Verdun, QC H4H 1R3, Canada
[2]Montreal Neurological Institute, 3801 University Street, Montreal, QC H3A 2B4, Canada
Full list of author information is available at the end of the article

Background

In vivo quantification of neurofibrillary tangles constitutes a new challenge in the field of Alzheimer's disease (AD) imaging research. It is expected that reliable imaging agents that are able to accurately quantify tangles in the human brain will complement the information provided by the existing amyloid-β tracers, allowing a more precise staging of AD. In addition, these imaging agents may prove to be crucial for the enrichment of clinical trial populations with tau-positive individuals and for monitoring the efficacy of disease-modifying interventions.

Over the last few years, three classes of tau tracers have appeared as candidates to selectively measure neurofibrillary tangles in the living human brain: the derivative of pyrido-indole ([^{18}F]AV1451) [1, 2], the derivatives of aryquinoline ([^{18}F]THK5117, [^{18}F]THK5317, and [^{18}F]THK5351) [3, 4], and the derivative of phenyl/pyridinyl-butadienyl-benzothiazoles/benzothiazolium ([^{11}C]PBB3) [5]. Although these tracers have shown affinity to neurofibrillary tangles, compelling evidence suggests that off-target binding heavily influences the signal of some of them, even in cortical brain regions that are considered a target for AD. For example, in a recent in vivo study, we have shown that the binding of [^{18}F]THK5351 in regions including the cingulate, temporal, and inferior parietal cortices is strongly driven by MAO-B availability [6]. Similarly, in vitro evidence suggests that MAO-A may influence the signal of [^{18}F]AV1451 [7] and that [^{11}C]PBB3 may bind to α-synuclein pathology [8]. Furthermore, most of these tracers have shown high binding in the striatum, which is not a region where the histopathological studies show a high density of tangles in AD [9]. Thus, a tau-imaging agent with low brain off-target binding remains an unmet need in the field of AD research.

The pyrrolopyridinyl isoquinoline amine derivative [^{18}F]MK-6240 has been recently developed by Merck. [^{18}F]MK-6240 is a tracer with a subnanomolar affinity and high selectivity for neurofibrillary tangles that showed excellent physicochemical properties in a preclinical observation [7]. [^{18}F]MK-6240 has shown characteristics with the potential to fulfill the criteria for a promising new-generation tau tracer, such as reduced brain off-target binding, fast brain penetration and kinetics, and the absence of brain permeable metabolite. Here, we aim to quantify [^{18}F]MK-6240 using gold standard methods with metabolite-corrected arterial input function. In addition, we aim to validate simplified methodologies that are capable of bypassing the need for invasive arterial sampling in young and elderly cognitively healthy (CN) individuals, mild cognitive impairment (MCI) patients, and AD patients.

Methods

[^{18}F]MK-6240 autoradiography

In vitro autoradiography with [^{18}F]MK-6240 was conducted in postmortem brain samples of patients with antemortem diagnosis of AD (Consortium to Establish a Registry for Alzheimer Disease (CERAD) positive) [10]) and CN subjects (CERAD negative) obtained from the Douglas-Bell Canada Brain Bank with the approval of the Brain Bank's scientific review and Douglas Institute's research ethics boards. In total, seven AD patients and seven CN individuals were studied. Six AD and six CN individuals had the cerebellum, hippocampus, and prefrontal regions assessed (one AD p and one CN individual did not have viable hippocampal sections). One AD patient and one CN individual had their whole hemisphere sections assessed. The postmortem delay ranged from 8.5 to 18.25 h and from 17.25 to 21.25 h in AD patients and CN individuals, respectively. Briefly, flash-frozen tissues were cut into 20 m thick sections and thawed on coated microscope slides using a freezing sliding microtome (Leica CM3050 S) at − 15 °C. The samples were then air-dried, warmed up to room temperature, and preincubated with 1% bovine serum albumin in a phosphate-buffered saline solution (pH 7.4) for 10 min to remove endogenous ligands. These samples were then once more air-dried and incubated with 20.4 MBq of [^{18}F]MK-6240 in 600 ml of phosphate-buffered saline solution for an additional 150 min. Subsequently, the tissues were dipped three times in the phosphate-buffered solution and, dipped in distilled water at 4 °C and dried under a stream of cool air. Finally, the samples were exposed to a radioluminographic imaging plate (Fujifilm BA SMS2025) for 20 min and the activity in photostimulated luminescence units per mm^2 was calculated using Image-Gauge software 4.0 (Fujifilm Medical Systems, Inc.). The activity in each individual's brain region was measured in three equidistant regions of interest (ROIs) placed by an experimenter blind to clinical diagnosis. Then, an averaged value of these three ROIs was used as the final region uptake. In order to correct for background noise and nonspecific activity, this uptake was normalized to the individual's cerebellar gray matter uptake. A t test assessed the difference in uptake across diagnostic groups. Further details regarding the in vitro autoradiography methods may be found elsewhere [11].

Participants

AD and MCI patients and young and aged CN individuals were recruited after extensive clinical assessments at the McGill University Research Centre for Studies in Aging. All participants underwent a detailed neuropsychological evaluation including the Clinical Dementia Rating (CDR) and Mini-Mental State Examination (MMSE) scales, an amyloid-PET scan with [^{18}F]AZD4694 in order to assess the presence of brain AD pathophysiology, and [^{18}F]MK-6240. CN individuals had no subjective or objective cognitive impairment and a CDR of 0. MCI patients had a CDR of 0.5, subjective and objective memory impairments, and essentially normal activities of daily living. AD dementia patients had CDR equal to or greater than 1 and met the National Institute on Aging and the Alzheimer's Association criteria for probable AD [12]. None of the individuals met the criteria for other neuropsychiatric disorders.

Radiosynthesis

[18F]Fluoride was produced via the $^{18}O(p,n)^{18}F$ reaction in a water target. The target filling was transferred with a steady stream of argon into a septum-closed vial inside a hot cell, where the synthesis of [18F]MK-6240 took place. After delivery of the radioactivity, the module transferred the fluoride anion onto a quaternary methyl amine (QMA) cartridge where it was retained, and the target water was transferred into a collection vial for recycling. [18F]Fluoride was then eluted off the QMA cartridge and into the reactor with a solution of 1.35 ml of acetonitrile containing 15 ± 1 mg tetraethyl ammonium carbonate. The solution was then evaporated to dryness repeatedly with additional acetonitrile at a temperature of 95 °C, a stream of nitrogen, and reduced pressure. After 15 min, a solution of 1 mg of the MK-6240 precursor in 1 ml dimethyl sulfoxide (DMSO) was added to the reactor and was heated stepwise to 150 °C for about 20 min. During this step, the deprotected final product [18F]MK-6240 was formed. The reactor was then cooled to 70 °C, and 1.5 ml of high-pressure liquid chromatography (HPLC) solvent (20 mM sodium phosphate/ CH3CN, 78/22) was added. The resulting mixture was transferred into the injector loop of the HPLC system and purified on a Luna C18 250 mm × 10 mm 5-μM HPLC column (Phenomenex Inc.), with a flow of 5 ml/min. The desired product eluted at a retention time of about 22-24 min. The product peak was collected with a 30-ml syringe containing 18 ml of water and 50 μl of ascorbic acid. The solution was passed through a C18 Sep-Pak cartridge (Waters Corp.). The cartridge was washed with an additional 10 ml of water. The product was then eluted from the cartridge into a round flask with 5 ml of ethanol. The flask was sealed off with a vacuum piece attached to a vacuum pump, and a water bath was raised to insert the flask into hot water. The HPLC solvent was evaporated to dryness under reduced pressure, and approximately 5 ml of ethanol was added to the flask via a three-way stopcock and a line attached to the vacuum piece. The ethanol was evaporated to dryness, and if any solvent remained visible, another 5 ml of ethanol USP (United States Pharmacopeia) was added and evaporated again. The dried [18F]MK-6240 was then dissolved in 0.5 ml of ethanol and then 9.5 ml of sterile saline, and transferred into a 10-ml syringe with an attached needle. The needle was then

removed and the syringe was inserted into the female Luer lock of a sterile filter, which is part of a preassembled bulk vial. Finally, the [18F]MK-6240 was sterile filtered into the product vial. [18F]MK-6240 had an average injected dose of 241 (standard deviation (SD) = 23) MBq with a specific activity at the time of injection of 629 (SD = 330) GBq/ μmol. [18F]AZD4694 was synthesized according to the previously published literature [13], with an average injected dose of 237 (SD = 19) MBq and an average specific activity at the time of injection of 325 (SD = 480) GBq/μmol.

PET acquisitions

PET scans were performed using the Siemens high-resolution research tomograph (HRRT) PET scanner. [18F]MK-6240 images were acquired dynamically and uninterruptedly in list mode files between 0 and 180 min after the intravenous bolus injection of the tracer. [18F]MK-6240 scans were reconstructed using an ordered-subsets expectation maximization (OSEM) algorithm on a 4D volume with 52 frames (12 × 6 s, 6 × 18 s, 4 × 30 s, 5 × 60 s, 5 × 120 s, 8 × 300 s, and 12 × 600 s) [14]. [18F]AZD4694 images were acquired 40–70 min after the intravenous bolus injection of the tracer, and the scans were reconstructed with the same OSEM algorithm on a 4D volume with three frames (3 × 600 s). A 6-min transmission scan was conducted with a rotating ^{137}Cs point source at the end of each dynamic acquisition for attenuation correction. All images were subsequently corrected for dead time, decay, and both random and scattered coincidences. A head holder was used to reduce head motion during the scan time. In addition, possible movements during the scanning procedure were corrected using a coregistration-based method that performs frame realignment and compensates for emission–transmission mismatches [15].

Image processing

All participants had an anatomical 3D T1-weighted magnetic resonance imaging (MRI) scan (3 T Siemens). The image analyses were performed using the Medical Image NetCDF software toolbox (www.bic.mni.mcgill.ca/ ServicesSoftware/MINC). In brief, the T1-weighted images were corrected for field distortions, segmented, nonuniformity corrected, and processed using the CIVET pipeline [16]. Subsequently, the T1-weighted images were linearly registered to the MNI reference template space [17], whereas the PET images were automatically coregistered to the individual's MRI space. Then, the final PET linear registration was performed using the transformations obtained from the MRI to MNI linear template and the PET to T1-weighted native image. PET images were then spatially smoothed to achieve a final resolution of 8-mm full-width at half maximum. ROIs were obtained from the MNI nonlinear ICBM atlas and subsequently reoriented to the individual's linear space [18]. The ROIs were tailored from the frontal, medial prefrontal, orbitofrontal, precuneus, anterior (ACC) and posterior cingulate (PCC), lateral and mediobasal temporal, inferior parietal, parahippocampus, hippocampus, insula, occipitotemporal, occipital pole, and cerebellar cortices as well as from the striatum, the pons, and the telencephalon white matter (cerebellar white matter not included). Subsequently, the ROIs were applied to the dynamic PET frames to obtain the time–activity curve data. The parametric images and the ROI standardized uptake value ratios (SUVRs) were measured for multiple different scan time frames and were generated using the cerebellar gray matter as the reference. Amyloid-PET positivity was determined visually by two raters blind to clinical diagnosis. Further information regarding the imaging methods pipeline may be found elsewhere [19, 20].

[^{18}F]MK-6240 metabolism

During the [^{18}F]MK-6240 scans, arterial blood samples were collected with an automatic blood sampling system (Swisstrace GmbH) throughout the full scanning procedure with a pump flow rate of 5 ml/min between 0 and 10 min and 0.65 ml/min between 11 and 180 min. Additional 5 ml samples for metabolite correction were collected manually at 5, 10, 20, 40, 60, 90, 120, and 180 min. A cross-calibrated gamma well counter (Caprac, Inc.) was used to measure the radioactivity in the whole blood and in the plasma. Briefly, the manual samples were collected with a 5-ml heparinized syringe and centrifuged at 4000 rpm for 5 min at 4 °C. Then, the plasma was separated from the blood cells, and 1 ml was diluted with 1 ml of acetonitrile. The samples were vortexed and once more centrifuged at 4000 rpm for 5 min at 4 °C. Then, the supernatant was separated and filtered using a Millipore GV 13-mm-diameter filter. This supernatant plasma was injected into the HPLC system (Waters 1525 Binary HPLC pump; Waters Corp.), connected to a UV/visible detector (Waters 2489 UV/Visible Detector) and a coincidence detector (Bioscan, Inc.), with a flow rate of 1 ml/min. This dedicated radio-HPLC system used an isocratic method with a C18 analytical column (XTerra MS C18 column, 5 μm, 4.6 mm 250 mm) and a mobile phase consisting of 55% sodium acetate and 45% acetonitrile in order to provide the parent-to-metabolite ratio. The radioactivity estimated with the radio-HPLC system was denoised to reduce the instability generated by its low levels in the later time frames. After background correction and cross-calibration with the PET scanner, the blood activity was multiplied by both the plasma-to-whole blood and the parent compound fractions in order to derive the metabolite-corrected plasma input function.

[^{18}F]MK-6240 kinetic modeling

The kinetic modeling was performed using KinFit (version 1.7) and PMOD (version 3.8) software. Using the metabolite-corrected plasma input function, the kinetic parameters of [^{18}F]MK-6240 were initially quantified using a reversible two-tissue compartment model with four parameters (2T-CM4k), assuming rapid kinetics between free and nonspecifically bound tracer. For the 2T-CM4k, the total distribution volume (V_T) was measured as $V_T = (K_1 / k_2).(1 + k_3 / k_4)$ (ml/cm^3), and the binding potential (BP) was directly measured as k_3 / k_4. In this equation, K_1 (ml/cm^3/min) and k_2 (1/min) represent the transport rates for the influx and efflux of the tracer across the blood–brain barrier, and the rate constants k_3 (1/min) and k_4 (1/min) represent the exchange from the nondisplaceable (ND; free and nonspecific tracer) to the specific binding compartment and return, respectively [21]. In addition, a one-tissue compartment model (1T-CM), an irreversible 2T-CM with three fitted parameters (2T-CM3k), and a Logan linear graphical method were performed [22]. The distribution volume ratio (DVR) was calculated by dividing the V_T from a target region by the distribution volume of a region assumed to contain only free and nonspecifically bound tracer (V_{ND}; cerebellar gray matter). We assumed a fractional tissue blood volume of 5% for the aforementioned models. The simplified reference tissue model (SRTM) and the reference Logan method, both using the cerebellar gray matter as the reference, were also fitted in order to obtain DVRs ($BP_{ND} + 1$) [23–25]. A k_2' value was estimated for each individual with the SRTM and used in the reference Logan method. The model's goodness of fit was assessed with R^2 and F test, while the Akaike information criterion (AIC) was used to compare the models [26]. A t test compared AIC values from different quantification methods. We tested the similarity between models with regression analysis based on all ROIs.

Determination of the optimal time window for the SUVR calculation

[^{18}F]MK-6240 secular and peak equilibria were used to guide the determination of the first time point used for the SUVR calculation. The shortest scan duration without compromising reliability was determined by analyzing the stability of SUVRs calculated using different time durations. Finally, we validated SUVR estimates against the gold standard 2T-CM4k with the metabolite-corrected plasma input function.

The time to reach the secular equilibrium was assumed as the point at which the curves representing the ratio of the target-to-reference region reached a plateau [27]. Similarly, the peak equilibrium was calculated using specific binding curves estimated as the difference between the target and the reference regions [13], where the equilibrium was defined when dCb(specific binding) / $d(t)$ = 0. The target region used in the analyses was a composite value from the regions with the highest ligand uptake (precuneus, posterior cingulate, inferior parietal, and lateral temporal cortices), whereas the reference region was the cerebellum gray matter. The time–activity curves were normalized for the injected tracer dose and the individual's weight.

In order to assess the optimal scan duration, we tested the stability of the coefficient of variation (CV) and the intraclass correlation coefficient (ICC) in SUVRs obtained with progressive longer durations (10, 20, 30, 40, 50, and 60 min) [28, 29]. The 95% confidence interval (CI) determined the absence of change in the CV and the ICC among the different SUVR durations. For each SUVR time duration, a subject's CV was determined as the average of CVs obtained within each ROI. ICCs were determined between SUVR time durations using all individuals' ROIs. In addition, ICCs were calculated between SUVR and 2T-CM4k DVR and BP (k_3 / k_4) estimates.

Finally, we estimated the slope, intercept, and R^2 between 2T-CM4k and SUVRs measured over the 52 reconstructed time frames in order to ascertain the points with an optimal equivalence between these two methods.

Results

In vitro [18F]MK-6240 autoradiography was performed in postmortem brain tissues from seven AD patients (mean age of death 72.5 (SD = 10) years, three males) and seven CN individuals (mean age of death 70 (SD = 13) years, three males). The total brain mass was 24% lower in AD patients (mean 977 (SD = 195) g) than CN subjects (mean 1221 (SD = 112) g) ($P = 0.03$). Autoradiographs showed greater [18F]MK-6240 uptake in AD patients than in CN individuals in brain regions that were expected to contain tangles such as prefrontal and hippocampal cortices, whereas similar uptake was found in the cerebellar gray matter ($P = 0.2$) (Fig. 1).

In vivo dynamic [18F]MK-6240 acquisitions were performed in 16 individuals (four AD patients, three MCI patients, six elderly CN individuals, and three young CN individuals). The demographics and key characteristics of the in vivo population are summarized in Table 1.

Time–activity curves revealed that the radioactivity appeared rapidly in the brain with an SUV peak between

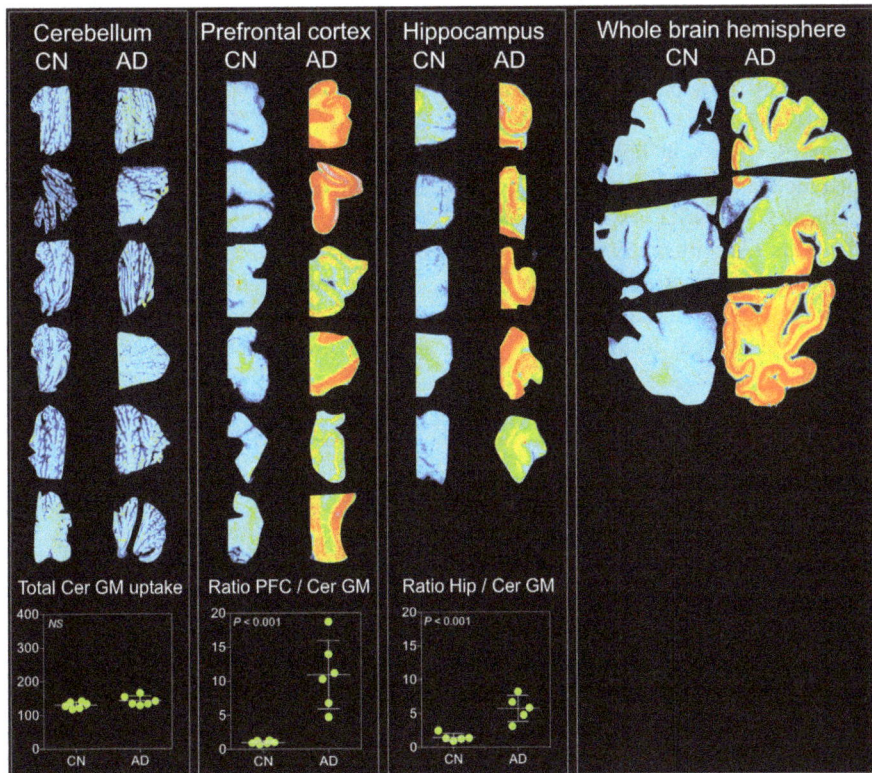

Fig. 1 [18F]MK-6240 autoradiographs of postmortem brain tissues of AD and CN individuals. In vitro autoradiography of postmortem brain tissue from prefrontal (PFC) and hippocampal (Hip) cortices as well as cerebellum and whole hemisphere of Alzheimer's disease (AD) patients and cognitively healthy (CN) individuals. Similar total uptake was found in cerebellar gray matter (Cer GM) of CN and AD individuals ($P = 0.2$). AD patients had higher relative uptake (ratio with Cer GM) than CN individuals in PFC and Hip cortices ($P < 0.001$). Total uptake was measured as photostimulated luminescence units per mm^2. NS not significant

Table 1 Demographics and key characteristics of the in vivo population

	Young CN individuals	Elderly CN individuals	MCI patients	AD patients
N	3	6	3	4
Age (years), mean (SD)	22.3 (1.5)	67.8 (8.5)	69 (3.4)	60.7 (6)
Male, n (%)	2 (67)	5 (83)	2 (67)	3 (75)
MMSE, mean (SD)	30 (0)	29.5 (0.5)	25 (2.6)	17.3 (5.8)
APOE ε4, n (%)	0 (0)	4 (67)	1 (33)	2 (50)
Amyloid-PET positive, n (%)	0 (0)	1 (17)	3 (100)	4 (100)

AD Alzheimer's disease, CN cognitively healthy, MCI mild cognitive impairment, MMSE Mini-Mental State Examination, PET positron emission tomography, SD standard deviation

2 and 5 min after the $[^{18}F]$MK-6240 injection. In young and elderly CN individuals, the time–activity curves had a uniform rapid washout and were similar in target and reference regions. In AD and MCI patients, the radio-activity showed a slower clearance in the regions that were expected to contain high concentrations of neuro-fibrillary tangles. Regional time–activity curves from selected brain regions of all individuals of the population are presented in Fig. 2.

Plasma analysis revealed that $[^{18}F]$MK-6240 has rapid clearance from the blood. The radio-metabolite analysis suggested only one metabolite, which is more polar than the parent compound. The metabolite peak was identified in the plasma eluting with a retention time of 4 min, whereas the parent compound appeared at 8 min. After 10 min, approximately 70% of the parent compound was metabolized (Fig. 3a).

The time–activity curves were well described by the 2T-CM4k across individuals and brain regions (Fig. 3b). The 2T-CM4k (AIC mean 11.39 (SD = 33)) provided a better fit than the 2T-CM3k (AIC mean 69.98 (SD = 45)) visually and statistically across subjects and regions (P < 0.0001, t test). The kinetic parameters derived from the preferred 2T-CM4k are presented in Table 2. The

cerebellar gray matter fitted the 2T-CM4k better, whereas the pons showed no difference in AIC between the fits with the 2T-CM4k and the 1T-CM. The Logan graphical model became linear approximately 80 min after the tracer injection in high binding regions (Fig. 3c).

The stabilization of specific binding (the difference between target and reference region) and total/ND binding (the ratio between target and reference region) was observed at 60 and 90 min for symptomatic individuals, respectively. In young and elderly CN individuals, specific binding and total/ND estimates were low, and the stabilization was reached earlier (Fig. 4).

The CV and ICC analyses performed after the total/ND binding reached equilibrium indicated that scan acquisitions from 90 to 110 min offer reliable measurements for the $[^{18}F]$MK-6240 SUVR calculation (Fig. 5). Additionally, ICCs between SUVRs measured from 90 to 110 min (SUVR$_{90-110}$) and 2T-CM4k DVRs and BPs (k_3 / k_4) were 0.993 (95% CI 0.99–0.995) and 0.791 (95% CI 0.7–0.857), respectively.

Using the cerebellar gray matter as the reference, the association between the SUVR and the 2T-CM4k showed progressively better goodness of fit and these

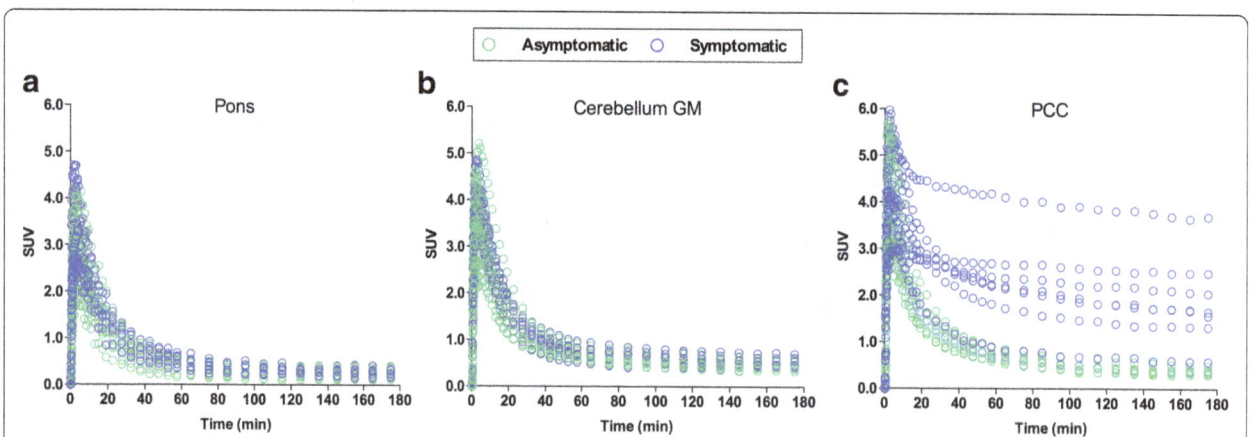

Fig. 2 Regional time–activity curves from selected brain regions for all participants. Regional standardized uptake value (SUV) time–activity curves of $[^{18}F]$MK-6240 in pons (**a**), cerebellar gray matter (GM) (**b**), and posterior cingulate cortex (PCC) (**c**) for all participants. Green dots represent young and elderly cognitively healthy individuals, blue dots represent MCI and Alzheimer's disease patients

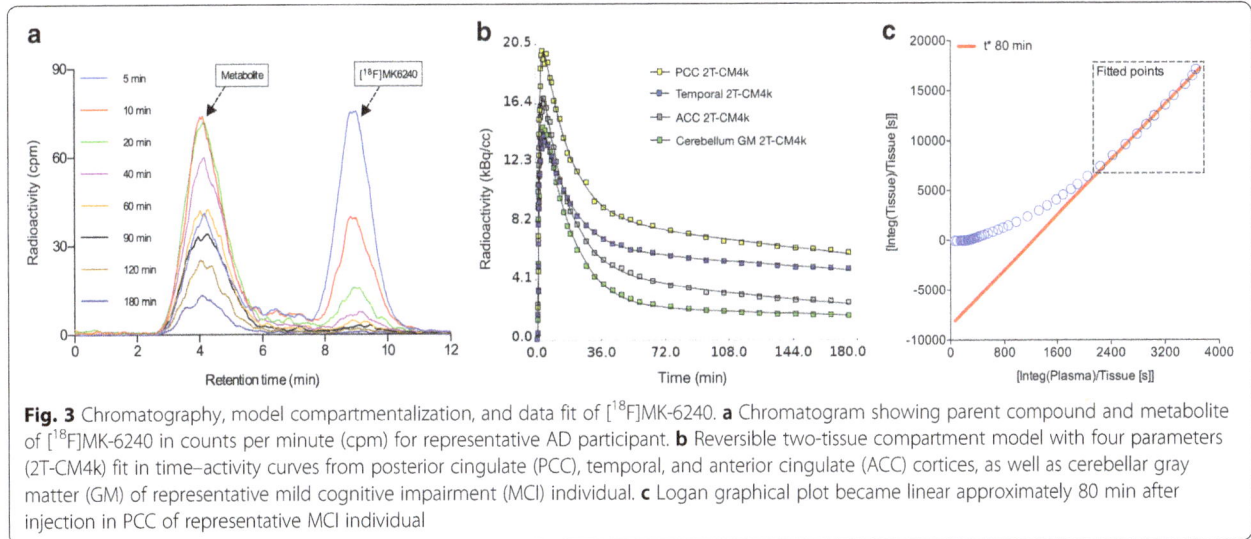

Fig. 3 Chromatography, model compartmentalization, and data fit of [^{18}F]MK-6240. **a** Chromatogram showing parent compound and metabolite of [^{18}F]MK-6240 in counts per minute (cpm) for representative AD participant. **b** Reversible two-tissue compartment model with four parameters (2T-CM4k) fit in time–activity curves from posterior cingulate (PCC), temporal, and anterior cingulate (ACC) cortices, as well as cerebellar gray matter (GM) of representative mild cognitive impairment (MCI) individual. **c** Logan graphical plot became linear approximately 80 min after injection in PCC of representative MCI individual

quantification methods showed progressively more similar estimates using progressively later time frames for the SUVR calculation, essentially approaching a plateau around 90 min (Fig. 6).

In addition, the 2T-CM4k DVRs were highly associated with the DVRs from the Logan method (slope = 0.9872, R^2 = 0.9953; Fig. 7a), the reference Logan method (slope = 0.8879, R^2 = 0.9864; Fig. 7b), and the SRTM (slope = 0.8658, R^2 = 0.9846; Fig. 7c). Moreover, DVRs using the reference Logan method (slope = 1.113, R^2 = 0.9915) and the SRTM (slope = 1.126, R^2 = 0.9807) were highly correlated with SUVR$_{90-110}$ (Fig. 7d, e).

2T-CM4k and Logan V_T estimates in the cerebellum gray matter and pons were the lowest and had the lowest variance between individuals and across diagnostic groups (Fig. 8a). DVR and SUVR$_{90-110}$ estimates showed a clear differentiation between MCI and AD from CN individuals (Fig. 8b, c). AD and MCI patients showed the highest binding in the PCC and the precuneus, where the binding in MCI and AD participants were on average around four and three times higher than in elderly CN individuals, respectively. [^{18}F]MK-6240 and

[^{18}F]AZD4694 SUVR parametric images from all individuals of the population are presented in Fig. 9.

Discussion

We have described here the first human evaluation of the novel PET ligand for neurofibrillary tangles [^{18}F]MK-6240 using full kinetic modeling and long scan acquisition duration. In this early observation, [^{18}F]MK-6240 was able to differentiate CN individuals from patients with MCI or AD, and valid binding estimates were obtained with simplified methods using a reference region such as the SUVR.

[^{18}F]MK-6240 showed fast brain penetration and kinetics after the injection, and one metabolite more polar than the parent compound was found. There were no clinically detectable side effects attributed to the [^{18}F]MK-6240 injection in our population. The fact that V_T values stabilized during the scan acquisition in humans, together with a previous preclinical observation, indirectly supports the notion that there is no radioactive metabolite gradually entering the brain at significant levels [7].

Table 2 Kinetic parameters obtained with the 2T-CM4k

Region	K_1	k_2	k_3	k_4	V_T	K_1/k_2	k_3/k_4	AIC	R^2
Asymptomatic individuals									
Cer GM	0.327 (0.08)	0.235 (0.00)	0.025 (0.03)	0.046 (0.04)	2 (0.1)	1.39 (0.36)	0.41 (0.3)	− 11 (2.8)	0.99 (0.00)
PCC	0.343 (0.03)	0.237 (0.04)	0.021 (0.01)	0.044 (0.01)	2.2 (0.1)	1.48 (0.42)	0.56 (0.52)	− 33.7 (4.3)	0.99 (0.00)
Symptomatic individuals									
Cer GM	0.230 (0.02)	0.125 (0.02)	0.009 (0.01)	0.01 (0.00)	3.4 (0.8)	1.88 (0.37)	0.86 (0.5)	− 2.0 (55)	0.99 (0.00)
PCC	0.246 (0.08)	0.099 (0.01)	0.052 (0.03)	0.01 (0.00)	14.2 (5.6)	2.45 (0.56)	5.11 (2.6)	− 3.7 (17)	0.99 (0.00)

Mean (standard deviation) of kinetic parameters obtained with the reversible two-tissue compartment model with four parameters (2T-CM4k) in the cerebellar gray matter (Cer GM) and posterior cingulate cortex (PCC) of asymptomatic (young and elderly cognitively healthy) and symptomatic (mild cognitive impairment and Alzheimer's disease) individuals who underwent arterial sampling

AIC Akaike information criterion, K_1 (ml/cm^3/min) transport rate for influx of tracer across blood–brain barrier, k_2 (1/min) transport rate for efflux of tracer across blood–brain barrier, k_3 (1/min) rate constant for exchange from nondisplaceable (free and nonspecific tracer) to specific binding compartment, k$_4$ (1/min) rate constant for exchange from specific binding compartment to nondisplaceable

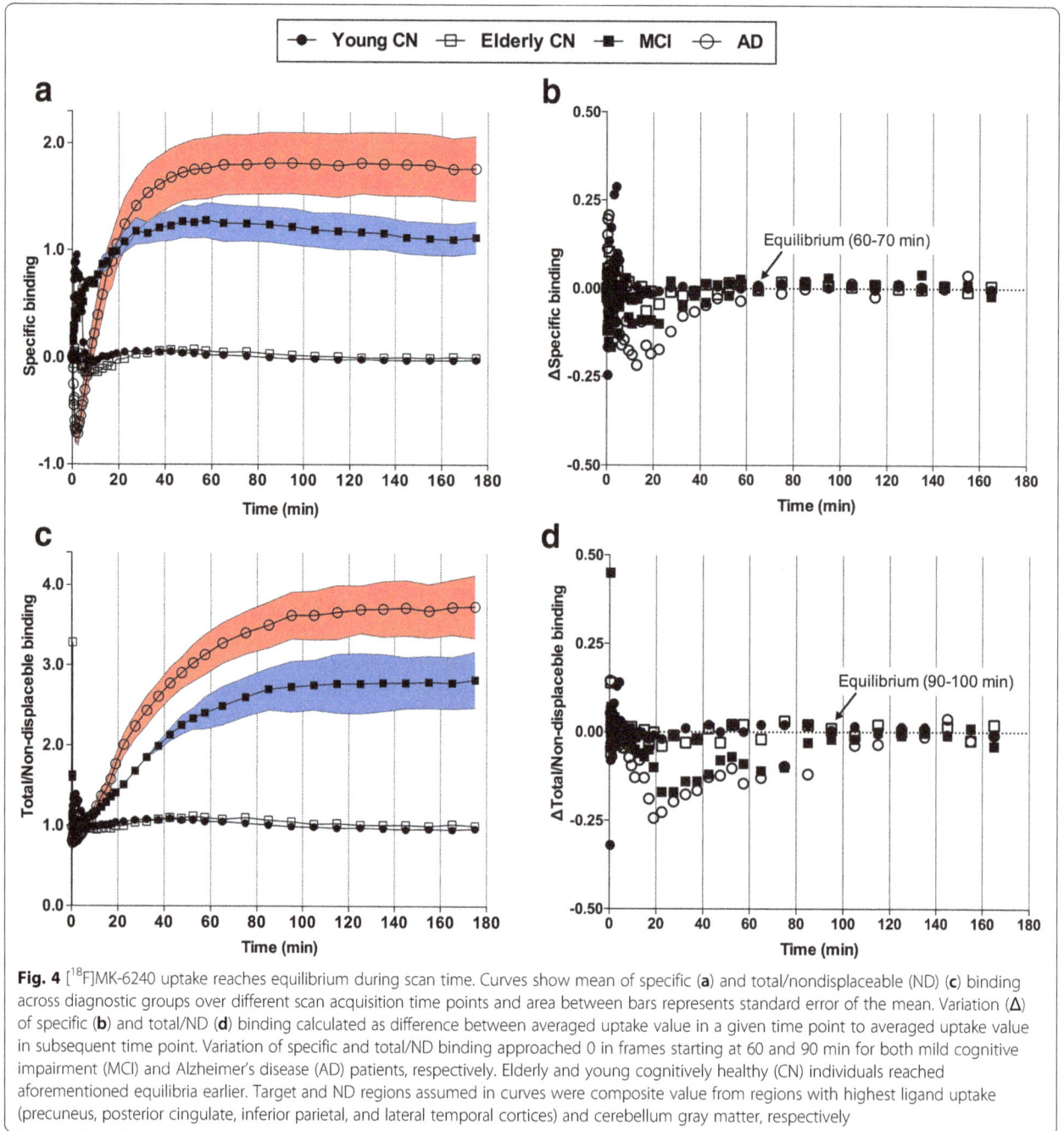

Fig. 4 [^{18}F]MK-6240 uptake reaches equilibrium during scan time. Curves show mean of specific (**a**) and total/nondisplaceable (ND) (**c**) binding across diagnostic groups over different scan acquisition time points and area between bars represents standard error of the mean. Variation (Δ) of specific (**b**) and total/ND (**d**) binding calculated as difference between averaged uptake value in a given time point to averaged uptake value in subsequent time point. Variation of specific and total/ND binding approached 0 in frames starting at 60 and 90 min for both mild cognitive impairment (MCI) and Alzheimer's disease (AD) patients, respectively. Elderly and young cognitively healthy (CN) individuals reached aforementioned equilibria earlier. Target and ND regions assumed in curves were composite value from regions with highest ligand uptake (precuneus, posterior cingulate, inferior parietal, and lateral temporal cortices) and cerebellum gray matter, respectively

The time–activity curves were well described with the 2T-CM4k, and the 2T-CM4k and the Logan graphical method using the plasma input function had similar estimates to the reference Logan method, SRTM, and SUVR. Moreover, reference region methods were highly correlated with each other. Together, these results further suggest that simplified reference methods offer valid estimates for the quantification of neurofibrillary tangles in the human brain using [^{18}F]MK-6240. Importantly, in our analysis, the estimates from reference methods underestimated the 2T-CM4k. Underestimation of the

2T-CM by reference methods has been observed for several other PET ligands such as [^{11}C]PIB, [^{18}F]AZD4694, and D2 receptor ligands, and the reasons suggested as underpinnings of this underestimation vary across ligands [13, 30–33].

V_T values were lowest in the cerebellar gray matter, pons, striatum, and white matter. The lowest variance between cognitively healthy and demented individuals was found in the cerebellar gray matter and pons, suggesting that these two regions have the highest potential to be used as a reference. Importantly, these regions are

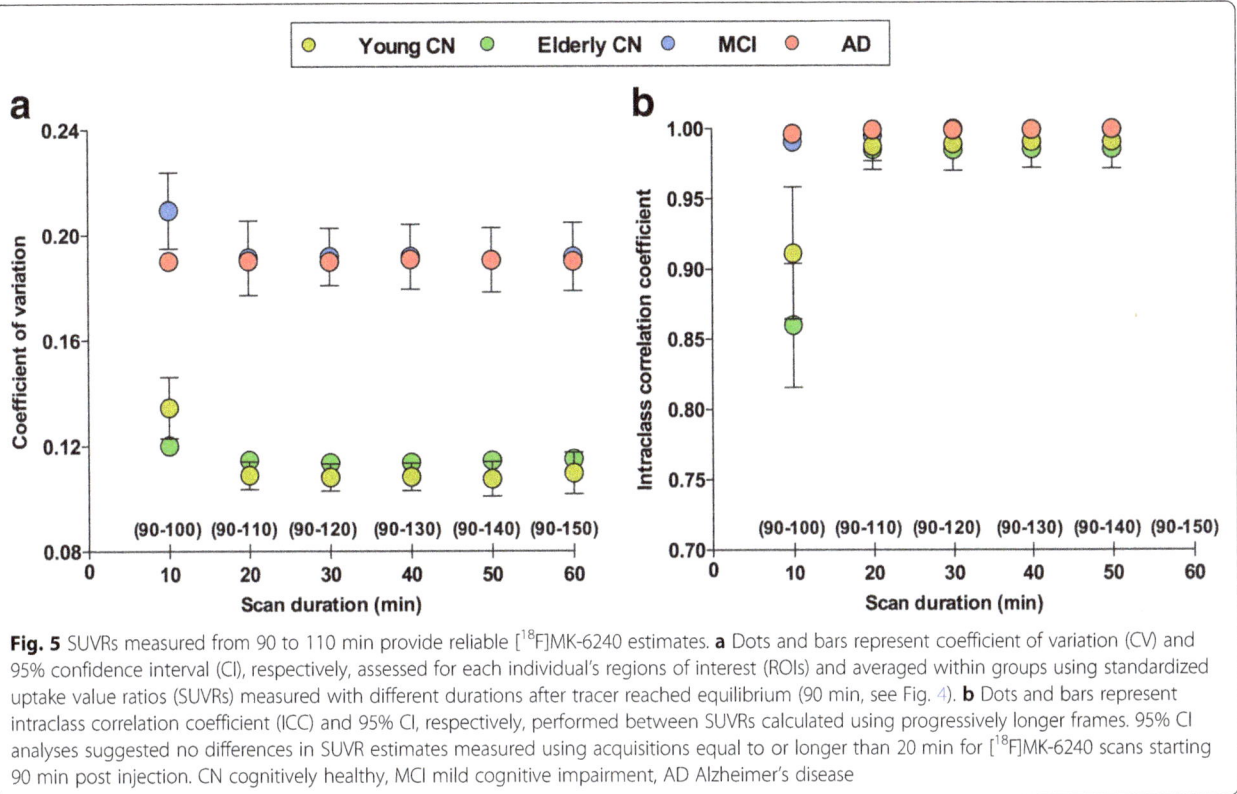

Fig. 5 SUVRs measured from 90 to 110 min provide reliable [^{18}F]MK-6240 estimates. **a** Dots and bars represent coefficient of variation (CV) and 95% confidence interval (CI), respectively, assessed for each individual's regions of interest (ROIs) and averaged within groups using standardized uptake value ratios (SUVRs) measured with different durations after tracer reached equilibrium (90 min, see Fig. 4). **b** Dots and bars represent intraclass correlation coefficient (ICC) and 95% CI, respectively, performed between SUVRs calculated using progressively longer frames. 95% CI analyses suggested no differences in SUVR estimates measured using acquisitions equal to or longer than 20 min for [^{18}F]MK-6240 scans starting 90 min post injection. CN cognitively healthy, MCI mild cognitive impairment, AD Alzheimer's disease

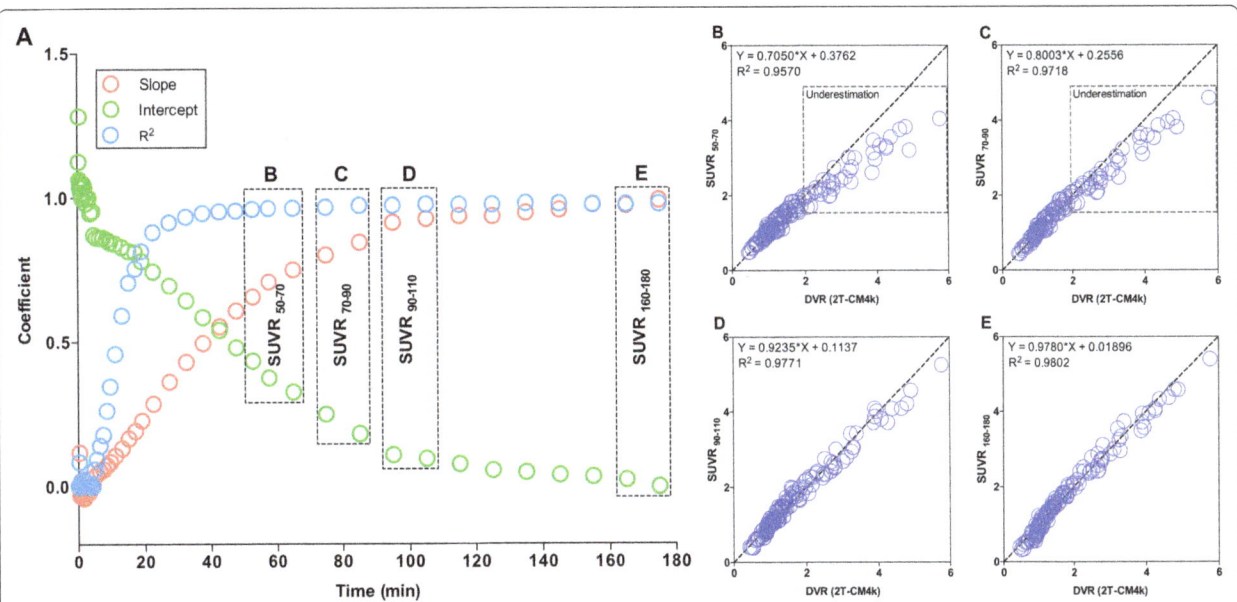

Fig. 6 SUVRs measured in later time frames had progressively more similar estimates than compartmental analysis. **a** Dots represent results of regressions between standardized uptake value ratios (SUVRs) obtained from different scan acquisition times and distribution volume ratio (DVR) obtained with reversible two-tissue compartment model (2T-CM4k) across subjects and brain regions. Association between SUVR and 2T-CM4k showed progressively better goodness of fit (R^2) and these quantification methods showed progressively more similar estimates (slope closer to 1 and intercept closer to 0) when using progressively later time frames for SUVR calculation. Although strength of the relationship showed constant increase until end of experiment, it approached the asymptote of the curve at 90 min post injection. Scatter plots show association between 2T-CM4k DVRs and SUVRs calculated from (**b**) 50 to 70 min, (**c**) 70 to 90 min, (**d**) 90 to 110 min, and (**e**) 160 to 180 min. SUVRs calculated before 90 min post injection underestimated 2T-CM4k in regions with moderate and high binding, but not in low binding regions

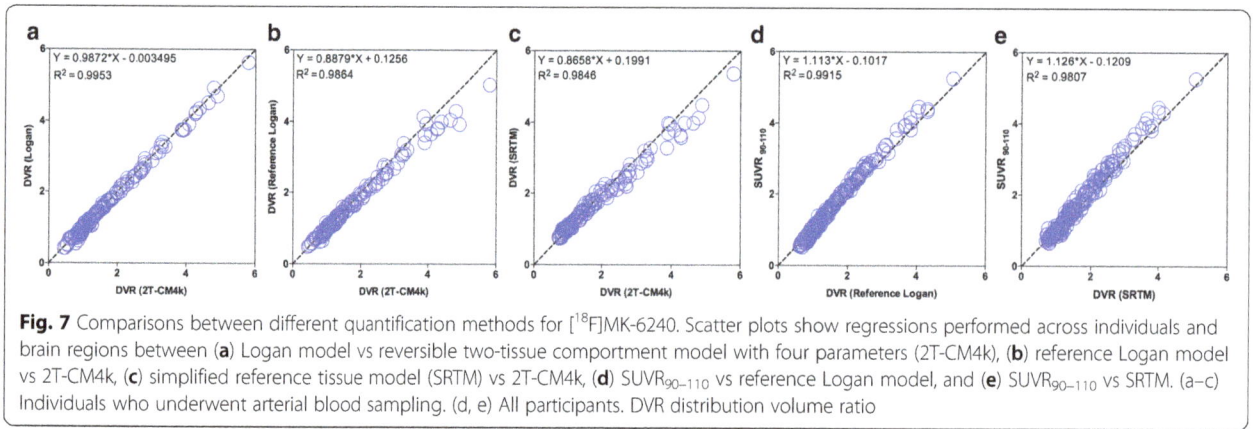

Fig. 7 Comparisons between different quantification methods for [^{18}F]MK-6240. Scatter plots show regressions performed across individuals and brain regions between (**a**) Logan model vs reversible two-tissue compartment model with four parameters (2T-CM4k), (**b**) reference Logan model vs 2T-CM4k, (**c**) simplified reference tissue model (SRTM) vs 2T-CM4k, (**d**) SUVR$_{90-110}$ vs reference Logan model, and (**e**) SUVR$_{90-110}$ vs SRTM. (a–c) Individuals who underwent arterial blood sampling. (d, e) All participants. DVR distribution volume ratio

reported to be relatively unaffected by neurofibrillary tangles in histopathological AD studies [9]. Since the time–activity curves in the cerebellar gray matter were more stable across subjects, which is expected since it is a larger region, this region was chosen as the reference region. In our analysis, the cerebellar gray matter fitted the 2T-CM4k. Similarly, the fact that more than one compartment is needed to describe a reference region has already been observed with other imaging agents for protein aggregates [13, 34]. In the case of [^{18}F]MK-6240, it is unclear whether the uptake in the cerebellar meninges may contribute to this finding. Although the BP (k_3 / k_4) values of the cerebellar gray matter overlapped across the diagnostic groups for some of the individuals, symptomatic individuals had a slightly higher V$_T$ than CN individuals, suggesting that future studies should assess the [^{18}F]MK-6240 binding in the reference regions.

The moment at which the specific binding peaks and the moment at which the target-to-reference region ratio approaches the plateau have been designated as the peak equilibrium [13] and the transient [33] or secular [27] equilibrium, respectively. Both of these parameters of equilibrium have been used for previous PET studies [13, 35, 36]. In the present study, averaged [^{18}F]MK-6240 cortical-to-cerebellar gray matter ratio curves showed a constant relative increase, reaching an asymptote after 90 min. Therefore, this parameter suggested 90 min as the earliest time point for the SUVR calculation, while the SUVR stability analysis suggested that there is no benefit in acquisitions longer than 20 min for scans starting 90 min post injection. Taking these observations together, we determined scans performed at 90–110 min post injection to have an optimal tradeoff between duration and reliability.

As a subnanomolar affinity tracer, [^{18}F]MK-6240 reached equilibrium earlier (60 min) in low as compared with medium and high binding regions, where the ratio between the total/ND binding stabilized after 90 min.

Therefore, SUVRs calculated with frames obtained earlier than 90 min lead to a progressively higher underestimation of tau pathology among low, medium, and high load regions. As a consequence, it is expected that SUVRs estimated earlier than 90 min will underestimate the rate of tau accumulation over time. In the context of anti-tau clinical trials, SUVRs obtained before 90 min will reduce the drug effect size since pretreatment estimates will present a higher underestimation than posttreatment estimates. Studies in other subnanomolar affinity tracers, such as the D2 receptor ligands, have already shown the pitfalls of using early time windows for binding estimation in tracers with distinct times to reach the equilibrium in regions with low and high-density receptors [35].

MCI and AD patients showed [^{18}F]MK-6240 uptake across the whole brain cortex, with the highest binding in the PCC, precuneus, inferior parietal, and lateral temporal cortices. Regional [^{18}F]MK-6240 bindings measured with arterial input function and simplified reference methods were able to distinguish MCI and AD patients from CN individuals. In vitro autoradiography further supported greater contrast of [^{18}F]MK-6240 uptake in AD patients than in age-matched CN individuals across the aforementioned regions. This regional uptake is consistent with the pattern of neurofibrillary tangle deposition that was previously described in postmortem studies of AD and supports [^{18}F]MK-6240 as a promising ligand for measuring neurofibrillary tangles in the human brain [9].

Apparent differences in binding sites between [^{18}F]MK-6240 and the other available tau tracers were observed in this evaluation. For example, in contrast to the other ligands for neurofibrillary tangles, [^{18}F]MK-6240 had minimum uptake in the striatum, which despite being known as a region with low tangles concentration is one of the major binding sites of the other available tau tracers [37]. Moreover, the time–activity curves and quantification methods suggested similarities in [^{18}F]MK-6240

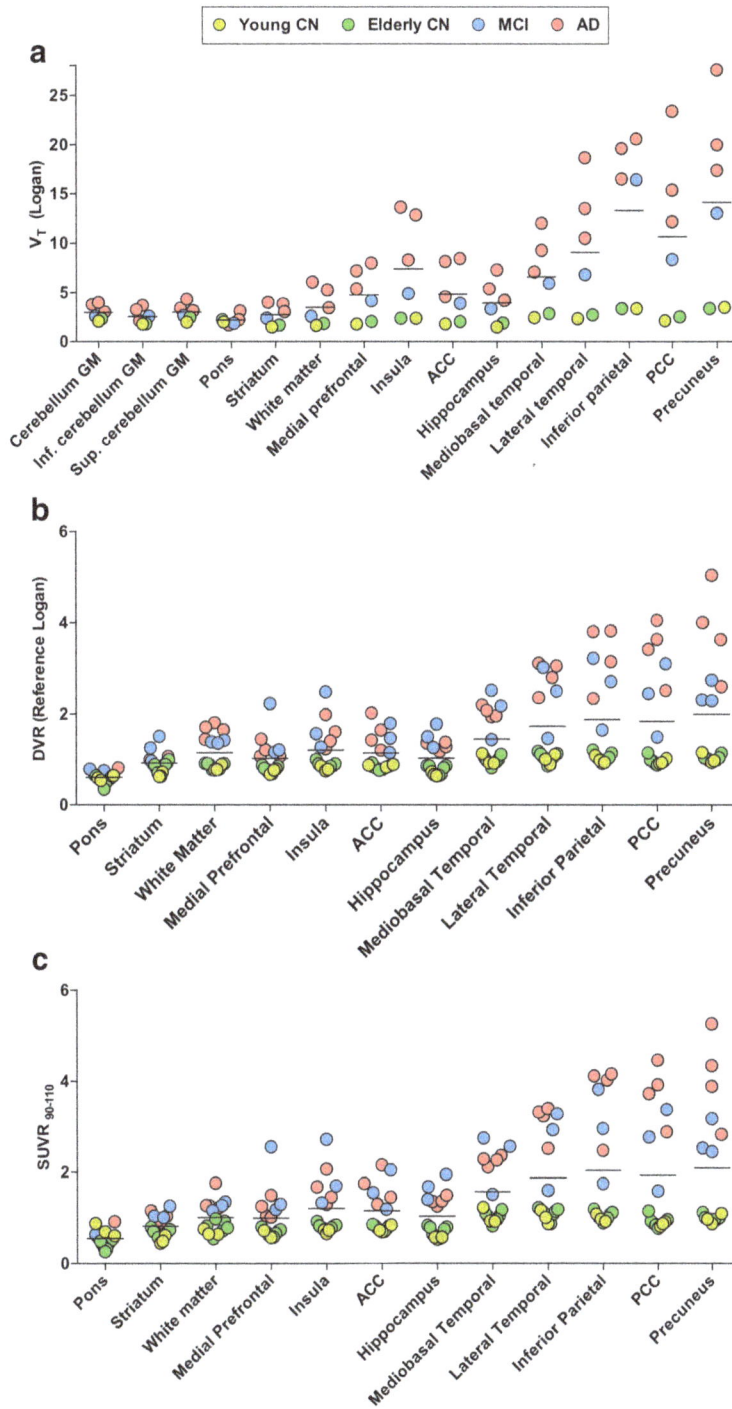

Fig. 8 Quantification estimates across clinical diagnosis and brain regions. Horizontal bar represents mean. **a** Total volume of distribution (V_T; ml/cm^3) values obtained with Logan graphical method using plasma input function in individuals who underwent arterial blood sampling. **b** Distribution volume ratio (DVR) values obtained with reference Logan method and (**c**) standardized uptake value ratio values measured between 90 and 110 min (SUVR$_{90-110}$) in all individuals, both using cerebellar gray matter (GM) as reference region. CN cognitively healthy, MCI mild cognitive impairment, AD Alzheimer's disease, Inf. inferior, Sup. superior, ACC anterior cingulate cortex, PCC posterior cingulate cortex

retention between young and elderly CN individuals within the associative neocortical brain regions that are expected to contain low tangle density in these populations. Together, these initial results support [^{18}F]MK-6240 as a ligand with high brain selectivity to neurofibrillary tangles. It is important to mention

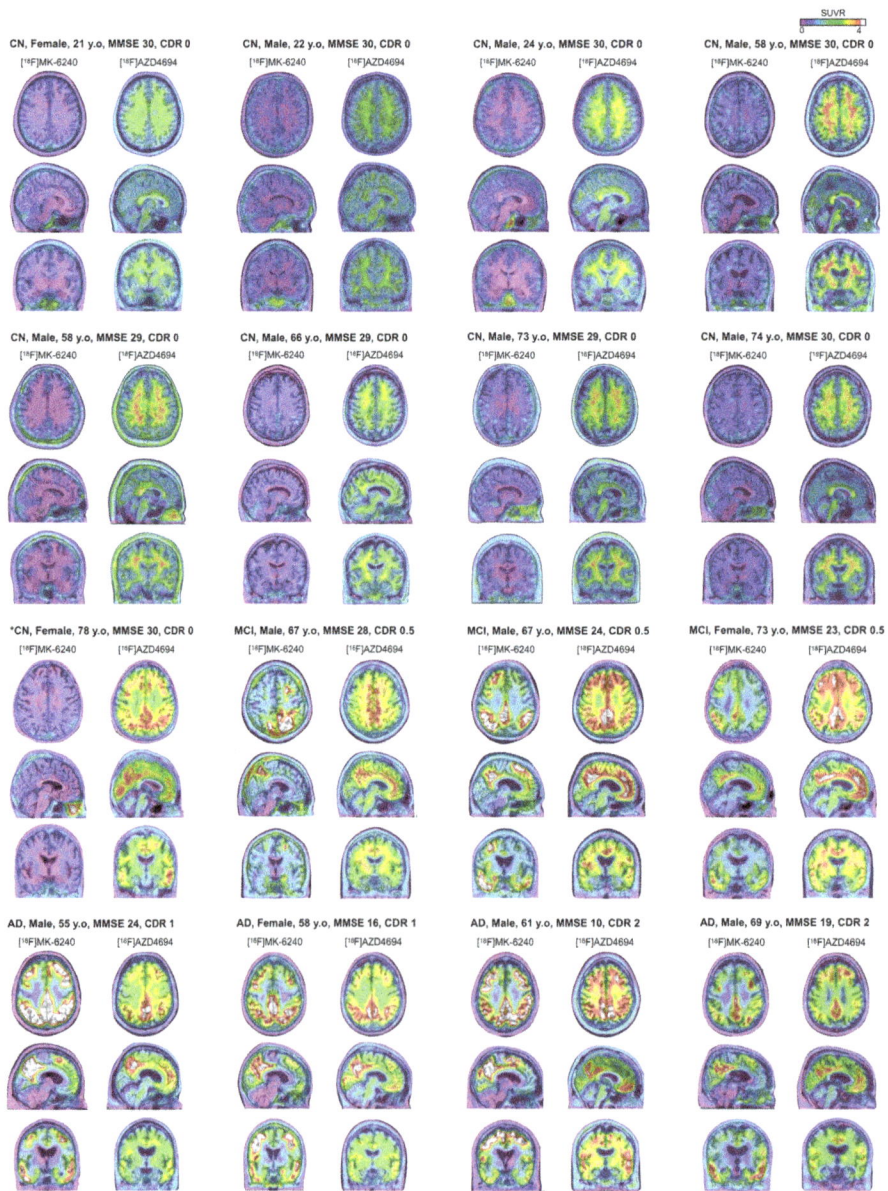

Fig. 9 [^{18}F]MK-6240 SUVR parametric images of all participants. [^{18}F]MK-6240 standardized uptake value ratio (SUVR) averaged between 90 and 110 min and [^{18}F]AZD4694 SUVR maps, overlaid on the individuals' structural MRI, of all individuals of the population. [^{18}F]MK-6240 images show clear visual differentiation between symptomatic (mild cognitive impairment (MCI) and Alzheimer's disease (AD)) and asymptomatic (cognitively healthy (CN) control) participants. All AD and MCI patients as well as one CN individual (*) were amyloid-β positive. CDR Clinical Dementia Rating, MMSE Mini-Mental State Examination, y.o years old

that possible off-target binding of [^{18}F]MK-6240 was observed in regions including the retina, ethmoid sinus, substantia nigra, and dura mater. However, since some of these findings were not consistent among participants, these observations require further validation.

This study has methodological limitations. The absence of confirmation of the presence of neurofibrillary tangles with specific antibodies is a limitation of our in vitro study. The small sample size is a limitation of our

in vivo study. However, the subjects studied here had a wide range of dynamic [^{18}F]MK-6240 uptake, which allowed the evaluation of the tracer kinetics in individuals with low and high binding. Future studies should address the test–retest reliability of [^{18}F]MK-6240 and definitively confirm whether the [^{18}F]MK-6240 radioactive metabolite does not appear in the brain in a significant amount. Since the HPLC has limited sensitivity in detecting low radioactivity counts [34], a further study using a more sensitive method of measuring the parent fraction is underway to completely define the limitations of quantifying [^{18}F]MK-6240 using simplified methods. [^{18}F]MK-6240 had the highest uptake in the precuneus and PCC. Previous postmortem observations did not relate these brain regions with the neurofibrillary tangles patterns typically found in AD [9]. In contrast, a recent PET study has shown that neurofibrillary tangle accumulation in the PCC is highly associated with AD pathophysiology [38]. This study highlights that the PCC may have been overlooked by postmortem observations that do not traditionally assess neurofibrillary tangles in this region [38]. Although we have focused on the PCC for some of our kinetic analysis, it is important to emphasize the importance of other brain regions such as the medial temporal cortex to the AD pathophysiological process. In addition, although our results suggest [^{18}F]MK-6240 binding as an indicator of AD-related tangles, it is important to mention that the association of this binding with the clinical staging and natural history of AD can be determined only by larger longitudinal studies. Since our population was limited to controls and individuals across the AD spectrum, more studies are needed to determine [^{18}F]MK-6240 binding properties associated with non-AD tauopathies.

Conclusions

[^{18}F]MK-6240 displayed favorable pharmacokinetics with rapid brain penetration and washout. In this early observation, [^{18}F]MK-6240 discriminated MCI and AD from controls using methods with plasma input function or simplified SUVR estimates. [^{18}F]MK-6240 is a promising new-generation tau radiotracer with the potential to be employed in the evaluation of disease-modifying therapies and future diagnostic use.

Abbreviations
2T-CM: Two-tissue compartment model; ACC: Anterior cingulate cortex; AD: Alzheimer's disease; AIC: Akaike information criterion; CDR: Clinical Dementia Rating; CERAD: Consortium to Establish a Registry for Alzheimer Disease; CI: Confidence interval; CN: Cognitively healthy; DVR: Distribution volume ratio; HPLC: High-pressure liquid chromatography; HRRT: High-resolution research tomograph; MCI: Mild cognitive impairment; MMSE: Mini-Mental State Examination; MNI: Montreal Neurological Institute; MRI: Magnetic resonance imaging; OSEM: Ordered-subsets expectation maximization; PCC: Posterior cingulate cortex; PET: Positron emission tomography; ROI: Region of interest; SD: Standard deviation; SRTM: Simplified reference tissue model; SUVR: Standardized uptake value ratio; V_T: Volume of distribution

Acknowledgements
The authors thank Alexey Kostikov, Dean Jolly, Karen Ross, Mehdi Boudjemeline, Sandy Li, and Monica Samoila-Lactatus for radiochemistry production.

Funding
This work was supported by the Weston Brain Institute, Canadian Institutes of Health Research (CIHR; MOP-11-51-31) (to PR-N), the Alzheimer's Association (NIRG-12-92090, NIRP-12-259245) (to PR-N), the Alzheimer Society Research Program (ASRP) and Canadian Consortium on Neurodegeneration in Aging (CCNA) scholarship (to TAP), and Fonds de Recherche du Québec—Santé

(FRQS; Chercheur Boursier) (to PR-N). SG and PR-N are members of the CIHR–CCNA Canadian Consortium of Neurodegeneration in Aging.

Authors' contributions
TAP, IB, SG, and PR-N conceived the study. RH and GM performed radiochemistry production and revised the manuscript. MS, MSK, MC, DC, JT, KPN, RB, H-HH, and ALB participated in acquisition of the PET data and revised the manuscript. TAP and SM performed the processing and quality control of the image data. TAP, SG, and PR-N performed the statistical analysis and interpreted the data. TAP, J-PS, SG, and PR-N prepared the figures and the table, and drafted the manuscript. All authors read and approved the final manuscript.

Consent for publication
Not applicable.

Competing interests
IB is a Merck & Co. employee. SG received honoraria for serving on the scientific advisory boards of Alzheon, Axovant, Lilly, Lundbeck, Novartis, Schwabe, and TauRx. The remaining authors declare that they have no competing interests.

Author details
[1]Translational Neuroimaging Laboratory, The McGill University Research Centre for Studies in Aging, 6825 LaSalle Boulevard, Verdun, QC H4H 1R3, Canada. [2]Montreal Neurological Institute, 3801 University Street, Montreal, QC H3A 2B4, Canada. [3]Translational Biomarkers, Merck & Co., Inc., 770 Sumneytown Pike, West Point, PA 19486, USA. [4]Douglas Hospital, McGill University, 6875 La Salle Blvd—FBC room 3149, Montreal, QC H4H 1R3, Canada.

References
1. Xia CF, Arteaga J, Chen G, Gangadharmath U, Gomez LF, Kasi D, Lam C, Liang Q, Liu C, Mocharla VP, et al. [(18)F]T807, a novel tau positron emission tomography imaging agent for Alzheimer's disease. Alzheimers Dement. 2013;9:666–76.
2. Chien DT, Bahri S, Szardenings AK, Walsh JC, Mu F, Su MY, Shankle WR, Elizarov A, Kolb HC. Early clinical PET imaging results with the novel PHF-tau radioligand [F-18]-T807. J Alzheimers Dis. 2013;34:457–68.
3. Harada R, Okamura N, Furumoto S, Furukawa K, Ishiki A, Tomita N, Hiraoka K, Watanuki S, Shidahara M, Miyake M, et al. [(18)F]THK-5117 PET for assessing neurofibrillary pathology in Alzheimer's disease. Eur J Nucl Med Mol Imaging. 2015;42:1052–61.
4. Stepanov V, Svedberg M, Jia Z, Krasikova R, Lemoine L, Okamura N, Furumoto S, Mitsios N, Mulder J, Langstrom B, et al. Development of [11C]/[3H]THK-5351—a potential novel carbon-11 tau imaging PET radioligand. Nucl Med Biol. 2017;46:50–3.
5. Hashimoto H, Kawamura K, Igarashi N, Takei M, Fujishiro T, Aihara Y, Shiomi S, Muto M, Ito T, Furutsuka K, et al. Radiosynthesis, photoisomerization, biodistribution, and metabolite analysis of 11C-PBB3 as a clinically useful PET probe for imaging of tau pathology. J Nucl Med. 2014;55: 1532–8.
6. Ng KP, Pascoal TA, Mathotaarachchi S, Therriault J, Kang MS, Shin M, Guiot MC, Guo Q, Harada R, Comley RA, et al. Monoamine oxidase B inhibitor, selegiline, reduces 18F-THK5351 uptake in the human brain. Alzheimers Res Ther. 2017;9:25.

7. Hostetler ED, Walji AM, Zeng Z, Miller P, Bennacef I, Salinas C, Connolly B, Gantert L, Haley H, Holahan M, et al. Preclinical characterization of 18F-MK-6240, a promising PET tracer for in vivo quantification of human neurofibrillary tangles. J Nucl Med. 2016;57:1599–606.

8. Koga S, Ono M, Sahara N, Higuchi M, Dickson DW. Fluorescence and autoradiographic evaluation of tau PET ligand PBB3 to alpha-synuclein pathology. Mov Disord. 2017;32:884–92.

9. Braak H, Braak E. Neuropathological stageing of Alzheimer-related changes. Acta Neuropathol. 1991;82:239–59.

10. Mirra SS, Heyman A, McKeel D, Sumi SM, Crain BJ, Brownlee LM, Vogel FS, Hughes JP, van Belle G, Berg L. The Consortium to Establish a Registry for Alzheimer's Disease (CERAD). Part II. Standardization of the neuropathologic assessment of Alzheimer's disease. Neurology. 1991;41:479–86.

11. Parent MJ, Bedard MA, Aliaga A, Minuzzi L, Mechawar N, Soucy JP, Schirrmacher E, Kostikov A, Gauthier SG, Rosa-Neto P. Cholinergic depletion in Alzheimer's disease shown by [(18)F]FEOBV autoradiography. Int J Mol Imaging. 2013;2013:205045.

12. McKhann GM, Knopman DS, Chertkow H, Hyman BT, Jack CR Jr, Kawas CH, Klunk WE, Koroshetz WJ, Manly JJ, Mayeux R, et al. The diagnosis of dementia due to Alzheimer's disease: recommendations from the National Institute on Aging-Alzheimer's Association workgroups on diagnostic guidelines for Alzheimer's disease. Alzheimers Dement. 2011;7:263–9.

13. Cselenyi Z, Jonhagen ME, Forsberg A, Halldin C, Julin P, Schou M, Johnstrom P, Varnas K, Svensson S, Farde L. Clinical validation of 18F-AZD4694, an amyloid-beta-specific PET radioligand. J Nucl Med. 2012;53:415–24.

14. Hudson HM, Larkin RS. Accelerated image reconstruction using ordered subsets of projection data. IEEE Trans Med Imaging. 1994;13:601–9.

15. Costes N, Dagher A, Larcher K, Evans AC, Collins DL, Reilhac A. Motion correction of multi-frame PET data in neuroreceptor mapping: simulation based validation. Neuroimage. 2009;47:1496–505.

16. Zijdenbos AP, Forghani R, Evans AC. Automatic "pipeline" analysis of 3-D MRI data for clinical trials: application to multiple sclerosis. IEEE Trans Med Imaging. 2002;21:1280–91.

17. Mazziotta JC, Toga AW, Evans A, Fox P, Lancaster J. A probabilistic atlas of the human brain: theory and rationale for its development. The International Consortium for Brain Mapping (ICBM). Neuroimage. 1995;2:89–101.

18. Mazziotta J, Toga A, Evans A, Fox P, Lancaster J, Zilles K, Woods R, Paus T, Simpson G, Pike B, et al. A probabilistic atlas and reference system for the human brain: International Consortium for Brain Mapping (ICBM). Philos Trans R Soc Lond Ser B Biol Sci. 2001;356:1293–322.

19. Pascoal TA, Mathotaarachchi S, Shin M, Benedet AL, Mohades S, Wang S, Beaudry T, Kang MS, Soucy JP, Labbe A, et al. Synergistic interaction between amyloid and tau plaques predicts the progression to dementia. Alzheimers Dement. 2017;13:644–53.

20. Pascoal TA, Mathotaarachchi S, Mohades S, Benedet AL, Chung CO, Shin M, Wang S, Beaudry T, Kang MS, Soucy JP, et al. Amyloid-beta and hyperphosphorylated tau synergy drives metabolic decline in preclinical Alzheimer's disease. Mol Psychiatry. 2017;22:306–11.

21. Gunn RN, Gunn SR, Cunningham VJ. Positron emission tomography compartmental models. J Cereb Blood Flow Metab. 2001;21:635–52.

22. Logan J, Fowler JS, Volkow ND, Wolf AP, Dewey SL, Schlyer DJ, MacGregor RR, Hitzemann R, Bendriem B, Gatley SJ, et al. Graphical analysis of reversible radioligand binding from time-activity measurements applied to [N-11C-methyl]-(–)-cocaine PET studies in human subjects. J Cereb Blood Flow Metab. 1990;10:740–7.

23. Wu Y, Carson RE. Noise reduction in the simplified reference tissue model for neuroreceptor functional imaging. J Cereb Blood Flow Metab. 2002;22:1440–52.

24. Lammertsma AA, Hume SP. Simplified reference tissue model for PET receptor studies. Neuroimage. 1996;4:153–8.

25. Logan J, Fowler JS, Volkow ND, Wang GJ, Ding YS, Alexoff DL. Distribution volume ratios without blood sampling from graphical analysis of PET data. J Cereb Blood Flow Metab. 1996;16:834–40.

26. Akaike H. A new look at the statistical model identification. IEEE Trans Autom Control. 1974;19:716–23.

27. Farde L, Eriksson L, Blomquist G, Halldin C. Kinetic analysis of central [11C]raclopride binding to D2-dopamine receptors studied by PET—a comparison to the equilibrium analysis. J Cereb Blood Flow Metab. 1989;9:696–708.

28. Bartko JJ. The intraclass correlation coefficient as a measure of reliability. Psychol Rep. 1966;19:3–11.

29. Quan H, Shih WJ. Assessing reproducibility by the within-subject coefficient of variation with random effects models. Biometrics. 1996;52:1195–203.

30. Yaqub M, Tolboom N, Boellaard R, van Berckel BN, van Tilburg EW, Luurtsema G, Scheltens P, Lammertsma AA. Simplified parametric methods for [11C]PIB studies. Neuroimage. 2008;42:76–86.

31. Gunn RN, Lammertsma AA, Hume SP, Cunningham VJ. Parametric imaging of ligand-receptor binding in PET using a simplified reference region model. Neuroimage. 1997;6:279–87.

32. Zhou Y, Sojkova J, Resnick SM, Wong DF. Relative equilibrium plot improves graphical analysis and allows bias correction of standardized uptake value ratio in quantitative 11C-PiB PET studies. J Nucl Med. 2012;53:622–8.

33. Carson RE, Channing MA, Blasberg RG, Dunn BB, Cohen RM, Rice KC, Herscovitch P. Comparison of bolus and infusion methods for receptor quantitation: application to [18F]cyclofoxy and positron emission tomography. J Cereb Blood Flow Metab. 1993;13:24–42.

34. Price JC, Klunk WE, Lopresti BJ, Lu X, Hoge JA, Ziolko SK, Holt DP, Meltzer CC, DeKosky ST, Mathis CA. Kinetic modeling of amyloid binding in humans using PET imaging and Pittsburgh compound-B. J Cereb Blood Flow Metab. 2005;25:1528–47.

35. Olsson H, Farde L. Potentials and pitfalls using high affinity radioligands in PET and SPET determinations on regional drug induced D2 receptor occupancy—a simulation study based on experimental data. Neuroimage. 2001;14:936–45.

36. Wong DF, Rosenberg PB, Zhou Y, Kumar A, Raymont V, Ravert HT, Dannals RF, Nandi A, Brasic JR, Ye W, et al. In vivo imaging of amyloid deposition in Alzheimer disease using the radioligand 18F-AV-45 (florbetapir [corrected] F 18). J Nucl Med. 2010;51:913–20.

37. Saint-Aubert L, Lemoine L, Chiotis K, Leuzy A, Rodriguez-Vieitez E, Nordberg A. Tau PET imaging: present and future directions. Mol Neurodegener. 2017;12:19.

38. Jack CR Jr, Wiste HJ, Schwarz CG, Lowe VJ, Senjem ML, Vemuri P, Weigand SD, Therneau TM, Knopman DS, Gunter JL, et al. Longitudinal tau PET in ageing and Alzheimer's disease. Brain. 2018;141:1517–28.

Clinical dementia severity associated with ventricular size is differentially moderated by cognitive reserve in men and women

Shraddha Sapkota[1]*(iD), Joel Ramirez[1], Donald T. Stuss[1,2,3,4], Mario Masellis[1,5] and Sandra E. Black[1,5]

Abstract

Background: Interindividual differences in cognitive reserve (CR) are associated with complex and dynamic clinical phenotypes observed in cognitive impairment and dementia. We tested whether (1) CR early in life (E-CR; measured by education and IQ), (2) CR later in life (L-CR; measured by occupation), and (3) CR panel (CR-P) with the additive effects of E-CR and L-CR, act as moderating factors between baseline ventricular size and clinical dementia severity at baseline and across 2 years. We further examined whether this moderation is differentially represented by sex.

Methods: We examined a longitudinal model using patients ($N = 723$; mean age = 70.8 ± 9.4 years; age range = 38–90 years; females = 374) from the Sunnybrook Dementia Study. The patients represented Alzheimer's disease ($n = 439$), mild cognitive impairment ($n = 77$), vascular cognitive impairment ($n = 52$), Lewy body disease ($n = 30$), and frontotemporal dementia ($n = 125$). Statistical analyses included (1) latent growth modeling to determine how clinical dementia severity changes over 2 years (measured by performance on the Dementia Rating Scale), (2) confirmatory factor analysis to establish a baseline E-CR factor, and (3) path analysis to predict dementia severity. Baseline age (continuous) and *Apolipoprotein E* status (ε4–/ε4+) were included as covariates.

Results: The association between higher baseline ventricular size and dementia severity was moderated by (1) E-CR and L-CR and (2) CR-P. This association was differentially represented in men and women. Specifically, men in only the low CR-P had higher baseline clinical dementia severity with larger baseline ventricular size. However, women in the low CR-P showed the (1) highest baseline dementia severity and (2) fastest 2-year decline with larger baseline ventricular size.

Conclusions: Clinical dementia severity associated with ventricular size may be (1) selectively moderated by complex and additive CR networks and (2) differentially represented by sex.

Keywords: Cognitive reserve, Ventricular size, Sex, Cognitive impairment, Dementia, Sunnybrook Dementia Study

Background

The spectrum of neurodegenerative pathologies in the aging brain in combination with cardiovascular risk factors has led to an increased prevalence and diagnosis of mixed neurodegenerative diseases (combination of proteinopathies and vasculopathies) [1]. A recent review examined 12 community-based neuropathology studies and identified that the frequency of Alzheimer's disease (AD) pathology was 19–67%,

Lewy body pathology was 6–39%, vascular pathologies was 28–70%, and mixed pathologies was 10–74% [2]. Combinations of neurodegenerative (e.g., proteinopathies) and non-neurodegenerative (e.g., metabolic-nutritional, vascular) pathologies may depict the multifaceted clinical manifestations observed in patients with dementia. In addition to the heterogeneity and complexity of pathologies, variability and differences in life experiences may further complicate the course of cognitive decline and clinical dementia severity. Identifying modifiable risk and protective proxies of cognitive reserve (CR) may lead to personalized interventions for those most at risk of accelerated cognitive impairment [3].

* Correspondence: shraddha.sapkota@sunnybrook.ca
[1]Hurvitz Brain Sciences Research Program, Sunnybrook Research Institute, Sunnybrook Health Sciences Centre, 2075 Bayview Avenue, M6-192, Toronto, ON M4N 3M5, Canada
Full list of author information is available at the end of the article

Cognitive resilience is another related and complementary hypothetical construct and term used in the literature [4].

CR is defined as the ability to compensate for neurological damage via recruitment of compensatory mechanisms [5, 6]. Diverse life experiences, including level of education [7], occupational attainment [8], involvement in leisure activities [9], and IQ, are commonly used as proxies to indirectly represent CR [10]. Many of these variables are intercorrelated; for example, higher IQ leads to more education [11]. However, independent associations have also been observed between each variable and cognitive decline [12]. Inconsistent findings between CR proxies and cognition imply a potentially elaborate CR network. Such intricate CR networks and pathology in the aging brain may be further convoluted by sex differences in AD [13], Parkinson's disease [14], vascular dementia [15], and frontotemporal dementia (FTD) [16]. For example, men diagnosed with AD show better performance on language, semantic and visuospatial tasks, and episodic memory than women after accounting for age, education, and dementia severity [17]. Estrogen deficiency in postmenopausal women may partly explain this disadvantage observed in women [18]. On the contrary, women may have an advantage in verbal memory even in the presence of hippocampal atrophy [19, 20].

In the present study, we examine whether the association between ventricular size and clinical dementia severity [21–23] is differentially moderated by CR in men and women across a large, heterogeneous sample of patients with cognitive impairment and dementia. We differentiate CR into two constructs: (1) CR acquired early in life (E-CR) measured with education and IQ as proxies and (2) CR acquired through maintenance or practice later in life (L-CR) measured with occupational attainment as a proxy, likely capturing what is referred to by some as "maintenance" [24, 25]. Our approach examines whether there are differences in CR moderation for (1) early life, (2) later life, and (3) the additive effects of E-CR + L-CR with the CR panel (CR-P). The synergistic associations of high E-CR and high L-CR may provide additional protection against neuropathological damage in cognitive impairment and dementia.

The rationale for differentiating the two constructs derive from studies focusing on occupation, education, and IQ separately as proxies for CR. Occupation has independently been linked to cognitive performance in multiple domains (memory, processing speed, attention) after accounting for potential confounding factors such as education, leisure activities, and sex differences [26]. Authors of a recent systematic review observed inconsistencies between occupation and general cognition in the presence of multiple brain pathologies in different clinical groups [27]. In men, higher intellectual and more engaging work was associated with better cognitive performance in late life independent of IQ or education [28]. Occupation, often characterized as nonformal education, is training in a particular skill set that can develop and evolve across the lifespan [29]. This suggests that the dynamic fluctuations and continually evolving proxy for CR across the lifespan is better represented by occupation, whereas IQ and education may be more accurate proxies for CR typically acquired in early life. We therefore examined (1) occupation as an independent factor contributing to the CR network to account for any changes, development, and skills acquired across the lifespan, including later in life (L-CR), and (2) education and IQ for CR acquired early in life that may not have been actively exercised or preserved in a stimulating work environment throughout the life course (E-CR).

In addition to commonly used CR proxies, CR has also been studied in the context of both functional and structural imaging. Functional imaging studies have commonly been used to capture CR by examining differential activation patterns [29, 30]. AD patients with high CR (indexed by education) may have higher functional connectivity in the posterior cingulate cortex. Specifically, higher activation of compensatory neural mechanisms in this region may mitigate the effects of greater AD pathology [31]. Structural imaging research has also shown that (1) lower socioprofessional attainment in midlife was associated with faster hippocampal atrophy [32], (2) interaction between white matter lesions and high CR predicted higher conversion rate of mild cognitive impairment (MCI) to AD [33], and (3) larger intracranial volume provided support for brain reserve hypothesis against AD pathology [34]. CR may account for discrepancies observed between sex, lifestyle factors, AD neuropathological changes, small-vessel vascular impairment, and dementia with Lewy bodies (DLB) [35].

Brain pathologies commonly represented by neuroimaging biomarkers (e.g., ventricular atrophy, white matter hyperintensities) provide a baseline to predict cognitive decline [36, 37] and risk of dementia [38]. We specifically focus on ventricular volume in the present study because previous research has shown that (1) ventricular volume is an important marker in predicting conversion from MCI to AD [39], (2) ventricular expansion is accelerated 24 months prior to signs of cognitive deficits in MCI participants [40], and (3) larger ventricular volumes may indicate higher risk of clinical dementia severity or related pathology [41]. However, the impact of a CR network and sex differences should be studied in conjunction with ventricular volume to understand the neural underpinnings associated with rate of cognitive deterioration in dementia. The present study includes a unique cohort of cognitive impairment and dementia patients recruited from a real-world tertiary clinical setting. The patients represent a wide clinical spectrum of typical neuropathology, including AD, MCI, vascular cognitive impairment (VCI), FTD, DLB, and combined pathologies (e.g., AD + VCI, AD + DLB, AD + VCI).

Research questions

We examined four main research questions. Overall, we tested whether ventricular size [40] (an overall global measure of atrophy [42, 43]) predicts clinical dementia severity using the Dementia Rating Scale (DRS) (a commonly used scale to stage clinical dementia severity [44, 45]) at baseline and over 2 years. A longitudinal design was used for baseline DRS scores and two follow-up visits at 12 months and 24 months. Any associations were further tested for CR moderation and stratified by sex (see Fig. 1).

Research question 1 (RQ1)

Does higher baseline ventricular size predict poorer baseline DRS performance and steeper 2-year decline? On the basis of previous research, we expected to first establish this association in our present dementia sample.

Research question 2 (RQ2)

Does E-CR moderate clinical dementia severity for ventricular size such that those with higher ventricular size and lower E-CR have poorer DRS performance and steeper decline than those with a higher level of E-CR? We also examined whether this association is magnified in women compared with men.

Research question 3 (RQ3)

Does L-CR moderate clinical dementia severity for ventricular size such that those with higher ventricular size and lower L-CR have poorer DRS performance and steeper decline than those with higher levels of L-CR? We also examined whether this moderation is magnified in women compared with men.

Research question 4 (RQ4)

Does CR-P moderate clinical dementia severity for ventricular size such that those with higher ventricular size in the low CR-P group have poorer DRS performance and steeper 2-year decline than those in the high CR-P

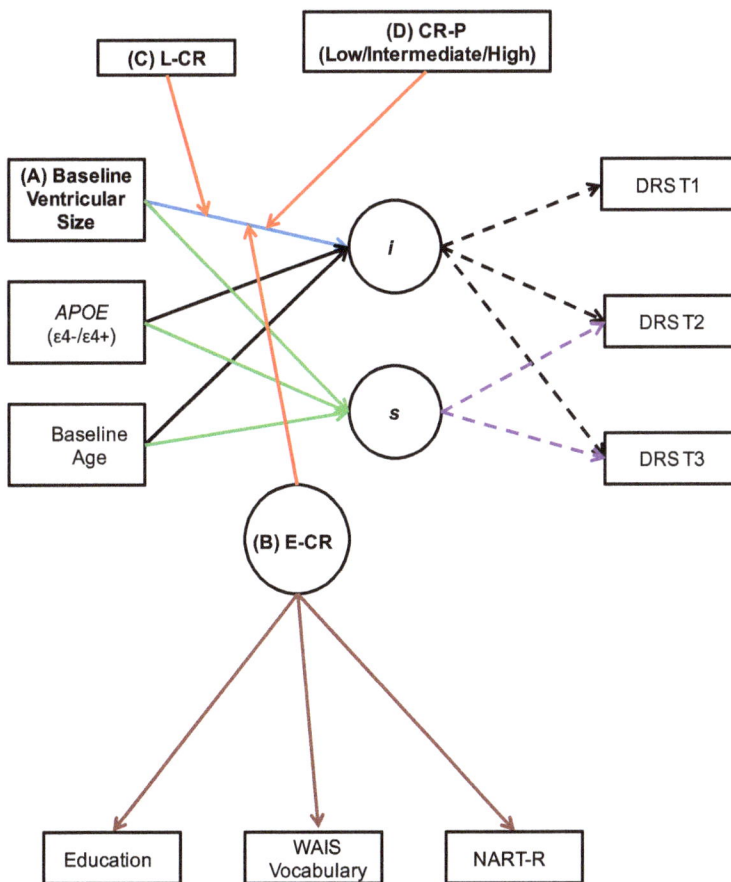

Fig. 1 Conceptual model for baseline ventricular size on baseline Dementia Rating Scale (DRS) performance and 2-year change (A) independently, (B) as moderated by early-life cognitive reserve (E-CR), (C) as moderated by later-life cognitive reserve (L-CR), and (D) as moderated by cognitive reserve panel (CR-P = E-CR + L-CR). Apolipoprotein E (APOE) genotype and baseline age are included as covariates in all analyses. i Intercept, s Slope, T Time point, WAIS Wechsler Adult Intelligence Scale, NART North American Reading Test-Revised

group? We also examined whether this moderation is differentially represented by sex. We expected that any moderating effects between higher baseline ventricular size and higher dementia severity and accelerated increase (steeper 2-year DRS decline) would be magnified in the low CR-P panel, particularly in women.

Methods

Participants

We used data from the Sunnybrook Dementia Study (SDS) [46], a large, longitudinal, observational, prospective cohort study (1994–present) of patients with dementia in Toronto, Canada, that includes clinical, standardized neuroimaging, neuropsychological, functional, mood, behavioral, and genetic assessments (ClinicalTrials.gov, NCT01800214). Patients and control subjects (N = 1498) were recruited from the Cognitive Neurology Clinic at Sunnybrook Health Sciences Centre, University of Toronto, Canada. All patients were enrolled through physician referrals and cognitively normal control individuals through word of mouth or advertisements. The recruited patients represented AD [47, 48], MCI [49, 50], VCI [51], DLB [52], FTD [53, 54], and mixed neurodegenerative diseases. Human/institutional research ethics guidelines were met in full for all SDS and ongoing data collection procedures. Written informed consent was obtained from all participants. For the present sample, we applied the following exclusionary criteria: (1) all cognitively normal control individuals, (2) participants who did not have data on the DRS, and (3) participants who did not have baseline ventricular size and total intracranial volume data. Accordingly, a total of 723 patients (age range = 38–90 years; mean age = 70.77 [9.42] years; females = 374) were included in this analysis. The patients represented were AD (n = 439), MCI (n = 77), VCI (n = 52), DLB (n = 30), and

FTD (n = 125) (Table 1). Any mixed neurodegenerative cases were grouped into the dominant clinical group.

Magnetic resonance imaging acquisition protocols and processing

Structural brain images were obtained using a 1.5-T Signa system (GE Healthcare Life Sciences, Milwaukee, WI, USA). Ventricular size was calculated as the ventricular cerebrospinal fluid compartment using the Lesion Explorer (LE) pipeline and Semi-Automatic Brain Region Extraction (SABRE) tools [55, 56]. Complete details on the LE pipeline and SABRE are available elsewhere [55, 57]. For the present study, all baseline ventricular size measurements were corrected with total intracranial volume (ICV) for each participant (baseline ventricular size/baseline ICV).

Cognitive reserve

We examined two standard and widely used measures of intelligence and years of education as proxies for E-CR factor [6, 10, 58, 59] and occupation [60] as proxy for L-CR.

Wechsler Adult Intelligence Scale vocabulary

This verbal IQ test [61] consists of a list of 35 words. Participants are asked the meaning of each word starting at item 4. Each item receives a score of 0 (incorrect meaning), 1 (a vague answer), or 2 (correct meaning). Participants receive 2 points each for items 1–3 if items 4–8 received a score of 1 or 2. The test is discontinued after five consecutive failures. The final score is out of 70, with higher scores representing better performance.

North American Adult Reading Test–Revised

This verbal IQ test [62] consists of 61 words in four columns. Participants are asked to read each word aloud,

Table 1 Baseline participant characteristics by clinical status

Characteristics	AD	MCI	VCI	FTD	DLB	Total
n	439	77	52	125	30	723
Age, years	71.7 (9.3)	70.3 (8.2)	71.1 (8.2)	66.9 (9.1)	73.2 (8.8)	70.8 (9.4)
Sex, F/M	233/206	47/30	20/32	64/61	10/20	374/349
MMSE	23.0 (4.8)	27.6 (1.9)	25.7 (3.9)	23.1 (6.0)	23.9 (4.4)	23.8 (4.9)
Ventricular size[a], cm^3	43.4 (19.9)	31.4 (17.2)	45.6 (24.5)	42.5 (21.2)	42.7 (20.0)	42.1 (20.5)
WMH[a], cm^3	7.8 (11.1)	3.3 (4.8)	13.2 (17.5)	4.6 (6.8)	7.2 (11.6)	7.1 (10.8)
TIV, cm^3	1213.6 (140.2)	1198.0 (121.8)	1225.1 (122.3)	1204.9 (121.1)	1269.5 (127.3)	1213.6 (133.7)
Dementia Rating Scale	117.8 (14.8)	133.5 (7.8)	126.4 (13.7)	115.7 (19.3)	118.7 (14.6)	119.9 (15.9)
NART-R	107.4 (9.9)	110.1 (9.1)	108.3 (10.3)	102.3 (11.0)	110.0 (10.4)	107.1 (10.3)
WAIS vocabulary	42.8 (14.1)	51.3 (9.8)	42.2 (12.5)	34.7 (18.2)	44.8 (13.3)	42.7 (14.5)
Education, years	13.8 (3.8)	14.0 (3.4)	13.7 (3.9)	14.1 (3.9)	13.9 (3.4)	13.9 (3.7)

Abbreviations: AD Alzheimer's disease, *DLB* Dementia with Lewy bodies, *FTD* Frontotemporal dementia, *MCI* Mild cognitive impairment, *MMSE* Mini Mental State Examination, *NART-R* National Adult Reading Test–Revised, *TIV* Total intracranial volume, *VCI* Vascular cognitive impairment, *WAIS* Wechsler Adult Intelligence Scale, *WMH* White matter hyperintensities
[a]Corrected for total intracranial volume

going down the list for the two columns on the first page and continuing on to the next page. The number of errors is recorded. The final scaled score is computed with the formula = 127.8–0.78 (number of errors), with higher scores representing better performance.

Education

Years of total education [63] completed was recorded and used as a continuous scale. Years of education ranged from 0 to 32. Higher number of years represented higher levels of education.

Hollingshead Index of Social Position

Participants were asked their current occupation. For the present study, we examined only the occupation scale [60], which has a total weight of 7, with lower scores representing higher executive and major professionals and higher scores for those with hard physical work/labor (*see* Additional file 1: Table S1).

Clinical dementia severity

Mattis Dementia Rating Scale

This test [64] is widely used to measure clinical dementia severity in older adults and dementia patients [44, 65, 66]. The test consists of five subscales: (1) attention - 37 points; (2) initiation and preservation - 37 points, (3) construction - 6 points, (4) conceptualization - 39 points, and (5) memory - 25 points. Participants are asked to correctly perform different tasks within each subscale. The final score is from 0 to 144, with lower scores reflecting poorer performance (i.e., higher dementia severity).

Statistical analyses

Structural equation modeling was used for all analyses with Mplus version 7.4 [67]. All missing values for E-CR measures were assumed to be missing at random and were estimated using maximum likelihood. Cases with missing predictor values were removed using list-wise deletion in Mplus 7.4.

First, we used confirmatory factor analysis to examine loadings of three manifest variables (Wechsler Adult Intelligence Scale [WAIS] vocabulary, North American Adult Reading Test–Revised [NART-R], and education) on the predicted one-factor E-CR latent variable. All three observed variables were tested to determine the best fit and parsimonious model. The best fit model was determined by examining several fit statistics. The chi-square test of model (χ^2; $p > 0.05$) allowed for an overall indication of good model fit. Additional absolute/comparative fit indices were also examined to determine a good model fit to the data [68]: root mean square error of approximation (RMSEA ≤ 0.05), comparative fit index (CFI ≥ 0.95), and standardized root mean square residual (SRMR ≤ 0.08).

Second, we used latent growth modeling to determine how DRS performance changes over 2 years. We adopted a model-building approach, started with a simple (null) model, and added parameters at each step to arrive at a baseline model of change. The null model assumes that there is no change over the three time points, followed by the addition of fixed intercepts, random intercepts, fixed slope, random slope, and fixed quadratic. In the null model, the variances for the intercepts were fixed across participants to 0. In the random intercepts model, individuals were allowed to vary in intercept variance by removing the fixed intercept at 0. A fixed linear slope was added to the baseline model by fixing the slope to 0 across all participants. The fixed linear slope assumed that all participants were changing in performance at the same rate. Participants were allowed to vary in their slope performance by removing the fixed linear slope constraint and adding a random intercept and random linear slope model of change. A fixed quadratic was added to the random intercept and random linear slope models, where both the intercepts and the slope were allowed to vary across individuals, but the curvilinear change was fixed across all participants. Following the examination of model fit, the χ^2 difference statistic was calculated to detect any improvement in fit with the addition of free parameters at each step.

Third, to examine moderating effects, we created interaction terms between E-CR and ventricular size to examine E-CR moderation (RQ2) and L-CR and ventricular size to examine L-CR moderation (RQ3). We further examined both interactions stratified by sex. To test CR-P moderation and account for any sex differences, we dichotomized E-CR and L-CR into low and high and summed accordingly for the CR-P groups. This stratification approach to test moderation in Mplus is common and widely accepted (see [69–72]). Specifically, we used the same cutoff for low and high E-CR and L-CR groups in both sexes. We dichotomized (1) E-CR factor score into low versus high by splitting at the overall mean factor score, (2) L-CR with a median split (3.5) of occupational status into high (less than 3.5) versus low (greater than 3.5) groups, and (3) CR-P by subtracting across all low versus high dichotomized groups with E-CR factor (0 = low; 1 = high) – L-CR (0 = high; 1 = low). All possible combination scores of – 1 (low E-CR + low L-CRCR), 0 (low E-CR + high L-CR or high E-CR + low L-CR), and 1 (high E-CR + high L-CR) were represented as low, intermediate, and high CR-P groups, respectively.

Fourth, the best DRS latent growth model was regressed on baseline ventricular size (RQ1) independently, (RQ2) with E-CR × ventricular size, E-CR, ventricular size and as stratified by sex, (RQ3) with L-CR × ventricular size, L-CR, ventricular size and as stratified by sex, and (RQ4) moderated by CR-P (low versus intermediate versus high) and as stratified by sex. Baseline age (continuous) and *APOE* (ε4−/ε4+) status [73–77] were included as covariates in all analyses. One hundred ninety-eight participants with missing values on apolipoprotein E (*APOE*) genotype and an additional fifteen participants with missing values on all three DRS time points were lost owing to list-wise deletion. For model fit statistics and significant results, we examined the regression estimate and $p < 0.05$.

Results

Descriptive characteristics for all participants by dementia classification are reported in Table 1. One-factor E-CR factor with WAIS vocabulary, NART-R, and education provided the best model fit [$\chi^2(df) = 1.121$ (1), $p = 0.299$; RMSEA (90% CI) = 0.013 (0.000–0.101); CFI = 1.000; SRMR = 0.062]. We computed factor scores for the E-CR latent factor, which was used in all succeeding analyses to examine moderation. For the DRS latent growth model, the random intercept and random slope model provided the best model fit (*see* Table 2) and was used in all subsequent analyses.

For RQ1, we observed that larger baseline ventricular size was associated with poorer DRS performance ($\beta = -0.202$, SE = 0.033, $p < 0.001$) and predicted steeper 2-year decline ($\beta = -0.085$, SE = 0.026, $p = 0.001$) in the overall group.

For RQ2, we observed two significant effects of E-CR moderation between baseline ventricular size and DRS performance. First, the negative impact of lower E-CR on DRS performance was more pronounced in patients with larger ventricular size ($\beta = -0.093$, SE = 0.032, $p = 0.004$). Second, when stratified by sex, this significant association was present only in men. Specifically, the negative impact of lower E-CR on DRS performance was present only in men with larger baseline ventricular size ($\beta = -0.104$, SE = 0.041, $p = 0.012$). We did not observe that E-CR moderated the association between baseline ventricular size and DRS performance or 2-year change in women.

For RQ3, we observed two significant effects of L-CR moderation. First, the negative impact of lower L-CR on DRS performance was more pronounced in patients with larger baseline ventricular size ($\beta = -0.052$, SE = 0.021, $p = 0.014$). Second, when stratified by sex, this significant association was present only in women. Specifically, the negative impact of lower L-CR on DRS performance was present only in women with larger baseline ventricular size ($\beta = -0.086$, SE = 0.034, $p = 0.012$). We did not observe that L-CR moderated the association between baseline ventricular size and DRS performance or 2-year change in men.

For RQ4, we observed three significant associations. First, CR-P moderated the association between baseline ventricular size and DRS performance and change. Specifically, larger baseline ventricular size was associated with poorer baseline DRS performance in the low ($\beta = -0.382$, SE = 0.064, $p < 0.001$) and intermediate ($\beta = -0.212$, SE = 0.052, $p < 0.001$) CR-P groups and steeper 2-year decline in the low ($\beta = -0.127$, SE = 0.055, $p = 0.020$) and high ($\beta = -0.089$, SE = 0.032, $p = 0.005$) CR-P group overall (Fig. 2). Second, when stratified by sex, larger baseline ventricular size in men was associated with poorer performance ($\beta = -0.323$, SE = 0.080, $p < 0.001$) only in the low CR-P group. Men in all three groups did not show 2-year DRS decline with larger baseline ventricular size. Third, in women, larger baseline ventricular size was associated with poorer performance in the low ($\beta = -0.455$, SE = 0.103, $p < 0.001$) and intermediate ($\beta = -0.308$, SE = 0.067, $p < 0.001$) CR-P groups (*see* Table 3; Fig. 3). For 2-year decline, women with larger baseline ventricular size showed steeper decline in the low ($\beta = -0.221$, SE = 0.098, $p = 0.024$), intermediate ($\beta = -0.178$, SE = 0.079, $p = 0.025$), and high ($\beta = -0.143$, SE = 0.065, $p = 0.027$) CR-P groups (*see* Table 3; Fig. 3).

Discussion

We examined whether the association between baseline ventricular size and clinical dementia severity (measured with DRS) is differentially moderated by CR in men and women. This is the first study to show that (1) CR-P (an

Table 2 Latent growth model fit statistics and chi-square difference test for Dementia Rating Scale

Model	$\chi^2_M(df_M)$	CFI	RMSEA (90% CI)	SRMR	χ^2_D (df_D)
Fixed intercept	587.826(5)**	0.000	0.409 (0.381–0.437)	0.801	–
Random intercept	264.295(4)**	0.535	0.306 (0.275–0.337)	0.577	323.531(1)**
Random intercept, fixed slope	76.559(3)**	0.869	0.188 (0.153–0.225)	0.402	187.736(1)**
Random intercept, random slope	0.967(1)	1.000	0.000 (0.000–0.099)	0.033	75.592(2)**
Random intercept, random slope, fixed quadratic	0.000(0)**	1.000	0.000 (0.000–0.000)	0.000	0.967(1)
Random intercept, random slope, random quadratic			No convergence		

χ^2_M Chi-square test of model fit, df_M Degrees of freedom for model fit, *RMSEA* Root mean square error of approximation, *CFI* Comparative fix index, *SRMR* Standardized root mean square residual, χ^2_D Chi-square test of difference, df_D Degrees of freedom for chi-square difference test
**$p < 0.001$

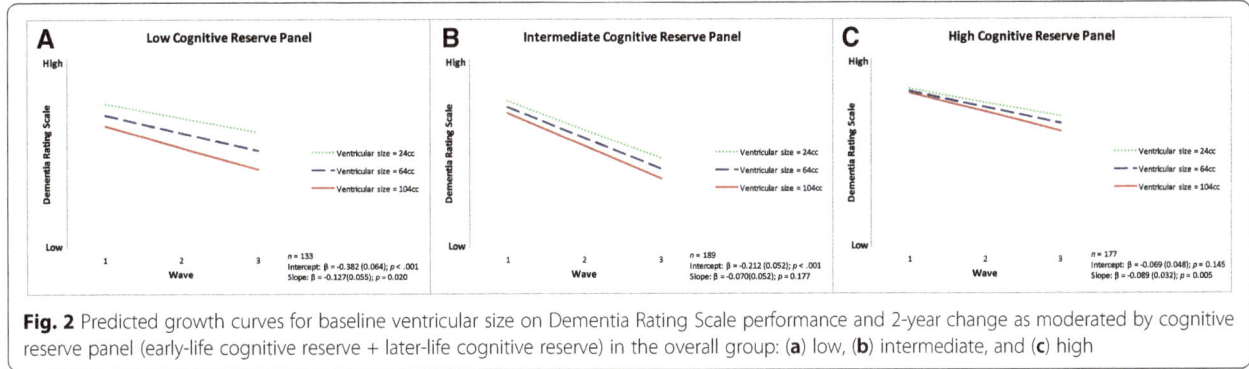

Fig. 2 Predicted growth curves for baseline ventricular size on Dementia Rating Scale performance and 2-year change as moderated by cognitive reserve panel (early-life cognitive reserve + later-life cognitive reserve) in the overall group: (**a**) low, (**b**) intermediate, and (**c**) high

additive panel of E-CR and L-CR) (2) moderates the association between baseline ventricular size and DRS performance and 2-year change (3) in a heterogeneous dementia population (AD, MCI, VCI, DLB, FTD, mixed pathologies). We observed two main findings. First, we established a baseline association between ventricular size and dementia severity in our mixed dementia sample. Specifically, higher baseline ventricular size was associated with poorer baseline DRS performance and steeper 2-year decline. Second, we observed that this association is moderated by (1) E-CR and L-CR (occupational attainment) in the overall group and differentially

Table 3 Unstandardized regression coefficients and model fit indices for all models examining baseline ventricular size on Dementia Rating Scale performance and 2-year change

Models	Intercept			Linear slope			Model fit indices			
	β	SE	p Value	β	SE	p Value	χ^2_M(df_M)	CFI	RMSEA (90% CI)	SRMR
Independent (n = 510)	− 0.202	0.033	0.000	− 0.085	0.026	0.001	13.258 (6), p = 0.039	0.986	0.049 (0.010–0.085)	0.034
E-CR moderation (n = 510)	− 0.093	0.032	0.004	− 0.049	0.028	0.079	5.582 (7), p = 0.589	1.000	0.000 (0.000–0.047)	0.013
E-CR moderation by sex										
Male (n = 254)	− 0.104	0.041	0.012	− 0.046	0.033	0.167	6.737 (7), p = 0.457	1.000	0.000 (0.000–0.075)	0.035
Female (n = 256)	− 0.076	0.054	0.159	− 0.046	0.052	0.378	5.499 (8), p = 0.703	1.000	0.000 (0.000–0.056)	0.045
L-CR moderation (n = 499)	− 0.052	0.021	0.014	0.016	0.015	0.296	7.308 (7), p = 0.398	0.999	0.009 (0.000–0.056)	0.012
L-CR moderation by sex										
Male (n = 252)	− 0.033	0.027	0.218	0.015	0.017	0.359	7.265 (7), p = 0.402	0.999	0.012 (0.000–0.079)	0.034
Female (n = 247)	− 0.086	0.034	0.012	0.010	0.033	0.764	7.200 (8), p = 0.515	1.000	0.000 (0.000–0.070)	0.024
CR-P moderation							31.751 (18), p = 0.024	0.973	0.068 (0.025–0.106)	0.058
(a) Low (n = 133)	− 0.382	0.064	0.000	− 0.127	0.055	0.020				
(b) Intermediate (n = 189)	− 0.212	0.052	0.000	− 0.070	0.052	0.177				
(c) High (n = 177)	− 0.069	0.048	0.145	− 0.089	0.032	0.005				
CR-P moderation by sex										
Male							32.143 (18), p = 0.021	0.941	0.097 (0.037–0.150)	0.141
(a) Low (n = 58)	− 0.323	0.080	0.000	− 0.094	0.069	0.171				
(b) Intermediate (n = 94)	− 0.107	0.074	0.151	0.011	0.068	0.875				
(c) High (n = 100)	− 0.107	0.063	0.091	− 0.048	0.032	0.130				
Female							12.656 (18), p = 0.817	1.000	0.000 (0.000–0.062)	0.078
(a) Low (n = 75)	− 0.455	0.103	0.000	− 0.221	0.098	0.024				
(b) Intermediate (n = 95)	− 0.308	0.067	0.000	− 0.178	0.079	0.025				
(c) High (n = 77)	− 0.026	0.075	0.727	− 0.143	0.065	0.027				

Abbreviations: β Regression estimate, χ^2_M Chi-square test of model fit, df_M Degrees of freedom for model fit, CFI Comparative fix index, CR-P Cognitive reserve panel (E-CR + L-CR), E-CR Early-life cognitive reserve, L-CR Later-life cognitive reserve, RMSEA Root mean square error of approximation, SRMR Standardized root mean square residual

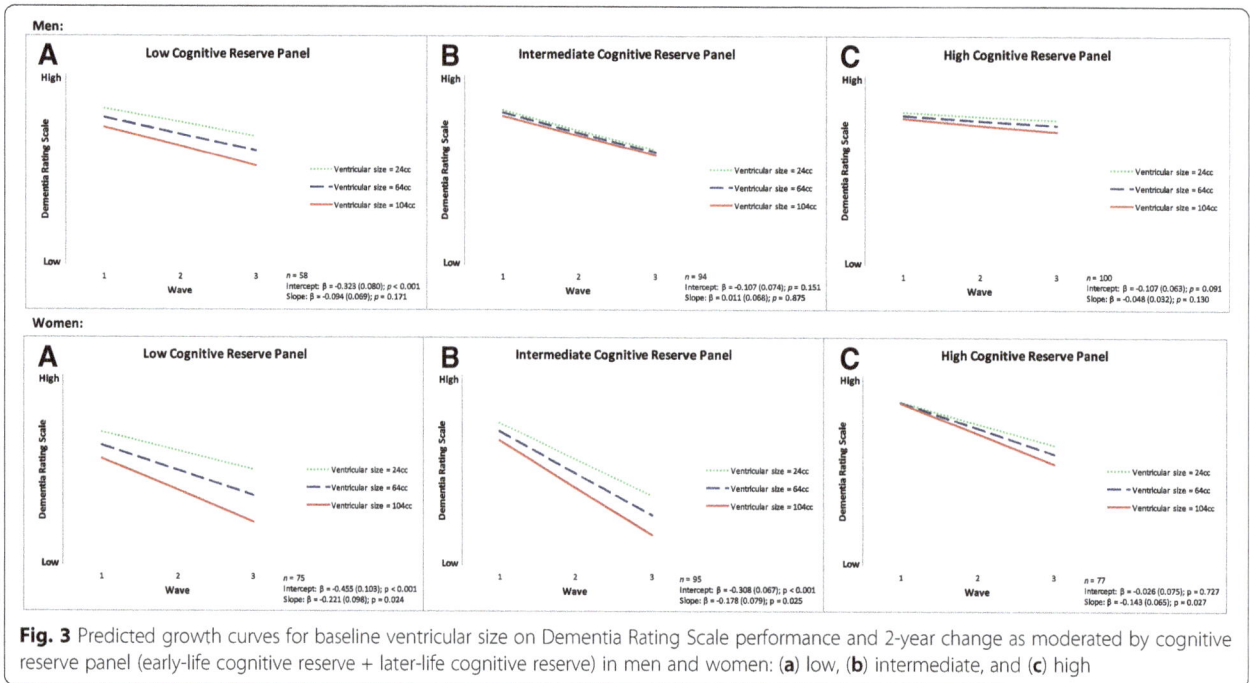

Fig. 3 Predicted growth curves for baseline ventricular size on Dementia Rating Scale performance and 2-year change as moderated by cognitive reserve panel (early-life cognitive reserve + later-life cognitive reserve) in men and women: (**a**) low, (**b**) intermediate, and (**c**) high

in men and women and (2) CR-P in the overall group and differentially in men and women. Specifically, women in all three CR-P groups had steeper 2-year DRS decline with larger baseline ventricular size, whereas men in the same groups were not declining at a significant rate.

Our novel approach and findings suggest that (1) it is imperative to account for both the independent and additive influences of E-CR and L-CR and sex differences in conjunction with clinical symptoms and neuroimaging biomarkers to understand the underlying neuropathology of clinical phenotypes in dementia and (2) understanding this complex synergistic association may lead to earlier detection and personalized interventions by identifying subgroups at high risk. Specific comments related to our findings by RQs follow.

For RQ1, the main result was that larger baseline ventricular size was associated with poorer DRS performance and steeper 2-year decline. As expected and observed in previous studies [78], this study establishes the link between subcortical atrophy (i.e., ventricular size [22]) and cognitive impairment in sampling across different dementias in the present sample. We observed that baseline ventricular size alone is an important predictor of cognitive impairment and dementia severity. Supporting recent findings with other brain structures include (1) hippocampal atrophy was associated with lower scores on the Montreal Cognitive Assessment [79], (2) white matter hyperintensities were associated with performance on the Boston Naming Test and the Trail

Making Test B [80], (3) ventricular size and hippocampal volume predicted dementia incidence [81], and (4) baseline volume of the right hippocampus and entorhinal cortex were associated with time to preclinical AD incidence [82]. Our findings extend previous literature on brain atrophy and cognition in normal aging older adults and pure dementia cases to a unique sample representing a range of dementias.

For RQ2, we observed that E-CR latent factor moderated the association between baseline ventricular size and baseline dementia severity in the overall group. However, when stratified by sex, the negative effect of lower E-CR on DRS performance was present only in men with larger baseline ventricular size. This suggests that CR typically obtained in early life (IQ and education) alone may not be an important independent moderator between ventricular size and dementia severity in both sexes. Because this is the first study to examine for interactive associations between E-CR factor and ventricular size sampling from different dementia groups, our goal was to test a general cognitive functioning domain. In this regard, we chose the DRS, which included subscales for memory, attention, preservation, construction, and conceptualization [64]. Future studies should consider examining moderation effects of E-CR between other neuroimaging biomarkers (e.g., hippocampal atrophy, white matter hyperintensities) and specific cognitive domains (e.g., memory, neurocognitive speed) in pure cognitive impairment and dementia cases (e.g., MCI or AD [80, 83]).

For RQ3, L-CR moderated the association between baseline ventricular size and DRS performance. Specifically, the negative effect of lower L-CR on DRS performance was more pronounced in patients with larger baseline ventricular size. When stratified by sex, this association was only present in women. This sex difference for L-CR suggests that women with lower occupational status may be more vulnerable to higher dementia severity than men. We examined occupation as a measure of L-CR that is obtained across the lifespan because previous work has shown that higher levels of occupational complexity among adults at risk for dementia and with similar levels of cognition were associated with lower hippocampal volume and higher overall brain atrophy [84]. Lower socioprofessional attainment in midlife and across the life course has also been linked to faster rate of hippocampal atrophy [32]. In the present study, this implies that adults with higher occupational status and complexity may be using CR accumulated across the lifespan. This interesting and novel finding implies that L-CR with occupation as a proxy may be more important for women in the context of larger baseline ventricular size. Previous work examining neuropathological changes in men and women has shown similar levels of AD- and FTD-related dementia severity, despite men having significantly reduced cerebral metabolic glucose rate (an indication of greater CR) [16, 85]. Future studies may benefit from examining sex differences when studying the influence of neuroimaging biomarkers on dementia severity as moderated by dynamic CR networks.

For RQ4, CR-P moderated the association between baseline ventricular size and DRS performance and 2-year decline. Specifically, larger baseline ventricular size was associated with poorer baseline DRS performance in the low and intermediate CR-P groups, as well as with steeper 2-year DRS decline in the low and high CR-P groups. Although we expected to observe significant decline only in the low L-CR group, our significant finding is consistent with the literature showing that older adults with higher CR show higher resilience and plasticity to cognitive impairment [86]. Patients with dementia with high CR factors are more likely to have greater brain pathology and vulnerability triggering a rapid deterioration in cognition once a critical threshold is reached [87]. This threshold effect may be more common in clinically diagnosed cases with the presence of additional neuronal pathologies than in cognitively normal older adults [80, 88]. Our finding demonstrates that the additive effects of E-CR and L-CR may differentially contribute to the complex clinical manifestations observed in dementia. Future studies should consider testing the relationship between E-CR and L-CR in patients with dementia to target intervention programs at a younger age.

Previous studies have observed that cognitively normal older adults with high IQ and high socioeconomic status show less cognitive impairment in the presence of hippocampal atrophy [79], and early education and intellectual activities may protect against amyloid beta deposition in late life [89]. Consistent with these other studies, we observed that dementia patients in the high CR-P group were protected from poorer baseline DRS performance with larger baseline ventricular size but showed steeper 2-year DRS decline. The protective effects of high CR-P were present at baseline, but this association was absent for change over time on the DRS. Two forms of underlying neural networks are commonly linked to CR: (1) neural reserve, reserve associated with preexisting cognitive networks, and (2) neural compensation, the ability to recruit compensatory mechanisms [87]. Findings on neural networks have observed that older adults with high CR may have reduced neural reserve and increased neural compensation compared with younger adults with high CR [87]. Our present findings extend this literature by (1) showing that clinically diagnosed older adults with high CR-P maybe recruiting more neural mechanisms at baseline to compensate for the higher baseline subcortical atrophy, whereas those with low CR-P are not able to perform at the same level, and (2) this protective association of high CR-P despite larger baseline ventricular size on DRS performance dissipates across 2 years, resulting in greater dementia severity.

We also observed differential interactions between the three CR-P groups and baseline ventricular size on DRS performance in men and women. Both men and women in the low CR-P groups showed greater dementia severity. However, only women in the intermediate group had greater dementia severity with larger baseline ventricular size, but men in the same group did not show this association. Regarding steeper 2-year decline, men did not show decline on the DRS with larger baseline ventricular size in any of the of three (low, intermediate, high) CR-P groups. However, women in all three CR-P groups had steeper 2-year DRS decline with larger baseline ventricular size. A major biological difference between older men and women is reduced estrogen levels in postmenopausal women, which may lead to increased dementia risk [18]. Estrogen, primarily produced by the corpus luteum and the placenta, influences receptors in the hippocampus, basal forebrain, and cerebral cortex. Estrogen has also been shown to be important for growth and survival of cholinergic neurons, antioxidant properties, and increased metabolism of amyloid precursor protein [18]. Future studies may benefit from studying the relationship between estrogen replacement therapy [17] and CR networks in older women at high risk of dementia to identify potential underlying mechanisms.

Furthermore, we observed that the longitudinal association between larger baseline ventricular size and steeper 2-year DRS decline in women was magnified in the low

CR-P group ($\beta = -0.221$) compared with the high group ($\beta = -0.143$) (Table 3; Additional file 1: Table S2). This implies a faster rate of decline for women with low CR-P than for women with high CR-P. This novel finding emphasizes the need to aim for sex-specific intervention programs.

We note several strengths and limitations of the present study. First, we examined overall baseline ventricular size, whereas future studies may benefit from examining differences in specific brain regions contributing to ventricular size as well as longitudinal change in ventricular size [90]. Future studies should also consider other neuroimaging biomarkers targeting specific clinical diagnoses, such as hippocampal atrophy as a potential biomarker for AD [91]. Second, previous studies have shown that age and *APOE* ε4 status may play a role in dementia [81]. We included both as covariates in all our analyses and performed post hoc analyses to examine whether *APOE* genotype (ε4− versus ε4+) predicted baseline ventricular volume in our sample. *APOE* genotype did not influence baseline ventricular size ($\beta = -1.074$, SE = 1.807, $p = 0.552$) in our sample (Additional file 1: Table S3). Future studies should consider looking at specific networks of genetic risks identified in recent genome-wide association studies and as stratified by *APOE* ε4 groups to investigate cognitive associations in both preclinical [71] and clinical cases. Third, traditionally, premorbid IQ is used as a proxy for CR [87], and we note this as a potential limitation in our study. IQ in the present study was measured at baseline when patients with mild dementia were recruited. Fourth, although we had a robust measure of occupational status (using the Hollingshead Index of Social Position), future studies should also include occupational complexity [84, 92] in addition to occupational status to examine L-CR and additive effects of other established proxies of reserve (e.g., lifestyle and physical activities, financial management [93]). Fifth, because we used the first three DRS measurements to examine change in dementia severity over a 2-year period, we acknowledge that additional time points may have resulted in a random quadratic or a different growth model [68]. Future studies should consider examining additional time points to address long-term changes in dementia severity.

There are also several strengths of the present study. First, our sample provides a unique representation of patients with dementia across a range of neurodegenerative diseases in a real-world tertiary clinic setting. We include this heterogeneous dementia population because the association of ventricular size with dementia severity may differ across all represented neurodegenerative conditions. As part of post hoc analyses, we excluded the MCI group to examine the association between ventricular size and dementia severity as moderated by CR-P in men and women. Similar to the overall group, this MCI-excluded group showed poorer baseline DRS

performance with larger ventricular size in the low ($p < 0.001$) and intermediate ($p = 0.001$) CR-P groups and steeper 2-year decline in the low ($p = 0.031$) and high ($p = 0.011$) CR-P groups. For men, we observed poorer baseline DRS performance with larger ventricular size in only the low ($p < 0.001$) CR-P group. For women, we observed poorer baseline DRS performance with larger ventricular size in the low ($p < 0.001$) and intermediate ($p < 0.001$) CR-P groups and steeper 2-year decline in the low ($p = 0.044$), intermediate (borderline significance: $p = 0.059$), and high ($p = 0.042$) CR-P groups. Second, we have a latent E-CR factor compared with other studies that have used only single variables (i.e., education) as a proxy for CR. This approach examines the common variances across two IQ variables (WAIS vocabulary, NART-R) and education to eliminate any measurement errors associated with testing procedures and single variables. In addition, our latent factor in Mplus by default accounts for missing data with maximum likelihood estimation to generate factor scores. Third, to the best of our knowledge, this is the first study to distinguish between E-CR versus L-CR, and importantly our results show that such distinction accounts for additive effects of CR that is accumulated throughout the lifespan. This has not always been emphasized in studies on CR. Fourth, compared with previous CR studies, we stratified by sex to examine differences in CR moderation of ventricular volume in men and women. Fifth, we examined a commonly used global measure of cognitive performance and decline. The DRS includes several subscales of cognitive domains, including executive function, memory, and attention, and is widely used to test clinical performance in dementia [44].

Conclusions

We examined independent and synergistic contributions of E-CR (education, IQ) and L-CR (occupation) on the association between neurodegeneration (ventricular volume) and dementia severity as stratified by sex. Larger baseline ventricular size was associated with poorer DRS baseline performance and steeper 2-year DRS decline in a heterogeneous neurodegenerative population (i.e., AD, VCI, combined). This association was moderated by E-CR (education and IQ), L-CR (occupation, which may represent a form of maintenance), and the additive effects (CR-P) of E-CR and L-CR. All moderations were differentially represented by sex. Specifically, E-CR significantly moderated the association between ventricular size and DRS performance in men and L-CR in women. Men with high CR-P were protected from the detrimental effects of poorer baseline and steeper 2-year DRS decline with larger baseline ventricular size. However, women with high CR-P showed steeper 2-year DRS decline with larger baseline ventricular size, and this rate of decline was magnified for women with low CR-P. Future studies should consider replicating this important contribution in other samples. In dementia, complex interactions between CR (in early life and across the life course) and neuroimaging biomarkers (i.e., ventricular atrophy) on cognitive impairment may be selective and differentially represented in men and women. Future research should focus on similar innovative methodological approaches to identify potential complex and dynamic CR mechanisms that may lead to personalized interventions across neurodegenerative diseases.

Abbreviations
β: Regression estimate; x^2_M: Chi-square test of model fit; df_M: Degrees of freedom for model fit; AD: Alzheimer's disease; *APOE: Apolipoprotein E*; CFI: Comparative fit index; CR: Cognitive reserve; CR-P: E-CR + L-CR; DLB: Dementia with Lewy bodies; DRS: Dementia Rating Scale; E-CR: Early-life cognitive reserve; FTD: Frontotemporal dementia; *i*: Intercept; ICV: Intracranial volume; L-CR: Later-life cognitive reserve; MCI: Mild cognitive impairment; NART-R: North American Adult Reading Test–Revised; RMSEA: Root mean square error of approximation; *s*: Slope; SDS: Sunnybrook Dementia Study; SRMR: Standardized root mean square residual; *T*: Time point; VCI: Vascular cognitive impairment; WAIS: Wechsler Adult Intelligence Scale; WMH: White matter hyperintensities

Acknowledgements
We gratefully acknowledge and thank all volunteer participants and the Sunnybrook Dementia Study (SDS) staff for their time and contributions.

Funding
This work was supported by a Canadian Institutes of Health Research (MOP 13129) grant to SEB, MM, and DTS. The authors also gratefully acknowledge financial support from the following sources. SEB receives salary support from the Toronto Dementia Research Alliance, University of Toronto, the Hurvitz Brain Sciences Research Program at Sunnybrook Research Institute, and the Department of Medicine at Sunnybrook Health Sciences Centre (SHSC). MM receives salary support from the Department of Medicine at SHSC and the University of Toronto, as well as from the Sunnybrook Foundation. JR acknowledges support from the LC Campbell Cognitive Neurology Research Institute and Ontario Neurodegeneration Research Initiative, Ontario Brain Institute. SS is supported by the Canadian Consortium of Neurodegeneration in Aging/Alzheimer Society of Canada Postdoctoral Fellowship. The funding sources did not have role in the study design; data collection; statistical analysis; or results interpretation, reporting, or submission decisions.

Authors' contributions
SS designed and planned the research and performed the statistical analyses. SS wrote drafts of the paper. JR, MM, DTS, and SEB designed and contributed to data collection, interpretation of data, critical revision of the manuscript for intellectual content, and approval for publication. All authors read and approved the final manuscript.

Consent for publication
Not applicable.

Competing interests
The authors declare that they have no competing interests.

Author details
[1]Hurvitz Brain Sciences Research Program, Sunnybrook Research Institute, Sunnybrook Health Sciences Centre, 2075 Bayview Avenue, M6-192, Toronto, ON M4N 3M5, Canada. [2]Departments of Medicine, University of Toronto, 190 Elizabeth Street, R. Fraser Elliot Building, 3-805, Toronto, ON M5G 2C4, Canada. [3]Department of Psychology, University of Toronto, 100 St. George Street, 4th Floor, Sidney Smith Hall, Toronto, ON M5S 3G3, Canada. [4]Rotman Research Institute of Baycrest Centre, 3560 Bathurst Street, Toronto, ON M6H 4A6, Canada. [5]Department of Medicine (Neurology), University of Toronto, 190 Elizabeth Street, R. Fraser Elliot Building, 3-805, Toronto, ON M5G 2C4, Canada.

References
1. Viswanathan A, Rocca WA, Tzourio C. Vascular risk factors and dementia: how to move forward? Neurology. 2009;72:368–74.
2. Rahimi J, Kovacs GG. Prevalence of mixed pathologies in the aging brain. Alzheimers Res Ther. 2014;6:82.
3. Windle G. What is resilience? A review and concept analysis. Rev Clin Gerontol. 2011;21:152–69.
4. Kaup AR, Nettiksimmons J, Harris TB, Sink KM, Satterfield S, Metti AL, et al. Cognitive resilience to apolipoprotein E ε4. JAMA Neurol. 2015;72:340.
5. Stern Y. An approach to studying the neural correlates of reserve. Brain Imaging Behav. 2017;11:410–6.
6. Jones RN, Manly J, Glymour MM, Rentz DM, Jefferson AL, Stern Y. Conceptual and measurement challenges in research on cognitive reserve. J Int Neuropsychol Soc. 2011;17:593–601.
7. Stern Y, Gurland B, Tatemichi TK, Tang MX, Wilder D, Mayeux R. Influence of education and occupation on the incidence of Alzheimer's disease. JAMA. 1994;271:1004–10.
8. Stern Y, Albert S, Tang MX, Tsai WY. Rate of memory decline in AD is related to education and occupation: cognitive reserve? Neurology. 1999;53:1942–7.
9. Scarmeas N, Stern Y. Cognitive reserve and lifestyle. J Clin Exp Neuropsychol. 2003;25:625–33.
10. M. Tucker A, Stern Y. Cognitive reserve in aging. Curr Alzheimer Res. 2011;8: 354–60.
11. Ceci S. How much does schooling influence general intelligence and its cognitive components? A reassessment of the evidence. Dev Psychol. 1991; 27:703–22.
12. Stern Y. Cognitive reserve: implications for assessment and intervention. Folia Phoniatr. Logop. NIH Public Access; 2013;65:49–54.
13. Andersen K, Launer LJ, Dewey ME, Letenneur L, Ott A, Copeland JR, et al. Gender differences in the incidence of AD and vascular dementia: the EURODEM studies. Neurology. 1999;53:1992–7.
14. Miller IN, Cronin-Golomb A. Gender differences in Parkinson's disease: clinical characteristics and cognition. Mov Disord. 2010;25:2695–703.
15. Ruitenberg A, Ott A, van Swieten JC, Hofman A, Breteler MM. Incidence of dementia: does gender make a difference? Neurobiol Aging. 2001;22:575–80.

16. Perneczky R, Diehl-Schmid J, Förstl H, Drzezga A, Kurz A. Male gender is associated with greater cerebral hypometabolism in frontotemporal dementia: evidence for sex-related cognitive reserve. Int J Geriatr Psychiatry. 2007;22:1135–40.

17. Laws KR, Irvine K, Gale TM. Sex differences in cognitive impairment in Alzheimer's disease. World J Psychiatry. 2016;6:54–65.

18. Janicki SC, Schupf N. Hormonal influences on cognition and risk for Alzheimer's disease. Curr Neurol Neurosci Rep. 2010;10:359–66.

19. Sundermann EE, Biegon A, Rubin LH, Lipton RB, Mowrey W, Landau S, et al. Better verbal memory in women than men in MCI despite similar levels of hippocampal atrophy. Neurology. 2006;86:1368–76.

20. Sundermann EE, Maki PM, Rubin LH, Lipton RB, Landau S, Biegon A, et al. Female advantage in verbal memory. Neurology. 2016;87:1916–24.

21. Breteler MMB, Van Amerongen NM, Van Swieten JC, Claus JJ, Grobbee DE, Van Gijn J, et al. Cognitive correlates of ventricular enlargement and cerebral white matter lesions on magnetic resonance imaging the Rotterdam study. Stroke. 1994;25:1109–15.

22. Nestor SM, Rupsingh R, Borrie M, Smith M, Accomazzi V, Wells JL, et al. Ventricular enlargement as a possible measure of Alzheimer's disease progression validated using the Alzheimer's disease neuroimaging initiative database. Brain. 2008;131:2443–54.

23. Luxenberg JS, Haxby JV, Creasey H, Sundaram M, Rapoport SI. Rate of ventricular enlargement in dementia of the Alzheimer type correlates with rate of neuropsychological deterioration. Neurology. 1987;37:1135–40.

24. Barulli D, Stern Y. Efficiency, capacity, compensation, maintenance, plasticity: emerging concepts in cognitive reserve. Trends Cogn Sci. 2013;17:502–9.

25. Yokoyama JS, Evans DS, Coppola G, Kramer JH, Tranah GJ, Yaffe K. Genetic modifiers of cognitive maintenance among older adults. Hum Brain Mapp. 2014;35:4556–65.

26. Ansiau D, Marquié JC, Soubelet A, Ramos S. Relationships between cognitive characteristics of the job, age, and cognitive efficiency. Int Congr Ser. 2005;1280:43–8.

27. Chapko D, McCormack R, Black C, Staff R, Murray A. Life-course determinants of cognitive reserve (CR) in cognitive aging and dementia – a systematic literature review. Aging Ment Health. 2017. https://doi.org/10.1080/13607863.2017.1348471.

28. Potter GG, Helms MJ, Plassman BL. Associations of job demands and intelligence with cognitive performance among men in late life. Neurology. 2008;70:1803–8.

29. Baldivia B, Baldivia B, Andrade VM, Francisco O, Bueno A. Contribution of education, occupation and cognitively stimulating activities to the formation of cognitive reserve. Dement Neuropsychol. 2008;2:173–82.

30. Stern Y. Cognitive reserve and Alzheimer disease. Alzheimer Dis Assoc Disord. 2006;20:112–7.

31. Bozzali M, Dowling C, Serra L, Spanò B, Torso M, Marra C, et al. The impact of cognitive reserve on brain functional connectivity in Alzheimer's disease. J Alzheimers Dis. 2015;44:243–50.

32. Elbejjani M, Fuhrer R, Abrahamowicz M, Mazoyer B, Crivello F, Tzourio C, et al. Life-course socioeconomic position and hippocampal atrophy in a prospective cohort of older adults. Psychosom Med. 2017;79:14–23.

33. Serra L, Musicco M, Cercignani M, Torso M, Spanò B, Mastropasqua C, et al. Cognitive reserve and the risk for Alzheimer's disease: a longitudinal study. Neurobiol Aging. 2015;36:592–600.

34. Negash S, Xie S, Davatzikos C, Clark CM, Trojanowski JQ, Shaw LM, et al. Cognitive and functional resilience despite molecular evidence of Alzheimer's disease pathology. Alzheimers Dement. 2013;9:e89–95.

35. Latimer CS, Keene CD, Flanagan ME, Hemmy LS, Lim KO, White LR, et al. Resistance to Alzheimer disease neuropathologic changes and apparent cognitive resilience in the Nun and Honolulu-Asia aging studies. J Neuropathol Exp Neurol. 2017;76:458–66.

36. Nettiksimmons J, Harvey D, Brewer J, Carmichael O, DeCarli C, Jack CR, et al. Subtypes based on cerebrospinal fluid and magnetic resonance imaging markers in normal elderly predict cognitive decline. Neurobiol Aging. 2010;31:1419–28.

37. Ruan Q, D'Onofrio G, Sancarlo D, Bao Z, Greco A, Yu Z. Potential neuroimaging biomarkers of pathologic brain changes in mild cognitive impairment and Alzheimer's disease: a systematic review. BMC Geriatr. 2016;16:104.

38. Ewers M, Sperling RA, Klunk WE, Weiner MW, Hampel H. Neuroimaging markers for the prediction and early diagnosis of Alzheimer's disease dementia. Trends Neurosci. 2011;34:430–42.

39. Jack CR, Shiung MM, Weigand SD, O'Brien PC, Gunter JL, Boeve BF, et al. Brain atrophy rates predict subsequent clinical conversion in normal elderly and amnestic MCI. Neurology. 2005;65:1227–31.

40. Carlson NE, Moore MM, Dame A, Howieson D, Silbert LC, Quinn JF, et al. Trajectories of brain loss in aging and the development of cognitive impairment. Neurology. 2008;70:828–33.

41. Carmichael OT, Kuller LH, Lopez OL, Thompson PM, Dutton RA, Lu A, et al. Ventricular volume and dementia progression in the cardiovascular health study. Neurobiol Aging. 2007;28:389–97.

42. Hua X, Hibar DP, Lee S, Toga AW, Jack CR Jr, Weiner MW, et al. Sex and age differences in atrophic rates: an ADNI study with N=1368 MRI scans. Neubiol Aging. 2010;31:1463–80.

43. Gutman BA, Hua X, Rajagopalan P, Chou YY, Wang Y, Yanovsky I, et al. Maximizing power to track Alzheimer's disease and MCI progression by LDA-based weighting of longitudinal ventricular surface features. Neuroimage. 2013;70:386–401.

44. Shay KA, Duke LW, Conboy T, Harrell LE, Callaway R, Folks DG. The clinical validity of the Mattis dementia rating scale in staging Alzheimer's dementia. Top Geriatr. 1991;4:18–25.

45. Rascovsky K, Salmon DP, Hansen LA, Galasko D. Distinct cognitive profiles and rates of decline on the Mattis Dementia Rating Scale in autopsy-confirmed frontotemporal dementia and Alzheimer's disease. J Int Neuropsychol Soc. 2008;14:373–83.

46. Nestor SM, Mišić B, Ramirez J, Zhao J, Graham SJ, NPLG V, et al. Small vessel disease is linked to disrupted structural network covariance in Alzheimer's disease. Alzheimers Dement. 2017;13:749–60.

47. McKhann GM, Knopman DS, Chertkow H, e a. The diagnosis of dementia due to Alzheimer's disease: recommendations from the National Institute on Aging-Alzheimer's Association workgroups on diagnostic. Alzheimers Dement. 2011;7:263–9.

48. McKhann G, Drachman D, Folstein M, Katzman R, Price D, Stadlan EM. Clinical diagnosis of Alzheimer's disease: report of the NINCDS-ADRDA work group under the auspices of Department of Health and Human Services Task Force on Alzheimer's disease. Neurology. 1984;34:939–44.

49. Petersen RC. Mild cognitive impairment as a diagnostic entity. J Intern Med. 2004;256:183–94.

50. Winblad B, Palmer K, Kivipelto M, Jelic V, Fratiglioni L, Wahlund LO, et al. Mild cognitive impairment - beyond controversies, towards a consensus: report of the international working group on mild cognitive impairment. J Intern Med. 2004;256:240–6.

51. Román GC, Tatemichi TK, Erkinjuntti T, Cummings JL, Masdeu JC, Garcia JH, et al. Vascular dementia: diagnostic criteria for research studies: report of the NINDS-AIREN international workshop. Neurology. 1993;43:250–60.

52. McKeith IG, Dickson DW, Lowe J, Emre M, O'Brien JT, Feldman H, et al. Diagnosis and management of dementia with Lewy bodies: third report of the DLB Consortium. Neurology. 2005;65:1863–72.

53. Gorno-Tempini ML, Hillis AE, Weintraub S, Kertesz A, Mendez M, Cappa SF, et al. Classification of primary progressive aphasia and its variants. Neurology. 2011;76:1006–14.

54. Rascovsky K, Hodges JR, Knopman D, Mendez MF, Kramer JH, Neuhaus J, et al. Sensitivity of revised diagnostic criteria for the behavioural variant of frontotemporal dementia. Brain. 2011;134:2456–77.

55. Ramirez J, Gibson E, Quddus A, Lobaugh NJ, Feinstein A, Levine B, et al. Lesion explorer: a comprehensive segmentation and parcellation package to obtain regional volumetrics for subcortical hyperintensities and intracranial tissue. Neuroimage. 2011;54:963–73.

56. Ramirez J, McNeely AA, Scott CJ, Stuss DT, Black SE. Subcortical hyperintensity volumetrics in Alzheimer's disease and normal elderly in the Sunnybrook Dementia Study: correlations with atrophy, executive function, mental processing speed, and verbal memory. Alzheimers Res Ther. 2014;6:49.

57. Dade LA, Gao FQ, Kovacevic N, Roy P, Rockel C, O'Toole CM, et al. Semiautomatic brain region extraction: a method of parcellating brain regions from structural magnetic resonance images. Neuroimage. 2004;22:1492–502.

58. Satz P, Cole MA, Hardy DJ, Rassovsky Y. Brain and cognitive reserve: mediator(s) and construct validity, a critique. J Clin Exp Neuropsychol. 2011;33:121–30.

59. Harada CN, Natelson Love MC, Triebel KL. Normal cognitive aging. Clin Geriatr Med. 2013;29:737–52.

60. Hollingshead. Four Factor Index of Socioeconomic Status. Yale J Sociol. 1975;8:21–52.

61. Wechsler D. Manual for the Wechsler Adult Intelligence Scale. Corp: New York: Psychological; 1955.

62. Nelson HE. The National Adult Reading Test (NART): test manual. Windsor: NFER-Nelson; 1982.

63. Springer MV, McIntosh AR, Winocur G, Grady CL. The relation between brain activity during memory tasks and years of education in young and older adults. Neuropsychology. 2005;19:181–92.

64. Mattis S. Dementia rating scale. Lutz: Psychological Assessment Resources; 1988.

65. Meiran N, Stuss DT, Guzman DA, Lafleche G, Willmer J. Diagnosis of dementia: methods for interpretation of scores of 5 neuropsychological tests. Arch Neurol. 1996;53:1043–54.

66. Monsch AU, Bondi MW, Salmon DP, Butters N, Thal LJ, Hansen LA, et al. Clinical validity of the Mattis Dementia Rating Scale in detecting dementia of the Alzheimer type: a double cross-validation and application to a community-dwelling sample. Arch. Neurol. 1995;52:899–904.

67. Muthén L, Muthén B. Mplus user's guide. 7th ed. Muthén & Muthén: Los Angeles, CA; 1998.

68. Kline RB. Principles and practice of structural equation modeling. 3rd ed. New York: Guilford Press; 2010.

69. McFall GP, Wiebe SA, Vergote D, Westaway D, Jhamandas J, Bäckman L, et al. ApoE and pulse pressure interactively influence level and change in the aging of episodic memory: protective effects among ε2 carriers. Neuropsychology. 2015;29:388–401.

70. McFall GP, Sapkota S, McDermott KL, Dixon RA. Risk-reducing apolipoprotein E and Clusterin genotypes protect against the consequences of poor vascular health on executive function performance and change in nondemented older adults. Neurobiol Aging. 2016;42:91–100.

71. Sapkota S, Bäckman L, Dixon RA. Executive function performance and change in aging is predicted by apolipoprotein E, intensified by catechol-O-methyltransferase and brain-derived neurotrophic factor, and moderated by age and lifestyle. Neurobiol Aging. 2017;52:81–9.

72. Sapkota S, Dixon RA. A network of genetic effects on non-demented cognitive aging: Alzheimer's genetic risk (CLU + CR1 + PICALM) intensifies cognitive aging genetic risk (COMT + BDNF) selectively for APOE 4 carriers. J Alzheimers Dis. 2018;62:887–900.

73. Risacher SL, Kim S, Nho K, Foroud T, Shen L, Petersen RC, et al. APOE effect on Alzheimer's disease biomarkers in older adults with significant memory concern. Alzheimers Dement. 2015;11:1417–29.

74. Liu CC, Liu CC, Kanekiyo T, Xu H, Bu G. Apolipoprotein E and Alzheimer disease: risk, mechanisms and therapy. Nat Rev Neurol. 2013;9:106–18.

75. Raber J, Huang Y, Ashford JW. ApoE genotype accounts for the vast majority of AD risk and AD pathology. Neurobiol Aging. 2004;25:641–50.

76. Brainerd CJ, Reyna VF, Petersen RC, Smith GE, Taub ES. Is the apolipoprotein e genotype a biomarker for mild cognitive impairment? Findings from a nationally representative study. Neuropsychology. 2011;25:679–89.

77. Brainerd CJ, Reyna VF, Petersen RC, Smith GE, Kenney AE, Gross CJ, et al. The apolipoprotein E genotype predicts longitudinal transitions to mild cognitive impairment but not to Alzheimer's dementia: findings from a nationally representative study. Neuropsychology. 2013;27:86–94.

78. Fotuhi M, Hachinski V, Whitehouse PJ. Changing perspectives regarding late-life dementia. Nat Rev Neurol. 2009;5:649–58.

79. Topiwala A, Allan CL, Valkanova V, Zsoldos E, Filippini N, Sexton CE, et al. Resilience and MRI correlates of cognitive impairment in community-dwelling elders. Br J Psychiatry. 2015;207:435–9.

80. Vemuri P, Weigand SD, Przybelski SA, Knopman DS, Smith GE, Trojanowski JQ, et al. Cognitive reserve and Alzheimer's disease biomarkers are independent determinants of cognition. Brain. 2011;134:1479–92.

81. Kuller LH, Lopez OL, Becker JT, Chang Y, Newman AB. Risk of dementia and death in the long-term follow-up of the Pittsburgh Cardiovascular Health Study–Cognition Study. Alzheimers Dement. 2016;12:170–83.

82. Soldan A, Pettigrew C, Lu Y, Wang MC, Selnes O, Albert M, et al. Relationship of medial temporal lobe atrophy, APOE genotype, and cognitive reserve in preclinical Alzheimer's disease. Hum Brain Mapp. 2015; 36:2826–41.

83. Schuff N, Woerner N, Boreta L, Kornfield T, Shaw LM, Trojanowski JQ, et al. MRI of hippocampal volume loss in early Alzheimer's disease in relation to ApoE genotype and biomarkers. Brain. 2008;132:1067–77.

84. Boots EA, Schultz SA, Almeida RP, Oh JM, Koscik RL, Dowling MN, et al. Occupational complexity and cognitive reserve in a middle-aged cohort at risk for Alzheimer's disease. Arch Clin Neuropsychol. 2015;30:634–42.

85. Perneczky R, Drzezga A, Diehl-Schmid J, Li Y, Kurz A. Gender differences in brain reserve. J Neurol. 2007;254:1395–400.

86. Li CY, Wu SC, Sung FC. Lifetime principal occupation and risk of cognitive impairment among the elderly. Ind Health. 2002;40:7–13.

87. Stern Y. Cognitive reserve in ageing and Alzheimer's disease. Lancet Neurol. 2012;11:1006–12.

88. Rusmaully J, Dugravot A, Moatti J-P, Marmot MG, Elbaz A, Kivimaki M, et al. Contribution of cognitive performance and cognitive decline to associations between socioeconomic factors and dementia: a cohort study. PLoS Med. 2017;14:e1002334.

89. Arenaza-Urquijo EM, Bejanin A, Gonneaud J, Wirth M, La Joie R, Mutlu J, et al. Association between educational attainment and amyloid deposition across the spectrum from normal cognition to dementia: neuroimaging evidence for protection and compensation. Neurobiol Aging. 2017;59:72–9.

90. Ramirez J, McNeely AA, Berezuk C, Gao F, Black SE. Dynamic progression of white matter hyperintensities in Alzheimer's disease and normal aging: results from the Sunnybrook dementia study. Front Aging Neurosci. 2016;8:62.

91. Murray AD, Staff RT, McNeil CJ, Salarirad S, Ahearn TS, Mustafa N, et al. The balance between cognitive reserve and brain imaging biomarkers of cerebrovascular and Alzheimer's diseases. Brain. 2011;134:3687–96.

92. Kroger E, Andel R, Lindsay J, Benounissa Z, Verreault R, Laurin D. Is complexity of work associated with risk of dementia? The Canadian Study of Health and Aging. Am J Epidemiol. 2008;167:820–30.

93. Berezuk C, Ramirez J, Black SE, Zakzanis KK, Alzheimer's Disease Neuroimaging Initiative. Managing money matters: managing finances is associated with functional independence in MCI. Int J Geriatr Psychiatry. 2018;33:517–22.

Non-beta-amyloid/tau cerebrospinal fluid markers inform staging and progression in Alzheimer's disease

Umesh Gangishetti[1], J. Christina Howell[1,2], Richard J. Perrin[3,4], Natalia Louneva[4], Kelly D. Watts[1^], Alexander Kollhoff[1], Murray Grossman[7,8,9], David A. Wolk[6,9], Leslie M. Shaw[10], John C. Morris[3,5], John Q. Trojanowski[6,7,10], Anne M. Fagan[3,5], Steven E. Arnold[6,7,11] and William T. Hu[1,2*] (iD)

Abstract

Background: Alzheimer's disease (AD) is a complex neurodegenerative disorder characterized by neuropathologic changes involving beta-amyloid (Aβ), tau, neuronal loss, and other associated biological events. While levels of cerebrospinal fluid (CSF) Aβ and tau peptides have enhanced the antemortem detection of AD-specific changes, these two markers poorly reflect the severity of cognitive and functional deficits in people with altered Aβ and tau levels. While multiple previous studies identified non-Aβ, non-tau proteins as candidate neurodegenerative markers to inform the A/T/N biomarker scheme of AD, few have advanced beyond association with clinical AD diagnosis. Here we analyzed nine promising neurodegenerative markers in a three-centered cohort using independent assays to identify candidates most likely to complement Aβ and tau in the A/T/N framework.

Methods: CSF samples from 125 subjects recruited at the three centers were exchanged such that each of the nine previously identified biomarkers can be measured at one of the three centers. Subjects were classified according to cognitive status and CSF AD biomarker profiles as having normal cognition and normal CSF ($n = 31$), normal cognition and CSF consistent with AD ($n = 13$), mild cognitive impairment and normal CSF ($n = 13$), mild cognitive impairment with CSF consistent with AD ($n = 23$), AD dementia ($n = 32$; CSF consistent with AD), and other non-AD dementia ($n = 13$; CSF not consistent with AD).

Results: Three biomarkers were identified to differ among the AD stages, including neurofilament light chain (NfL; $p < 0.001$), fatty acid binding protein 3 (Fabp3; $p < 0.001$), and interleukin (IL)-10 ($p = 0.033$). Increased NfL levels were most strongly associated with the dementia stage of AD, but increased Fabp3 levels were more sensitive to milder AD stages and correlated with both CSF tau markers. IL-10 levels did not correlate with tau biomarkers, but were associated with rates of longitudinal cognitive decline in mild cognitive impairment due to AD ($p = 0.006$). Prefreezing centrifugation did not influence measured CSF biomarker levels.

Conclusion: CSF proteins associated with AD clinical stages and progression can complement Aβ and tau markers to inform neurodegeneration. A validated panel inclusive of multiple biomarker features (etiology, stage, progression) can improve AD phenotyping along the A/T/N framework.

Keywords: Biomarkers, Fatty acid binding protein, Interleukin-10, Mild cognitive impairment, Neurofilament light chain

* Correspondence: william.hu@emory.edu
^Deceased
[1]Department of Neurology, Emory University, 615 Michael Street, 505F, Atlanta, GA 30322, USA
[2]Department of Alzheimer's Disease Research Center, Emory University, Atlanta, GA, USA
Full list of author information is available at the end of the article

Background

The clinicopathologic description of Alzheimer's disease (AD) underwent recent revisions to better characterize, on parallel continuums, the cognitive and neuropathologic features associated with beta-amyloid (Aβ) deposition, tau hyperphosphorylation, and neurodegeneration [1–5]. This A/T/N framework has the advantage of providing a multi-dimensional view of AD, although accurate antemortem detection of all three features remains an obstacle in early diagnosis and clinical trial design. AD biomarkers, including cerebrospinal fluid (CSF) [6] or positron emission tomography (PET) [7, 8] measures of amyloid and tau proteins, correlate well with postmortem amyloid and tau (A/T) pathology, but their levels have not been shown to accurately track disease progression [9, 10] to provide information on neurodegeneration. We and others have previously identified CSF proteins which accompany altered amyloid and tau biomarkers in large discovery cohorts, and these non-Aβ, non-tau (NANT) markers are candidate markers of neurodegeneration [11–17]. However, successful replication of these markers' association with AD has been challenging. This may be due to many issues, including recruitment bias [18], processing artifacts when assays are performed by commercial vendors [19], and different antibodies, and few of them have been replicated across cohorts and assay platforms to undergo further standardization and application.

CSF is a ready source for simultaneously testing multiple markers reflecting AD core pathology, copathology (ischemia, Lewy bodies), neurodegeneration, common biological alterations (e.g., neuroinflammation), and unique exposures (e.g., environmental toxins) [20]. We previously sought to identify NANT biomarkers through single-center studies [12, 14, 19], and subsequently determined that some replication failures resulted from biases in recruitment, diagnosis, preanalytical handling, and analytical algorithms [18]. To validate the association between AD pathology, neurodegeneration, and the top NANT biomarkers, we adapted a round-robin design [21] involving subjects recruited from three Alzheimer's disease centers, and collaboratively measured levels of nine analytes to correlate with AD biomarkers and clinical AD stages.

Methods

Standard protocol approvals, registrations, and patient consents

The protocols were approved by the Institutional Review Boards (IRB) at Emory University (Emory), University of Pennsylvania (Penn), and Washington University (WU). Banked CSF samples were used for this study, and all subjects had previously consented to the long-term storage and subsequent analysis of CSF samples. Frozen CSF samples were exchanged among the centers under six bilateral material transfer agreements.

Subjects and preanalytical processing

Demographic (age, sex, education), diagnostic (syndrome, global Clinical Dementia Rating (CDR), Mini-Mental State Examination (MMSE)), and APOE allelic information were collected by each center (Table 1). At Emory, CSF was collected via syringe between 08.00 and 12.00 without overnight fasting using 24-G Sprotte needles, placed in polypropylene tubes, and immediately aliquoted without centrifugation, labeled, and frozen at –80 °C. At Penn, CSF was collected by gravity or syringe without overnight fasting in the morning using 24-G Sprotte needles, placed in polypropylene tubes, transferred locally, aliquoted without centrifugation, labeled, and frozen at –80 °C. At WU, CSF was collected at 08.00 following overnight fasting via gravity using 22-G Sprotte needles, placed in polypropylene tubes, centrifuged at low speed to pellet any cellular debris, aliquoted, and frozen at –80 °C. All samples were shipped to the two external sites overnight on dry ice and immediately placed at –80 °C until analysis.

Subject grouping

Each subject was categorized according to clinical diagnosis (normal cognition (NC), mild cognitive impairment/very mild dementia/CDR 0.5 (MCI), AD dementia, and other non-AD dementia (OD)), and those with NC or MCI were further stratified according to CSF AD biomarkers. In all subjects, CSF levels of Aβ42, total tau (t-Tau), and tau phosphorylated at threonine 181 (p-Tau$_{181}$) had been previously measured using INNO-BIA Alzbio3 (Emory [6], Penn [22]) or INNOTEST® (WU) [23] following the manufacturer's protocols (Fujirebio US, Malvern, PA). All three centers included subjects with NC without CSF biomarkers consistent with AD (NC$^-$), MCI with CSF consistent with AD (MCI$^+$), and AD dementia. In addition, Emory and WU included NC subjects with CSF biomarkers consistent with AD (NC$^+$), and Emory and Penn included MCI subjects with CSF not consistent with AD (MCI$^-$) as well as subjects with OD (Table 1). The diagnosis for OD includes behavioral variant frontotemporal dementia ($n = 5$), semantic variant of primary progressive aphasia ($n = 1$), progressive supranuclear palsy ($n = 2$), and dementia with Lewy bodies ($n = 5$).

NANT biomarker assays

Nine NANT analytes were selected by WTH, AMF, and SEA for validation based on previous biomarker discovery studies, and assay development and performance took place at Emory (interleukin (IL)-7, IL-10, fractalkine, tumor necrosis factor (TNF)-α), Penn (fatty acid binding protein 3 (Fabp3), insulin-like growth factor binding protein 2 (IGF-BP2), neurofilament light chain (NfL)), and WU (monocyte chemotactic protein 1 (MCP1), chitinase-3-like protein 1 (YKL-40)). At Emory, IL-7, IL-10, fractalkine, and TNF-α levels (Milliplex MAP Human Cytokine Panel,

Table 1 Demographic features of subjects included in the current study

	$NC^-(n=31)$	$NC^+(n=13)$	$MCI^-(n=13)$	$MCI^+(n=23)$	AD dementia$(n=32)$	$OD(n=13)$
Female, n (%)	19 (61%)	9 (69%)	7 (54%)	13 (56%)	21 (66%)	5 (39%)
Age (years)	69.1 ± 6.3	74.6 ± 6.9	70.1 ± 5.0	70.6 ± 6.2	72.8 ± 7.1	65.4 ± 4.5
Caucasian, n (%)	28 (90%)	13 (100%)	12 (92%)	23 (100%)	30 (94%)	13 (100%)
Has at least one *APOE* ε4 allele, %	26%	38%	3/10 (30%)	52%	72%	31%
Education (years)	15.7 ± 3.3	15.4 ± 3.2	15.5 ± 3.2	15.0 ± 2.8	14.7 ± 3.8	15.4 ± 1.7
MMSE	28.9 ± 1.8	28.5 ± 1.8	27.4 ± 2.1	26.4 ± 2.5	21.7 ± 4.9	23.2 ± 6.3
Recruiting center, n						
Emory	9	3	7	7	10	8
Penn	12	0	6	6	12	5
WU	10	10	0	10	10	0
Emory AD biomarkers (Luminex)						
Aβ42 (pg/mL)	301.3 ± 106.6	189.1 ± 134.8	306.3 ± 98.5	184.1 ± 68.6	171.3 ± 37.6	232.2 ± 114.9
t-Tau (pg/mL)	48.5 ± 22.4	77.3 ± 53.3	63.8 ± 27.9	150.4 ± 81.6	148.8 ± 52.3	90.8 ± 106.0
p-Tau$_{181}$ (pg/mL)	28.0 ± 10.1	53.4 ± 26.9	32.5 ± 6.9	63.3 ± 19.3	74.7 ± 16.6	27.6 ± 15.7
Penn AD biomarkers (Luminex)						
Aβ42 (pg/mL)	262.6 ± 72.5	N/A	242.1 ± 53.1	119.6 ± 18.0	121.9 ± 35.0	310.6 ± 72.9
t-Tau (pg/mL)	54.4 ± 13.1	N/A	76.9 ± 34.8	96.6 ± 64.9	117.9 ± 41.4	66.2 ± 28.3
p-Tau$_{181}$ (pg/mL)	19.3 ± 14.4	N/A	33.9 ± 34.2	36.6 ± 21.1	45.6 ± 22.6	15.2 ± 4.5
WU AD biomarkers (ELISA)						
Aβ42 (pg/mL)	736.9 ± 152.7	369.2 ± 87.5	N/A	349.0 ± 121.8	291.7 ± 74.4	N/A
t-Tau (pg/mL)	282.8 ± 115.7	359.5 ± 230.3	N/A	615.2 ± 177.7	628.2 ± 363.1	N/A
p-Tau$_{181}$ (pg/mL)	54.4 ± 19.1	74.7 ± 40.7	N/A	107.4 ± 52.3	90.7 ± 52.7	N/A

Values are shown as mean ± standard deviation unless otherwise indicated

Aβ beta-amyloid, *AD* Alzheimer's disease, *ELISA* enzyme-linked immunosorbent assay, *Emory* Emory University, *MCI* mild cognitive impairment, *MMSE* Mini-Mental State Examination, *N/A* not available, *NC* normal cognition, *OD* other non-AD dementia, *Penn* University of Pennsylvania, *p-Tau$_{181}$* phosphorylated tau, *t-Tau* total tau, *WU* Washington University

HCYTOMAG-60 K, EMD Millipore, Billerica, MA) were measured in a Luminex 200 platform following the manufacturer's protocol except that two 100-μL aliquots of CSF were used for duplicates. At Penn, plate-based enzyme-linked immunosorbent assays (ELISAs) were performed according to the manufacturer's instructions for human IGFBP-2 (Sigma, St. Louis, MO; cat. no. RAB0233), human FABP3 (EMD Millipore; cat. no. EZFABP3-38 K), and human neurofilament-light RUO (IBL International, Hamburg, Germany; cat. no. UD51001). At WU, MCP1 levels were analyzed in a Luminex 200 platform (Milliplex MAP Human Adipocyte Panel, HADCYMAG-61 K; EMD Millipore, Billerica, MA), and YKL-40 levels were measured using ELISA (MicroVue YKL-40 EIA Kit, Quidel, San Diego, CA) [11]. All operators were blinded to the diagnosis, and final assay results were collected at Emory for analysis.

Effects of centrifugation
Because CSF samples were centrifuged after collection at WU but not centrifuged at Emory and Penn, we performed prospective experiments at Emory to determine the effect of prefreezing centrifugation. Specifically, after CSF was collected from 16 subjects, CSF samples were immediately divided into two equal portions. One portion was centrifuged at 2000 g and 4 °C for 10 min while the other portion was kept on ice. The supernatant from the centrifuged portion was carefully aliquoted, labeled, and frozen at −80 °C until analysis, and the noncentrifuged portion was similarly aliquoted, labeled, and frozen at −80 °C until analysis. Levels of two analytes whose levels varied according to center (IL-7, IL-10) and one analyte whose level did not vary according to center (NfL) were analyzed in samples with and without centrifugation.

Statistical analysis
Statistical analysis was performed by IBM-SPSS 24 (Chicago, IL) at Emory. For baseline comparison among the three centers, Chi-squared tests for categorical variables and analysis of variance (ANOVA) for continuous variables were used to determine differences. *APOE* genotyping was not available for 3 MCI⁻ subjects from Emory. Since MCI⁻ and OD were included for comparative purposes, these

missing genotypes did not influence the study's main analysis.

For biomarker levels, ANOVA showed that three analytes (IL-7, IL-10, and MCP-1) differed significantly among the recruiting centers. To standardize data handling and to account for these center-associated differences, a site-specific Z score was created for each analyte using the mean and standard deviation of the combined NC^- and AD dementia cohort. After Z transformation, the levels of each analyte were confirmed to be normally distributed by Kolmogorov-Smirnov tests. Student's t tests were then performed to identify analytes whose levels differed between NC^- and AD dementia, with a false discovery rate (FDR) threshold of 0.10 to account for multiple comparisons. Student's t tests were also used to determine whether prefreezing centrifugation affected biomarker levels.

Analysis of covariance (ANCOVA) was used to determine biomarkers that can differentiate among the four theoretical stages of AD development (NC^-, NC^+, MCI^+, AD dementia), adjusting for age, sex, $APOE\ \varepsilon 4$ status, and recruiting center. A threshold of 0.10 for FDR was selected to account for multiple comparisons. Pearson's correlation was then used to analyze the relationships between established CSF AD biomarkers ($A\beta 42$, t-Tau, p-Tau$_{181}$) and the three biomarkers identified through ANCOVA.

Finally, for correlation between baseline IL-10 levels and rates of longitudinal cognitive decline, mixed linear modeling was used to determine whether IL-10 levels were associated with faster rates of cognitive decline. Z scores for executive, memory, language, and visual spatial domains were calculated as previously described. In the mixed linear model, domain-specific Z scores were entered as the dependent variable; gender, race, t-Tau (previously found to influence rates of cognitive decline) [24], IL-10, time, time $\times$ IL-10, age, and education were entered as fixed variables, and time was also entered as a random variable. IL-10 was considered to significantly influence the rates of longitudinal decline if the interaction term time $\times$ IL-10 was associated with domain-specific Z scores at $p < 0.01$ to adjust for multiple comparisons.

Results

The overall cohort included 125 subjects, including 31 NC^-, 13 NC^+, 12 MCI^-, 24 MCI^+, 32 AD dementia, and 13 OD. Subjects were younger (68.7 vs. 73.4 years, $p = 0.003$) and more educated (15.7 vs. 14.0 years, $p = 0.025$) at Emory than WU. Neither site differed from Penn. All three sites were otherwise similar for sex ($p = 0.564$), race ($p = 0.418$), and $APOE\ \varepsilon 4$ status ($p = 0.445$).

NANT biomarkers associated with AD dementia
Since prior NANT biomarker studies sought biomarkers that distinguished between subjects with NC (NC^- with or without NC^+) and AD dementia, we first analyzed

whether levels of the nine candidate biomarkers differed between NC^- and AD dementia. This identified three analytes (NfL, Fabp3, and YKL-40) associated with AD dementia after adjusting for FDR of 5% (Fig. 1). None of the other analytes differed between NC^- and AD dementia (adjusted p value range of 0.252 to 0.977). Controlling for age, sex, center of recruitment, and $APOE\ \varepsilon 4$ status slightly diminished the significance of YKL-40 ($p = 0.062$) but showed similar results for NfL ($p < 0.001$) and Fabp3 ($p < 0.001$). Thus, NfL and Fabp3 best distinguished between the two extreme categories (NC^- and AD dementia).

NANT biomarkers associated with AD stages
Since the clinical manifestation of AD neuropathology is hypothesized to progress through the presymptomatic, MCI, and dementia stages, we next examined in this cross-sectional cohort whether levels of the candidate analytes differed among NC^-, NC^+, MCI^+, and AD dementia through ANCOVA adjusting for age, sex, education, and presence of $APOE\ \varepsilon 4$ allele. This confirmed NfL (F(3,94) = 9.455, $p < 0.001$) and Fabp3 (F(3,94) = 5.869, $p < 0.001$) to be associated with AD stages. Specifically, NfL levels were higher in AD dementia than NC^-, NC^+, or MCI^+ (Fig. 2a), and Fabp3 levels were higher in AD dementia than NC^- and NC^+, and higher in MCI^+ than NC^- (Fig. 2b). Furthermore, IL-10 (F(3,94) = 3.034, $p = 0.033$) showed stage-associated differences, with NC^+ having lower IL-10 levels than NC^-, but AD dementia having higher IL-10 levels than NC^+ or MCI^+ (Fig. 2c). No biomarkers significantly differed in their level between NC^+ and MCI^+ (Fig. 2d).

NfL and Fabp3 levels associated with CSF tau biomarkers
As emerging AD therapeutics often target amyloid and tau, levels of established CSF AD biomarkers ($A\beta 42$, t-Tau, and p-Tau$_{181}$) may serve better to inform target engagement than treatment-associated downstream effects. We therefore analyzed if CSF NfL, Fabp3, and IL-10 correlated with the established CSF AD biomarkers ($A\beta 42$, t-Tau, and p-Tau$_{181}$) to serve as downstream markers. Analyzing samples from Emory and Penn (where established biomarker assays had been performed on identical Luminex platforms) together, both CSF NfL and Fabp3 levels correlated strongly with CSF t-Tau levels ($p < 0.001$), and CSF Fabp3 ($R^2 = 0.348$, $p < 0.001$) levels better correlated with CSF p-Tau$_{181}$ levels than CSF NfL levels ($R^2 = 0.069$, $p = 0.035$, not significant after correction for multiple comparisons; Fig. 3). A similar trend was seen in samples from WU (where established biomarker assays were performed by ELISA), with Fabp3 levels correlating with t-Tau ($p < 0.001$) and p-Tau ($p < 0.001$), and NfL levels correlating better with t-Tau ($p < 0.001$) than p-Tau$_{181}$ ($p = 0.074$). None of the NANT biomarkers correlated with CSF $A\beta 42$, and diagnosis did not influence the relationship between tau

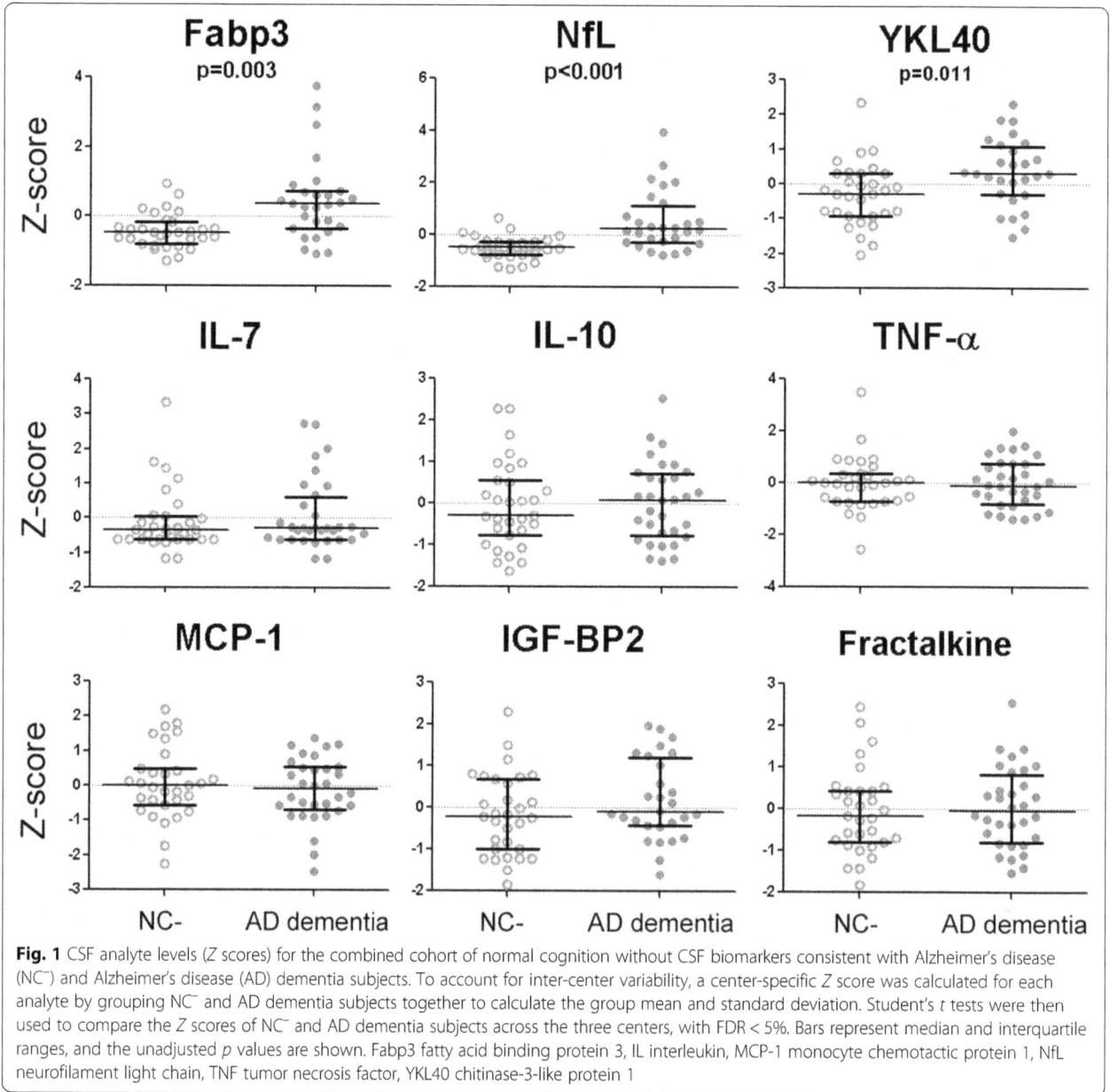

Fig. 1 CSF analyte levels (*Z* scores) for the combined cohort of normal cognition without CSF biomarkers consistent with Alzheimer's disease (NC⁻) and Alzheimer's disease (AD) dementia subjects. To account for inter-center variability, a center-specific *Z* score was calculated for each analyte by grouping NC⁻ and AD dementia subjects together to calculate the group mean and standard deviation. Student's *t* tests were then used to compare the *Z* scores of NC⁻ and AD dementia subjects across the three centers, with FDR < 5%. Bars represent median and interquartile ranges, and the unadjusted *p* values are shown. Fabp3 fatty acid binding protein 3, IL interleukin, MCP-1 monocyte chemotactic protein 1, NfL neurofilament light chain, TNF tumor necrosis factor, YKL40 chitinase-3-like protein 1

biomarkers and the two novel biomarkers (Fabp3 and NfL).

IL-10 associated with rates of longitudinal cognitive decline in MCI⁺

Because CSF IL-10 levels did not correlate with t-Tau or p-Tau$_{181}$, we then analyzed if CSF IL-10 levels correlated with rates of decline in MCI⁺ subjects since clinicians often consider longitudinal decline as an important feature of MCI⁺. This may introduce bias into the selection of MCI⁺ subjects, especially when IL-10 levels did not differ between NC⁻ and AD. Mixed linear modeling showed that, in a group of 51 MCI⁺ subjects longitudinally followed at Emory (median follow-up 36 months,

range 18–78 months), lower IL-10 levels were associated with greater rates of decline in memory *Z* scores ($p = 0.006$ for time × IL-10 levels; Table 2 and Fig. 4a), but not in executive ($p = 0.270$), language ($p = 0.246$), or visual spatial ($p = 0.975$) *Z* scores. In comparison, higher CSF t-Tau levels were associated with worse memory *Z* scores, but neither CSF t-Tau nor p-Tau$_{181}$ influenced the rates of memory decline.

NANT biomarker levels not associated with prefreezing CSF centrifugation

Finally, we sought to determine whether prefreezing CSF centrifugation (performed at WU) represented another bias in measured NANT levels since centrifuged samples

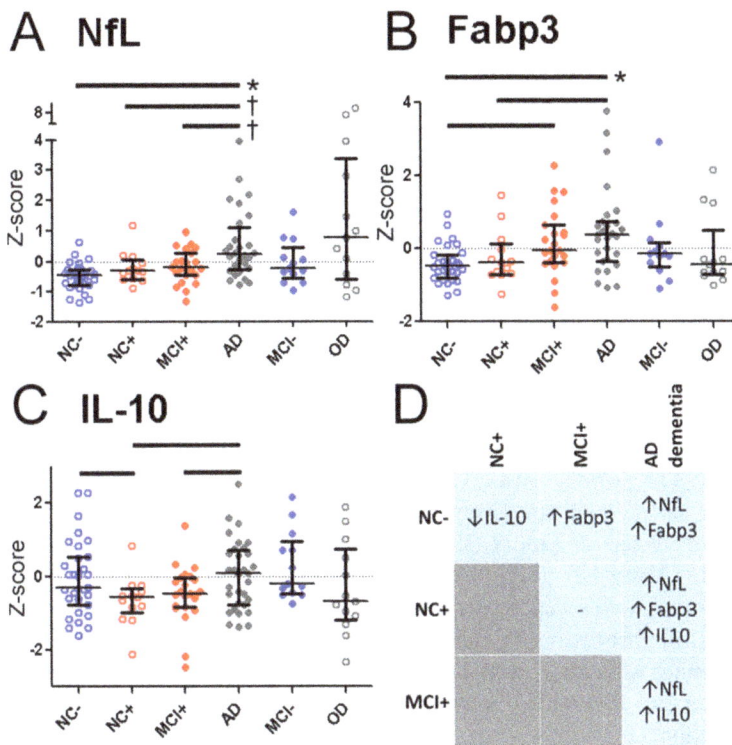

Fig. 2 CSF levels (Z scores) of neurofilament light chain (NfL) (**a**), fatty acid binding protein 3 (Fabp3) (**b**), and interleukin (IL)-10 (**c**) in subjects with normal cognition (NC), mild cognitive impairment (MCI), Alzheimer's disease (AD) dementia, and other non-AD dementia (OD). (*$p < 0.001$; [†]$p < 0.005$; $p < 0.05$ for other comparisons indicated). Differences between different subgroups are summarized in **d**, with direction of change reflecting the stage with more severe pathology or cognitive impairment

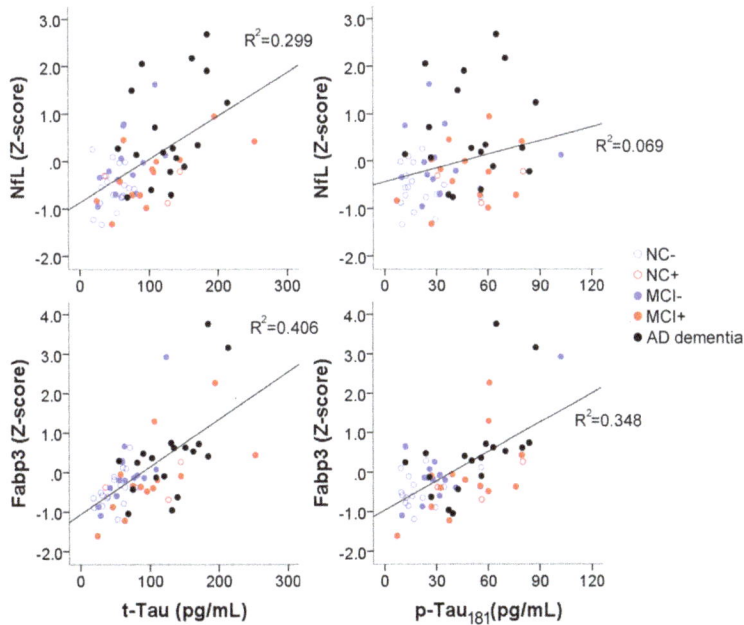

Fig. 3 Correlations between CSF tau-related proteins and neurofilament light chain (NfL) and fatty acid binding protein 3 (Fabp3) levels. Fabp3 levels correlated strongly with total tau (t-Tau) and phosphorylated tau (p-Tau$_{181}$) levels, while NfL levels correlated better with t-Tau than p-Tau$_{181}$ levels. AD Alzheimer's disease, MCI mild cognitive impairment, NC normal cognition

Table 2 Mixed linear model analysis of memory Z scores in MCI$^+$ subjects longitudinally characterized at Emory ($n = 51$)

	Coefficient (95% confidence interval)	p
Age	0.020 (−0.011, 0.051)	0.210
Male gender	0.613 (0.148, 1.078)	0.011
Minority race	0.210 (−0.647, 1.067)	0.625
Education (years)	0.029 (−0.057, 0.116)	0.505
t-Tau (pg/mL)	−0.002 (−0.005, −0.001)	0.073
IL-10 level (pg/mL)	−0.035 (−0.139, 0.069)	0.510
Time (months)	−0.043 (−0.060, −0.026)	< 0.001
Time × IL-10 (months × pg/mL)	0.003 (0.001, 0.005)	0.006

IL interleukin, *MCI* mild cognitive impairment, *t-Tau* total tau

represented 77% of NC$^+$ and 43% of MCI$^+$ cases. Centrifuged and noncentrifuged samples prospectively collected from the same individuals at Emory showed similar absolute levels of IL-10 and NfL (Fig. 4b), suggesting that their association with AD stages was independent of the preanalytical processing differences between the centers. In keeping with this, levels of IL-7 (which showed a large inter-site difference) were also not influenced by centrifugation.

Discussion

Reproducible NANT biomarkers associated with AD pathogenesis or progression have the potential for complementing existing cognitive/functional assessments and improving clinical trial designs. Here we used multicentered samples and independent assays to confirm CSF Fabp3 and NfL as stage-dependent biomarkers in AD. The levels of these two markers also correlated with t-Tau (both) and p-Tau$_{181}$ (Fabp3) in the CSF, and can be prospectively tested as surrogate markers of response in future clinical trials targeting tau. Furthermore, we found a complex relationship between CSF IL-10 levels, AD, and cognition, but associated lower CSF IL-10 levels to faster cognitive decline in MCI. Altogether, these findings point to a set of unique biochemical events associated with cumulative and on-going cognitive decline in AD, and add a suite of NANT biomarkers to the A/T/N scheme.

Previous work—including our own—has primarily focused on NANT biomarkers whose levels differed between NC$^-$ and AD dementia. Subjects with normal cognition but abnormal AD biomarkers (CSF or PET) were variably included with or excluded from those whose cognition and AD biomarkers were both normal, and the distinction between MCI$^+$ and AD dementia could be based on the number of impaired neuropsychological domains, functional independence, or consensus. Aside from these study design biases, our current study showed that analyzing only the two extreme groups overlooked at least one biologically meaningful marker,

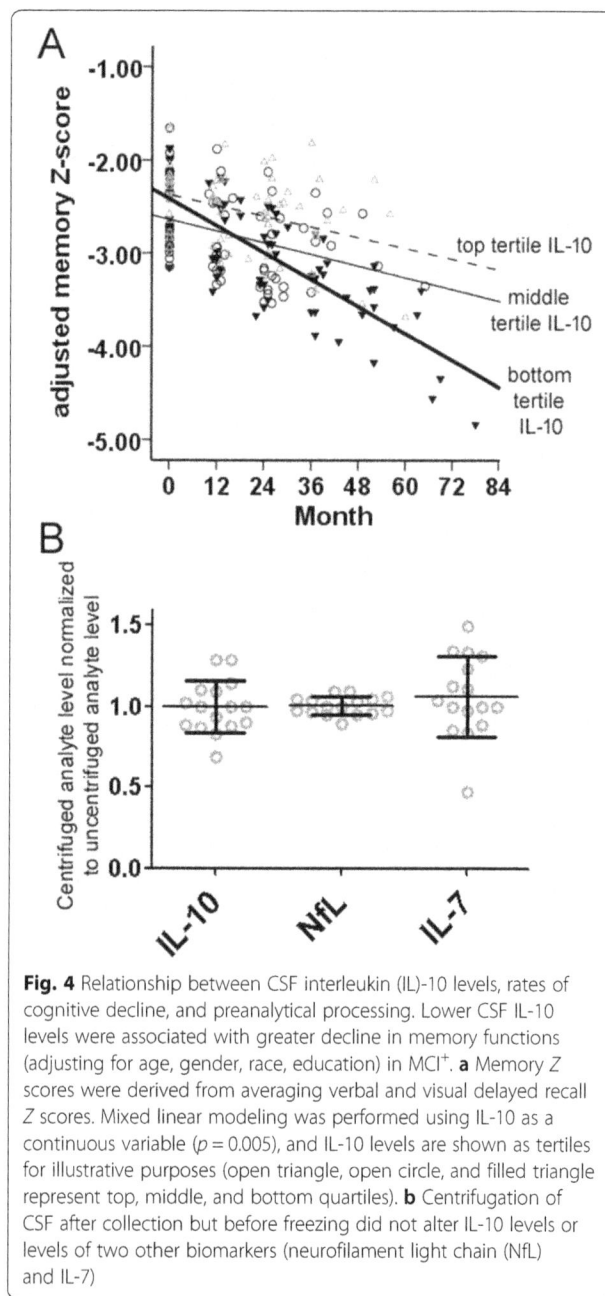

Fig. 4 Relationship between CSF interleukin (IL)-10 levels, rates of cognitive decline, and preanalytical processing. Lower CSF IL-10 levels were associated with greater decline in memory functions (adjusting for age, gender, race, education) in MCI$^+$. **a** Memory Z scores were derived from averaging verbal and visual delayed recall Z scores. Mixed linear modeling was performed using IL-10 as a continuous variable ($p = 0.005$), and IL-10 levels are shown as tertiles for illustrative purposes (open triangle, open circle, and filled triangle represent top, middle, and bottom quartiles). **b** Centrifugation of CSF after collection but before freezing did not alter IL-10 levels or levels of two other biomarkers (neurofilament light chain (NfL) and IL-7)

IL-10. At the same time, levels of the most commonly cited candidate staging marker—NfL, a neuronal cytoskeletal protein associated with axonal injury—were most elevated in the dementia stage of AD, but did not sufficiently distinguish between the earlier stages (NC$^-$, NC$^+$, MCI$^+$) nor correlate strongly with p-Tau$_{181}$. The difference in NfL observed here is in line with findings from the Alzheimer's Disease Neuroimaging Initiative (ADNI) and favors NfL more as a marker of staging/progression in neurodegenerative disorders with faster progression (e.g., frontotemporal dementia) than typical AD. Similarly, the difference in YKL-40 levels (a glycoprotein secreted by astrocytes and infiltrating macrophages) was consistent with previously reported ranges [11].

Fabp3 levels better distinguished between different AD stages than NfL and YKL-40 [11], and may serve as a good neurodegenerative biomarker since its levels correlated well with CSF t-Tau and p-Tau$_{181}$ levels. Fabp3 is a small soluble protein expressed in neurons, astrocytes, and brain endothelial cells [25–27]. It is involved in the intracellular transport of polyunsaturated fatty acid [28] as well as modulation of acetylcholine and glutamate release [29]. Brains with AD and schizophrenia were found to have reduced Fabp3 levels [30, 31], and serum Fabp3 levels are elevated in multiple dementia and brain injury syndromes [32–34]. Data from the ADNI and other studies have shown that CSF Fabp3 levels do not differ between NC$^-$ and NC$^+$ [35, 36], but do increase in the symptomatic AD stages [36, 37] and with progressive entorhinal atrophy [38]. Consistent with these prior findings, we also found similar Fabp3 levels in MCI$^+$ and AD dementia. Thus, whereas increased NfL levels may reflect sufficient neurodegeneration to result in functional decline [39], Fabp3 may be a more sensitive marker to predementia neurodegeneration.

We found IL-10 levels to differ between clinical AD stages but not between NC$^-$ and AD dementia. This came as counter-intuitive for us, which led to further experiments related to IL-10. CSF IL-10 levels were variably linked with AD in previous discovery-based studies [12, 14]. Among potential explanations for these discrepant findings, we eliminated analytical and preanalytical variabilities as confounds in our study since IL-10 levels were all measured at a single site and did not differ in a prospective follow-up study targeting the effects of pre-freezing centrifugation. At the same time, selection bias in banked biospecimens may account for reduced IL-10 levels in MCI$^+$ compared with AD as lower IL-10 levels were associated with greater rates of memory decline, a feature often considered when MCI samples are selected retrospectively. This is supported by our follow-up study where MCI subjects with the lowest CSF IL-10 levels tended to experience greater memory decline. At the same time, there exist potential biological explanations for lower IL-10 levels in NC$^+$ and MCI$^+$. IL-10 has often been considered an anti-inflammatory cytokine, but it is released by proinflammatory, anti-inflammatory, and regulatory T helper cells. Its release and effects are thus complex, and IL-10 does not exist or act in isolation. Lower IL-10 levels in NC$^+$ may be interpreted as a failure in anti-inflammatory processes associated with onset of pathologic AD, or alternatively balanced anti- and proinflammatory responses in asymptomatic AD (e.g., we previously showed complement activation to accompany the MCI$^+$ to AD transition [18]). Similarly, higher IL-10 levels in AD than NC$^+$ and MCI$^+$ may represent exaggerated anti-inflammatory responses or

appropriate IL-10 response to AD-related neuroinflammation. These challenges call for the simultaneous measurements of cytokines representing different pro- and anti-inflammatory pathways in future studies, as well as immunophenotyping analysis in the CSF. This approach will also better explain why reduced IL-10 levels may predict faster rates of decline in MCI.

Instead of measuring promising AD biomarkers only at a single site (academic or commercial), we show here that a collaborative model of replication moves the most promising NANT biomarkers towards further development. It enables a greater number of candidate markers to undergo simultaneous validation in subjects recruited from each center in a head-to-head design, identifies analytes with inter-site variabilities, and permits follow-up experiments to empirically determine the effects of different preanalytical procedures. At the same time, our study is limited by the sample size, as yet unidentified factors to account for center-to-center variations, genetic background of populations at the three geographically separate sites, and imperfect matching of some diagnostic categories among centers (NC$^+$, OD). We did not include CSF biomarkers for non-beta-amyloid/tau neurodegenerative processes (e.g., a-synuclein, phosphorylated TDP-43 levels) as they are less mature, and accounting for them may help explain variability across centers and AD stages. We also did not analyze the NANT biomarker levels in a large group of OD since cases with high confidence pathology (through autopsy confirmation or, less preferably, mutation because of the mutations' potential direct impact on inflammation) are limited in number. Translation of promising markers validated here into the A/T/N biomarker suite will need to prospectively determine the impact of biological, preanalytical, and analytical variabilities on the levels and stability of these markers, and the A/T/N scheme itself may need future revision to account for copathology and other contributors.

Conclusion

In summary, we successfully confirmed three proteins (Fabp3, NfL, and IL-10) as potentially informative biomarkers to complement established AD biomarkers (Aβ and tau) through a three-centered, North American, non-ADNI study. Importantly, we used assays easily accessible to investigators who can further optimize their development and translation.

Abbreviations

Aβ: Beta-amyloid; AD: Alzheimer's disease; ADNI: Alzheimer's Disease Neuroimaging Initiative; ANCOVA: Analysis of covariance; ANOVA: Analysis of variance; CDR: Clinical Dementia Rating; CSF: Cerebrospinal fluid; ELISA: Enzyme-linked immunosorbent assay; Emory: Emory University; Fabp3: Fatty acid binding protein 3; FDR: False discovery rate; IGF-BP2: Insulin-like growth factor binding protein 2; IL: Interleukin; MCI: Mild cognitive impairment; MCP1: Monocyte chemotactic protein 1; MMSE: Mini-Mental State Examination; NANT: Non-beta-amyloid, non-tau; NC: Normal cognition; NfL: Neurofilament light chain; OD: Other non-Alzheimer's disease dementia; Penn: University of Pennsylvania; PET: Positron emission tomography; p-Tau$_{181}$: Tau phosphorylated at threonine 181; TNF: Tumor necrosis factor; t-Tau: Total tau; WU: Washington University; YKL-40: Chitinase-3-like protein 1 (Chi3-l1)

Acknowledgements
The authors wish to acknowledge Allan I. Levey, MD, PhD, James J. Lah, MD, PhD, David M. Holtzman, MD, Jason H. Karlawish, MD, and Vivianna Van Deerlin, MD, PhD, and the National Alzheimer's Coordinating Center for funding, collecting data, and general support.

Funding
This work was supported by the National Institutes of Health (AG43885, AG42856, AG25688, AG10124, AG17586, AG05681, AG26276, AG03991, AG16976).

Authors' contributions
UG, RJP, LMS, JCM, JQT, AMF, SEA, and WTH were responsible for conception and design of the study; UG, JCH, RJP, NL, KDW, AK, MG, DAW, LMS, JCM, JQT, AMF, SEA, and WTH were responsible for acquisition, analysis, and interpretation of data; UG, JCH, JQT, AMF, SEA, and WTH were responsible for drafting the manuscript and revising it critically for important intellectual content. All authors read and approved the final manuscript.

Consent for publication
Not applicable.

Competing interests
LMS has received personal compensation for activities with Roche Diagnostics which produces CSF amyloid and tau assays. AMF is on the Scientific Advisory Boards for Roche Diagnostics which produces CSF amyloid and tau assays. WTH consults for ViveBio, LLC., which manufactures lumbar puncture trays; has a patent (assignee: Emory University) on the use of CSF p/t-Tau ratio in the evaluation of FTLD; has received research support from Fujirebio USA and Avid Pharmaceuticals; has received travel support from Hoffman La Roche and Abbvie. The remaining authors declare that they have no competing interests.

Author details
[1]Department of Neurology, Emory University, 615 Michael Street, 505F, Atlanta, GA 30322, USA. [2]Department of Alzheimer's Disease Research Center, Emory University, Atlanta, GA, USA. [3]Knight Alzheimer's Disease Research Center, Washington University, St. Louis, MO, USA. [4]Department of Pathology, Washington University, St. Louis, MO, USA. [5]Department of Neurology, Washington University, St. Louis, MO, USA. [6]Penn Memory Center, University of Pennsylvania, Philadelphia, PA, USA. [7]Center for Neurodegenerative Disease Research, University of Pennsylvania, Philadelphia, PA, USA. [8]Penn FTD Center, University of Pennsylvania, Philadelphia, PA, USA. [9]Department of Neurology, University of Pennsylvania, Philadelphia, PA, USA. [10]Department of Pathology and Laboratory Medicine, University of Pennsylvania, Philadelphia, PA, USA. [11]Present Address: Massachusetts General Hospital, Boston, MA, USA.

References
1. Sperling RA, Aisen PS, Beckett LA, Bennett DA, Craft S, Fagan AM, Iwatsubo T, Jack CR Jr, Kaye J, Montine TJ, et al. Toward defining the preclinical stages of Alzheimer's disease: recommendations from the National Institute on Aging-Alzheimer's Association workgroups on diagnostic guidelines for Alzheimer's disease. Alzheimers Dement. 2011;7:280–92.
2. Albert MS, DeKosky ST, Dickson D, Dubois B, Feldman HH, Fox NC, Gamst A, Holtzman DM, Jagust WJ, Petersen RC, et al. The diagnosis of mild cognitive impairment due to Alzheimer's disease: recommendations from the National Institute on Aging-Alzheimer's Association workgroups on diagnostic guidelines for Alzheimer's disease. Alzheimers Dement. 2011;7:270–9.
3. McKhann GM, Albert MS, Grossman M, Miller B, Dickson D, Trojanowski JQ. Clinical and pathological diagnosis of frontotemporal dementia: report of the Work Group on Frontotemporal Dementia and Pick's Disease. Arch Neurol. 2001;58:1803–9.
4. Hyman BT, Phelps CH, Beach TG, Bigio EH, Cairns NJ, Carrillo MC, Dickson DW, Duyckaerts C, Frosch MP, Masliah E, et al. National Institute on Aging-Alzheimer's Association guidelines for the neuropathologic assessment of Alzheimer's disease. Alzheimers Dement. 2012;8:1–13.
5. Jack CR Jr, Bennett DA, Blennow K, Carrillo MC, Dunn B, Haeberlein SB, Holtzman DM, Jagust W, Jessen F, Karlawish J, et al. NIA-AA research framework: toward a biological definition of Alzheimer's disease. Alzheimers Dement. 2018;14:535–62.
6. Hu WT, Watts KD, Shaw LM, Howell JC, Trojanowski JQ, Basra S, Glass JD, Lah JJ, Levey AI. CSF beta-amyloid 1-42—what are we measuring in Alzheimer's disease? Ann Clin Transl Neurol. 2015;2:131–9.
7. Clark CM, Schneider JA, Bedell BJ, Beach TG, Bilker WB, Mintun MA, Pontecorvo MJ, Hefti F, Carpenter AP, Flitter ML, et al. Use of florbetapir-PET for imaging beta-amyloid pathology. Jama. 2011;305:275–83.
8. Marquie M, Siao Tick Chong M, Anton-Fernandez A, Verwer EE, Saez-Calveras N, Meltzer AC, Ramanan P, Amaral AC, Gonzalez J, Normandin MD, et al. [F-18]-AV-1451 binding correlates with postmortem neurofibrillary tangle Braak Staging. Acta Neuropathol. 2017;134(4):619-28.
9. Bertens D, Knol DL, Scheltens P, Visser PJ, Alzheimer's Disease Neuroimaging Initiative. Temporal evolution of biomarkers and cognitive markers in the asymptomatic, MCI, and dementia stage of Alzheimer's disease. Alzheimers Dement. 2015;11:511–22.
10. Shokouhi S, McKay JW, Baker SL, Kang H, Brill AB, Gwirtsman HE, Riddle WR, Claassen DO, Rogers BP, Alzheimer's Disease Neuroimaging Initiative. Reference tissue normalization in longitudinal (18)F-florbetapir positron emission tomography of late mild cognitive impairment. Alzheimers Res Ther. 2016;8:2.
11. Craig-Schapiro R, Perrin RJ, Roe CM, Xiong C, Carter D, Cairns NJ, Mintun MA, Peskind ER, Li G, Galasko DR, et al. YKL-40: a novel prognostic fluid biomarker for preclinical Alzheimer's disease. Biol Psychiatry. 2010;68:903–12.
12. Hu WT, Chen-Plotkin A, Arnold SE, Grossman M, Clark CM, Shaw LM, Pickering E, Kuhn M, Chen Y, McCluskey L, et al. Novel CSF biomarkers for Alzheimer's disease and mild cognitive impairment. Acta Neuropathol. 2010;119:669–78.
13. Hu WT, Holtzman DM, Fagan AM, Shaw LM, Perrin R, Arnold SE, Grossman M, Xiong C, Craig-Schapiro R, Clark CM, et al. Plasma multianalyte profiling in mild cognitive impairment and Alzheimer disease. Neurology. 2012;79:897–905.
14. Craig-Schapiro R, Kuhn M, Xiong C, Pickering EH, Liu J, Misko TP, Perrin RJ, Bales KR, Soares H, Fagan AM, Holtzman DM. Multiplexed immunoassay panel identifies novel CSF biomarkers for Alzheimer's disease diagnosis and prognosis. PLoS One. 2011;6:e18850.
15. Abdi F, Quinn JF, Jankovic J, McIntosh M, Leverenz JB, Peskind E, Nixon R, Nutt J, Chung K, Zabetian C, et al. Detection of biomarkers with a multiplex quantitative proteomic platform in cerebrospinal fluid of patients with neurodegenerative disorders. J Alzheimers Dis. 2006;9:293–348.
16. Castano EM, Roher AE, Esh CL, Kokjohn TA, Beach T. Comparative proteomics of cerebrospinal fluid in neuropathologically-confirmed Alzheimer's disease and non-demented elderly subjects. Neurol Res. 2006;28:155–63.
17. Hendrickson RC, Lee AY, Song Q, Liaw A, Wiener M, Paweletz CP, Seeburger JL, Li J, Meng F, Deyanova EG, et al. High resolution discovery proteomics reveals candidate disease progression markers of Alzheimer's disease in human cerebrospinal fluid. PLoS One. 2015;10:e0135365.
18. Hu WT, Watts KD, Tailor P, Nguyen TP, Howell JC, Lee RC, Seyfried NT, Gearing M, Hales CM, Levey AI, et al. CSF complement 3 and factor H are staging biomarkers in Alzheimer's disease. Acta Neuropathol Commun. 2016;4:14.

19. Hu WT, Watts K, Grossman M, Glass J, Lah JJ, Hales C, Shelnutt M, Van Deerlin V, Trojanowski JQ, Levey AI. Reduced CSF p-Tau181 to Tau ratio is a biomarker for FTLD-TDP. Neurology. 2013;81:1945–52.

20. Richardson JR, Roy A, Shalat SL, von Stein RT, Hossain MM, Buckley B, Gearing M, Levey AI, German DC. Elevated serum pesticide levels and risk for Alzheimer disease. JAMA Neurol. 2014;71:284–90.

21. Pannee J, Gobom J, Shaw LM, Korecka M, Chambers EE, Lame M, Jenkins R, Mylott W, Carrillo MC, Zegers I, et al. Round robin test on quantification of amyloid-beta 1-42 in cerebrospinal fluid by mass spectrometry. Alzheimers Dement. 2016;12:55–9.

22. Shaw LM, Vanderstichele H, Knapik-Czajka M, Clark CM, Aisen PS, Petersen RC, Blennow K, Soares H, Simon A, Lewczuk P, et al. Cerebrospinal fluid biomarker signature in Alzheimer's disease neuroimaging initiative subjects. Ann Neurol. 2009;65:403–13.

23. Fagan AM, Roe CM, Xiong C, Mintun MA, Morris JC, Holtzman DM. Cerebrospinal fluid tau/beta-amyloid(42) ratio as a prediction of cognitive decline in nondemented older adults. Arch Neurol. 2007;64:343–9.

24. Ben Bouallegue F, Mariano-Goulart D, Payoux P, Alzheimer's Disease Neuroimaging Initiative. Comparison of CSF markers and semi-quantitative amyloid PET in Alzheimer's disease diagnosis and in cognitive impairment prognosis using the ADNI-2 database. Alzheimers Res Ther. 2017;9:32.

25. Veerkamp JH, Paulussen RJ, Peeters RA, Maatman RG, van Moerkerk HT, van Kuppevelt TH. Detection, tissue distribution and (sub)cellular localization of fatty acid-binding protein types. Mol Cell Biochem. 1990;98:11–8.

26. Owada Y, Yoshimoto T, Kondo H. Spatio-temporally differential expression of genes for three members of fatty acid binding proteins in developing and mature rat brains. J Chem Neuroanat. 1996;12:113–22.

27. Teunissen CE, Veerhuis R, De Vente J, Verhey FR, Vreeling F, van Boxtel MP, Glatz JF, Pelsers MA. Brain-specific fatty acid-binding protein is elevated in serum of patients with dementia-related diseases. Eur J Neurol. 2011;18:865–71.

28. Offner GD, Brecher P, Sawlivich WB, Costello CE, Troxler RF. Characterization and amino acid sequence of a fatty acid-binding protein from human heart. Biochem J. 1988;252:191–8.

29. Shioda N, Yamamoto Y, Watanabe M, Binas B, Owada Y, Fukunaga K. Heart-type fatty acid binding protein regulates dopamine D2 receptor function in mouse brain. J Neurosci. 2010;30:3146–55.

30. Cheon MS, Kim SH, Fountoulakis M, Lubec G. Heart type fatty acid binding protein (H-FABP) is decreased in brains of patients with Down syndrome and Alzheimer's disease. J Neural Transm Suppl. 2003;67:225-34.

31. Hamazaki K, Maekawa M, Toyota T, Iwayama Y, Dean B, Hamazaki T, Yoshikawa T. Fatty acid composition and fatty acid binding protein expression in the postmortem frontal cortex of patients with schizophrenia: a case-control study. Schizophr Res. 2016;171:225–32.

32. Mollenhauer B, Steinacker P, Bahn E, Bibl M, Brechlin P, Schlossmacher MG, Locascio JJ, Wiltfang J, Kretzschmar HA, Poser S, et al. Serum heart-type fatty acid-binding protein and cerebrospinal fluid tau: marker candidates for dementia with Lewy bodies. Neurodegener Dis. 2007;4:366–75.

33. O'Bryant SE, Xiao G, Edwards M, Devous M, Gupta VB, Martins R, Zhang F, Barber R, Texas Alzheimer's R, Care C. Biomarkers of Alzheimer's disease among Mexican Americans. J Alzheimers Dis. 2013;34:841–9.

34. Park SY, Kim MH, Kim OJ, Ahn HJ, Song JY, Jeong JY, Oh SH. Plasma heart-type fatty acid binding protein level in acute ischemic stroke: comparative analysis with plasma S100B level for diagnosis of stroke and prediction of long-term clinical outcome. Clin Neurol Neurosurg. 2013;115:405–10.

35. Hoglund K, Kern S, Zettergren A, Borjesson-Hansson A, Zetterberg H, Skoog I, Blennow K. Preclinical amyloid pathology biomarker positivity: effects on tau pathology and neurodegeneration. Transl Psychiatry. 2017;7:e995.

36. Harari O, Cruchaga C, Kauwe JS, Ainscough BJ, Bales K, Pickering EH, Bertelsen S, Fagan AM, Holtzman DM, Morris JC, et al. Phosphorylated tau-Abeta42 ratio as a continuous trait for biomarker discovery for early-stage Alzheimer's disease in multiplex immunoassay panels of cerebrospinal fluid. Biol Psychiatry. 2014;75:723–31.

37. Chiasserini D, Parnetti L, Andreasson U, Zetterberg H, Giannandrea D, Calabresi P, Blennow K. CSF levels of heart fatty acid binding protein are altered during early phases of Alzheimer's disease. J Alzheimers Dis. 2010;22:1281–8.

38. Desikan RS, Thompson WK, Holland D, Hess CP, Brewer JB, Zetterberg H, Blennow K, Andreassen OA, McEvoy LK, Hyman BT, et al. Heart fatty acid binding protein and Abeta-associated Alzheimer's neurodegeneration. Mol Neurodegener. 2013;8:39.

39. Merluzzi AP, Carlsson CM, Johnson SC, Schindler SE, Asthana S, Blennow K, Zetterberg H, Bendlin BB. Neurodegeneration, synaptic dysfunction, and gliosis are phenotypic of Alzheimer dementia. Neurology. 2018.

Modifiable dementia risk score to study heterogeneity in treatment effect of a dementia prevention trial: a post hoc analysis in the preDIVA trial using the LIBRA index

Tessa van Middelaar[1,2]* [iD], Marieke P. Hoevenaar-Blom[1], Willem A. van Gool[1], Eric P. Moll van Charante[3], Jan-Willem van Dalen[1], Kay Deckers[4], Sebastian Köhler[4] and Edo Richard[1,2]

Abstract

Background: Selecting high-risk participants for dementia prevention trials based on a modifiable dementia risk score may be advantageous, as it increases the opportunity for intervention. We studied whether a multi-domain intervention can prevent all-cause dementia and cognitive decline in older people across three different levels of a modifiable dementia risk score.

Methods: Prevention of Dementia by Intensive Vascular Care (preDIVA) is a randomised controlled trial studying the effect of multi-domain vascular care during 6–8 years on incident all-cause dementia in community-dwelling people aged 70–78 years. For this post hoc analysis, we stratified preDIVA participants in tertiles based on their baseline LIfestyle for BRAin Health (LIBRA) index, a modifiable dementia risk score. With Cox proportional hazards regression, the intervention effect on dementia was assessed. The effect on cognition was measured every 2 years with the Mini-Mental State Examination and Visual Association Test.

Results: Dementia developed in 220 of 3274 (6.7%) participants. In participants with a low, intermediate and high LIBRA index, the hazard ratio (HR) of the intervention on incident dementia was respectively 0.71 (95% CI 0.45–1.12), 1.06 (95% CI 0.66–1.69) and 1.02 (95% CI 0.64–1.62). Also, when adding the non-modifiable risk factors age, education and sex to the index, results were comparable (respectively HR 0.88, 95% CI 0.54–1.43; HR 0.91, 95% CI 0.57–1.47; HR 0.92, 95% CI 0.59–1.41). There was no statistically significant intervention effect on cognition during follow-up across the LIBRA groups.

Conclusions: In the preDIVA study population aged 70–78 years, the LIBRA modifiable dementia risk score did not identify a (high-)risk group in whom the multi-domain intervention was effective in preventing dementia or cognitive decline.

Keywords: Dementia, Prevention, Prognosis, Risk factors, Randomised controlled trial, Patient selection

* Correspondence: t.vanmiddelaar@amc.uva.nl
[1]Department of Neurology, Academic Medical Center (AMC), Meibergdreef 9, 1105, AZ, Amsterdam, the Netherlands
[2]Department of Neurology, Donders Institute for Brain, Cognition and Behaviour, Radboud University Medical Center, Nijmegen, the Netherlands
Full list of author information is available at the end of the article

Background

The number of dementia cases worldwide is anticipated to double over the coming two decades [1, 2]. Up to a third of Alzheimer's disease cases may be attributable to potentially modifiable risk factors, including several vascular risk factors such as diabetes mellitus, midlife hypertension and physical inactivity [3]. This offers a window of opportunity for prevention strategies. However, selection of the optimal target population when designing a randomised controlled trial (RCT) to prevent dementia remains a challenge [4]. Results from recent RCTs suggest that interventions may be most effective in those individuals at increased risk of dementia based on the presence of one or more dementia risk factors [5–7]. In such an at-risk population the potential to improve modifiable risk factors such as hypertension and physical inactivity, and thereby prevent dementia, is higher. In addition, the higher dementia incidence rates in high-risk populations increase the study power, decreasing the total number of participants required to demonstrate a treatment effect.

A dementia risk score could be a useful tool to recruit a high-risk population for prevention trials. Most risk scores that have been developed are, however, heavily dependent on non-modifiable risk factors such as age, sex and education [8]. The LIfestyle for BRAin Health (LIBRA) index is the first, and so far only, validated dementia risk score predominantly supported by modifiable health and lifestyle factors [9]. It consists of the following 12 risk and protective factors: depression, hypertension, obesity, smoking, hypercholesterolemia, diabetes, renal dysfunction, physical inactivity, coronary heart disease, low/moderate alcohol use, cognitive activity and adherence to the Mediterranean diet. As the index reflects an individual's potential for dementia prevention, it may identify those most responsive to an intervention.

Prevention of Dementia by Intensive Vascular Care (preDIVA) is a cluster RCT evaluating the effect of 6–8 years of nurse-led intensive vascular care on incident dementia in community-dwelling older people aged 70–78 years [5]. Overall, no preventive effect of the intervention was found. The intervention seemed more beneficial in a subgroup of individuals with untreated hypertension who adhered to the intervention. As the preDIVA intervention targets several vascular risk factors, our hypothesis was that a risk score capturing several modifiable risk factors may function even better at selecting those individuals responsive to the intervention.

Hence, our aim was to study whether a multi-domain intervention can prevent all-cause dementia and cognitive decline in older people across three different levels of a modifiable dementia risk score.

Methods

The current study is a post hoc analysis in the preDIVA trial, which was published previously [5]. In short, the intervention comprised 4-monthly visits to a practice nurse who gave individually tailored lifestyle advice on smoking, diet, physical activity, weight and blood pressure (BP). If indicated, pharmacological treatment was started or optimised according to the prevailing guidelines on cardiovascular risk management [10]. The control condition was standard care. All community-dwelling older people aged 70–78 years registered at participating Dutch general practices were invited to participate. The only exclusion criteria were a diagnosis of dementia and/or any condition likely to hinder long-term follow-up (such as terminal illness or alcoholism). The trial is registered at the International Standard Randomised Controlled Trial Number registry (ISRCTN29711771).

LIBRA index

The LIBRA index has been designed based on a systematic review and Delphi consensus, and has been validated in several cohorts, including a cohort aged 70–79 years [9, 11, 12]. In preDIVA, 10 out of 12 LIBRA factors were measured at baseline (Table 1). Similar to one of the previously mentioned validation studies [11], there was no information on cognitive activity or adherence to the Mediterranean diet. Data on medical history, medication use, history of smoking and alcohol use were self-reported and cross-referenced with the electronic medical record of the general practitioner. BP, weight and height (to calculate the body mass index (BMI)) were measured using standard protocols. A blood sample was drawn to measure cholesterol and creatinine levels. The 15-item Geriatric Depression Scale was used to measure depressive symptoms and the LASA Physical Activity Questionnaire to measure physical activity [13, 14]. The measures corresponding to the 10 LIBRA items (Table 1) were aligned to the previously published validation studies [9, 11]. Each item was assigned the appropriate score (Table 1) and the sum of these items formed the LIBRA index (with a maximum potential range of – 1.0 to + 12.7). Only participants with all 10 items available to calculate the LIBRA index were included in the analysis. For a secondary analysis, the LIBRA index was extended with the non-modifiable risk factors age, sex and education (Table 1), in order to make it more comparable to other available dementia risk indices [15]. This was also done in the previously published studies on the LIBRA index [9, 11].

Table 1 Definition of risk/protective factors in the LIBRA index and corresponding scores [11]

	Definition	Score
Modifiable risk factors		
Depression	Score ≥ 5 on the 15-item Geriatric Depression Scale	+ 2.1
Hypertension	SBP ≥ 140 mmHg, DBP ≥ 90 mmHg and/or use of antihypertensive medication	+ 1.6
Obesity	BMI ≥ 30	+ 1.6
Smoking	Current smoker	+ 1.5
	Hypercholesterolemia	Total
cholesterol ≥ 6.2 mmol/L or use of cholesterol-lowering medication	+ 1.4	
Diabetes	Diabetes mellitus[a]	+ 1.3
Renal dysfunction	Estimated glomerular filtration rate < 60 ml/min/1.73 m² [b]	+ 1.1
Physical inactivity	Not fulfilling World Health Organisation criteria for physical activity as measured with LASA Physical Activity Questionnaire[c]	+ 1.1
Coronary heart disease	Cardiovascular disease (defined as myocardial infarction, angina or peripheral arterial disease)[a]	+ 1.0
Low/moderate alcohol use	Alcohol use 1–14 units per week for males and 1–7 for females [21]	−1.0
Non-modifiable risk factors		
Age	Males: 70–74 years	+ 5.2
	Male: 75–78 years	+ 6.8
	Females: 70–74 years	+ 6.2
	Female: 75–78 years	+ 9.2
Education	High: ≥ 13 years	0
	Medium: 7–13 years	+ 1.4
	Low: ≤ 7 years	+ 2.7

LIBRA LIfestyle for BRAin Health, *SBP* systolic blood pressure, *DBP* diastolic blood pressure, *BMI* body mass index
[a]Data self-reported and cross-checked with electronic health records
[b]Estimated glomerular filtration rate calculated with the creatinine-based Chronic Kidney Disease–Epidemiology Collaboration equation [27]
[c]World Health Organisation criteria for physical activity defined as ≥ 150 min/week moderate intensity or ≥ 75 min/week vigorous intensity or an equivalent combination

Primary and secondary outcomes

The primary outcome was all-cause dementia, according to the *Diagnostic and Statistical Manual of Mental Disorders* IV [16]. An independent outcome adjudication committee validated all dementia diagnoses, including a 1-year follow-up period in incident cases to assure there were no false positive diagnoses. Cognition was the secondary outcome measure, which was measured every 2 years with the Mini-Mental State Examination (MMSE) and the Visual Association Test (VAT) [17, 18].

Participants attending at least one follow-up visit were included in the analyses on cognition.

Statistical analysis

We first assessed the association between the LIBRA index in the preDIVA population and incident dementia with Cox proportional hazards regression. We then divided the study population into participants with a low, intermediate and high LIBRA index based on tertiles of the index [11]. In each group, the crude effect of the intervention on all-cause dementia was assessed with Cox proportional hazards regression (model 1). The years from randomisation to dementia diagnosis or censoring date were used as the timescale. To assess whether the LIBRA index is more useful as a selection tool when containing both modifiable and major non-modifiable risk factors, we repeated our analysis with the LIBRA index expanded with education (model 2) and additionally with age and sex (model 3) [11]. As history of coronary heart disease is not modifiable, we removed it from the LIBRA index in a sensitivity analysis (model 4). Our primary analysis was crude and in a secondary analysis we adjusted for baseline imbalances between the intervention and control groups. We also assessed the effect of adjusting for education, as this is an important risk factor for dementia and is associated with many of the risk/protective factors included in the LIBRA index [3]. The proportional hazards assumption was tested using Schoenfeld residuals and was assessed graphically [19].

Because of the cluster-randomised design we additionally performed a multi-level analysis to account for clustering within general practices and health care centres. To account for competing risk of death, we assessed the intervention effect on mortality in the LIBRA groups, and, when appropriate, performed a competing risk analysis according to the cause-specific hazard method [20]. We added a per-protocol analysis to assess whether the results were influenced by adherence to the intervention or control condition. In the per-protocol analysis, we excluded intervention participants who had on average less than two visits per year and inadvertent crossover control participants who had on average more than two visits per year. As the LIBRA index is more sensitive in a younger cohort [11], we performed a pre-defined subgroup analysis on age (dichotomised at the median). In the primary preDIVA analyses, the intervention seemed to be effective in those individuals with untreated hypertension who adhered to the intervention. However, the LIBRA definition of hypertension is rather crude (dichotomously defined as systolic BP ≥ 140 mmHg, diastolic BP ≥ 90 mmHg and/or use of antihypertensive medication). Therefore, we added subgroup analyses on World Health Organisation hypertension grades (i.e.

normotension, systolic BP < 140 mmHg and/or diastolic BP < 90 mmHg; grade I hypertension, systolic BP 140–160 mmHg and/or diastolic BP 90–100 mmHg; grade II or III hypertension, systolic BP ≥ 160 mmHg and/or diastolic BP ≥ 100 mmHg) and use of antihypertensive medication [21]. In the Netherlands, people with a history of cardiovascular disease (CVD) and diabetes visit a practice nurse as part of standard care, potentially diluting an intervention effect [22]. We therefore added analyses in subgroups based on history of CVD and type 2 diabetes. To assess whether the intervention led to an improvement of cardiovascular risk factors, as a proxy for treatment effect, we compared decline in systolic BP, BMI and total cholesterol between baseline and the last available follow-up visit, across the three LIBRA groups.

To assess whether individual changes in cognition vary over time between treatment groups, we used a multilevel growth model stratified for participants with a low, intermediate and high LIBRA index [23]. In this linear mixed-effect model each participant and time in years were considered random effects and a time × randomisation interaction variable was included. Since absolute values of the MMSE and VAT, or logarithmic transformation of these values, were not normally distributed, change in MMSE/VAT since baseline, which was normally distributed, was used as an outcome variable in the model. We performed our analyses in R studio version 3.2 using the survival and nlme packages [24].

Results

Of the 3526 preDIVA participants at baseline, 3339 (94.7%) had all 10 LIBRA items available at baseline and could be included in the analyses (Additional file 1: Figure S1). The median LIBRA score at baseline was 3.1. Participants with the highest LIBRA index were slightly older (low 74.2 years, intermediate 74.3 years, high 74.5 years; $p < 0.01$) and more often had a low education level (low 19.2%, intermediate 22.1%, high 29.9%; $p < 0.01$; Table 2). Systolic BP was highest in the intermediate LIBRA group (low 151.5 mmHg, intermediate 157.5 mmHg, high 156.7 mmHg; $p < 0.01$). The baseline characteristics of the intervention and control groups within each LIBRA group were well balanced, except for small differences in total cholesterol (respectively, 5.3 vs 5.5 mmol/L; $p = 0.03$) in the intermediate LIBRA group and mean systolic BP (157.9 vs 155.3 mmHg; $p = 0.04$) and sex (37.3% vs 44.2%; $p = 0.02$) in the high LIBRA group (Additional file 1: Table S1).

All-cause dementia was diagnosed in 220 (6.7%) participants; 76 of 1091 participants (7.0%) participants with a low LIBRA index, 71 of 1081 (6.6%) with an intermediate LIBRA index and 73 of 1102 participants (6.6%) with a high LIBRA index. The LIBRA index (model 1) was not associated with incident dementia (crude hazard

ratio (HR) 1.02 per point increase in LIBRA index, 95% confidence interval (CI) 0.96–1.09). Adding education to the LIBRA index (model 2) did not change these results (HR 1.06; 95% CI 0.90–1.24). The LIBRA index including education, age and sex (model 3) was significantly associated with incident dementia (HR 1.07, 95% CI 1.02–1.12).

The HR of the effect of intensive vascular care on incident all-cause dementia was 0.71 (95% CI 0.45–1.12) in the low, 1.06 (95% CI 0.66–1.69) in the intermediate and 1.02 (95% CI 0.64–1.62) in the high LIBRA groups (model 1; Fig. 1; Table 3). The interaction between randomisation and LIBRA index divided into tertiles was not significant. Also, when including age, sex and education in (models 2 and 3) or excluding coronary heart disease from (model 4) the LIBRA index and stratifying our study population based on this modified LIBRA index, the intervention was not effective in any of the groups (Table 3). Adjustment for baseline imbalances or education did not significantly influence the results, nor did accounting for clustering within general practices and health care centres (Additional file 1: Table S2). The results were similar in the per-protocol analysis (Additional file 1: Table S2). Mortality risk increased with increasing LIBRA index, but the intervention effect on mortality was not significantly different in the LIBRA groups (Additional file 1: Table S3). In all secondary analyses, the HR was lowest, albeit non-significant, in participants with the lowest LIBRA index (Additional file 1: Table S2). Subgroup analyses showed a significant interaction ($p = 0.03$) between age and randomisation in the intermediate LIBRA group with a lower HR in younger participants aged < 74.3 years (HR 0.55; 95% 0.26–1.17) compared to older participants (HR 1.65; 95% CI 0.88–3.09) (Additional file 1: Table S4). We found an interaction with diabetes in the high LIBRA group ($p = 0.03$), with a lower HR in participants with diabetes (HR 0.61; 95% CI 0.32–1.15) in comparison to those without (HR 1.78; 95% CI 0.87–3.64). We found no other interactions in the subgroup analyses. Participants with a higher LIBRA index had on average more decline in systolic BP (respectively in the low, intermediate and high LIBRA groups − 2.3, − 5.9 and − 5.8; $p < 0.01$), less decline in total cholesterol (− 0.3, − 0.3 and − 0.1; $p < 0.01$) and more decline in BMI (− 0.5, − 0.5 and − 0.9; $p < 0.01$). The intervention led to a significant decline in systolic BP in the low (intervention vs control − 3.9 vs − 0.5; $p = 0.03$) and intermediate (− 7.4 vs − 4.2; $p = 0.04$) LIBRA groups, but not in the high LIBRA group (− 7.1 vs − 4.3; $p = 0.09$; Additional file 1: Table S5). The intervention did not significantly reduce cholesterol or BMI in any of the LIBRA groups (Additional file 1: Table S5).

A total of 2674 participants had at least one valid MMSE score and 2671 participants at least one valid

Table 2 Baseline characteristics by LIBRA group

	Low LIBRA index	Intermediate LIBRA index	High LIBRA index	p value
Total number of participants	1091	1081	1102	
Range in LIBRA index	−1.0 to 2.6	2.6 to 4.2	4.2 to 11.6	
Demographics				
Age (years)	74.2 (2.5)	74.3 (2.5)	74.5 (2.5)	< 0.01
Sex (male)	528 (48.4%)	519 (48.0%)	445 (40.4%)	< 0.01
Education				< 0.01
Low (< 7 years)	209 (19.2%)	239 (22.1%)	330 (29.9%)	
Medium (7–12 years)	695 (63.7%)	671 (62.1%)	660 (59.9%)	
High (> 12 years)	179 (16.4%)	161 (14.9%)	101 (9.2%)	
Race (white)	1057 (96.9%)	1042 (96.4%)	1054 (95.6%)	< 0.01
Medical history				
CVD (excluding stroke or TIA)	66 (6.0%)	372 (34.4%)	526 (47.7%)	< 0.01
Stroke or TIA	60 (5.5%)	95 (8.8%)	169 (15.3%)	< 0.01
Cardiovascular risk factors				
Systolic BP (mmHg)	151.5 (22.0)	157.5 (20.8)	156.7 (20.6)	< 0.01
Diastolic BP (mmHg)	81.0 (10.9)	82.0 (10.9)	81.3 (11.0)	0.09
Total cholesterol (mmol/L)	5.4 (0.9)	5.4 (1.1)	4.9 (1.2)	< 0.01
LDL cholesterol (mmol/L)	3.3 (0.8)	3.2 (1.0)	2.8 (1.0)	< 0.01
Body mass index (kg/m^2)	25.9 (3.1)	26.7 (3.6)	29.6 (4.6)	< 0.01
Type 2 diabetes	30 (2.7%)	103 (9.5%)	460 (41.7%)	< 0.01
Smoking (currently)	46 (4.2%)	113 (10.5%)	265 (24.0%)	< 0.01
Alcohol use (units/week)	3 (0–7)	4 (0–14)	0 (0–10)	< 0.01
Physically active (WHO)	1065 (97.6%)	990 (91.6%)	784 (71.1%)	< 0.01
Creatinine (μmol/L)	77 (68–88)	80 (68–93)	82 (71–97)	< 0.01
Medication use				
Antihypertensive medication	332 (30.4%)	631 (58.4%)	838 (76.0%)	< 0.01
Cholesterol-lowering medication	77 (7.1%)	370 (34.2%)	664 (60.3%)	< 0.01
Disability and neuropsychiatric assessment				
Mini-Mental State Examination	29 (28–30)	28,5 (27–29)	28 (27–29)	< 0.01
Visual Association Test	6 (5, 6)	6 (5, 6)	6 (5, 6)	0.05
Geriatric Depression Scale	1 (0–1)	1 (0–2)	2 (0–4)	< 0.01

Data presented as number (percentage), mean (standard deviation) or median (interquartile range)
LIBRA LIfestyle for BRAin Health, *CVD* indicates cardiovascular disease *TIA* transient ischemic attack, *BP* blood pressure, *LDL* low-density lipoprotein, *WHO* World Health Organisation

VAT score after baseline and could be included in the analyses on cognitive decline (Additional file 1: Figure S1). Participants excluded from these analyses were on average older, had a higher cardiovascular risk and had a lower baseline MMSE and VAT (Additional file 1: Table S6). After 3 years, decline in MMSE did not significantly differ between the intervention and control groups among participants with a low (mean difference (MD) − 0.08; 95% CI − 0.28 to 0.13), intermediate (MD 0.07; 95% CI − 0.14 to 0.27) or high (MD − 0.06; 95% CI − 0.30 to 0.18; Fig. 2a, Additional file 1: Table S7) LIBRA index. Decline in VAT also did not differ between treatment

groups in the low (MD 0.03; 95% CI − 0.09 to 0.14), intermediate (MD − 0.04; 95% CI − 0.16 to 0.08) or high (MD 0.07; 95% CI − 0.05 to 0.19; Fig. 2b, Additional file 1: Table S7) LIBRA groups.

Discussion

In the preDIVA study population, aged 70–78 years, the LIBRA index did not identify a high-risk group in whom the multi-domain intervention was effective in preventing dementia or cognitive decline. On the contrary, there was a trend for a preventive effect in the subgroup with a low LIBRA index. Results were

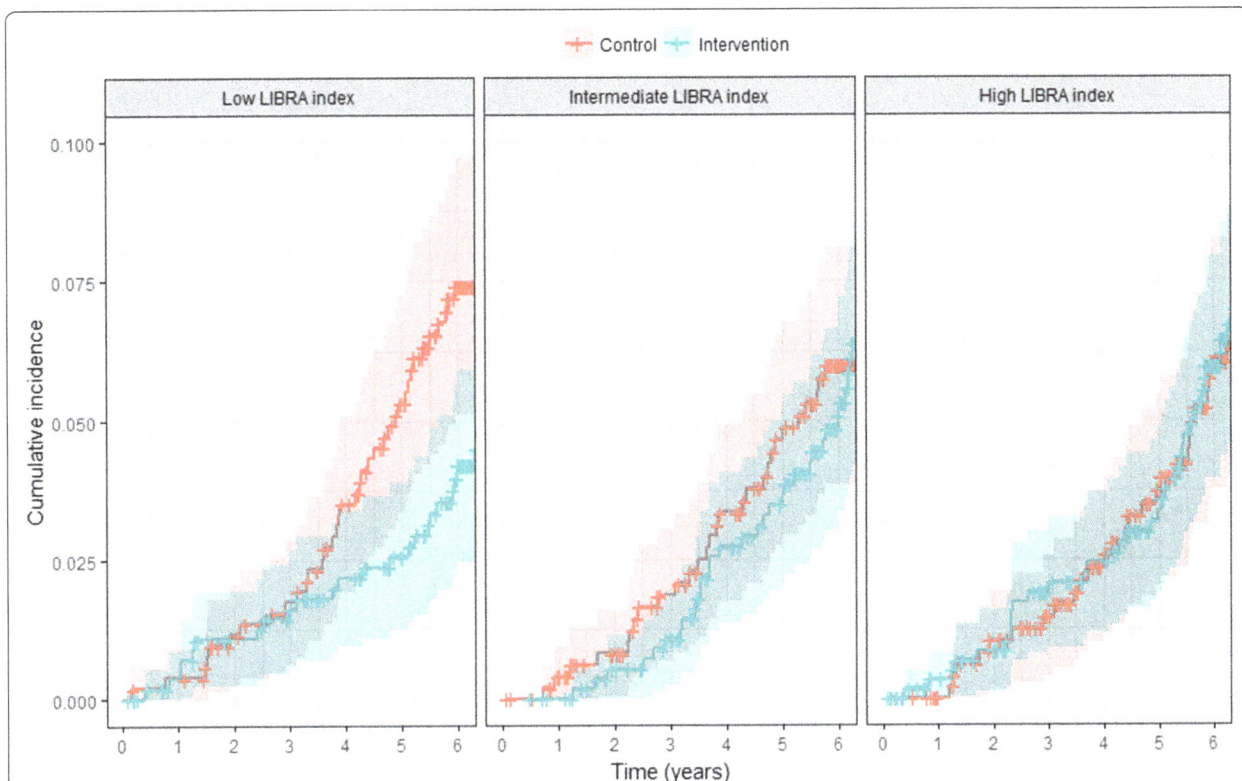

Fig. 1 Cumulative incidence curves of risk of dementia comparing intervention and control groups in participants with low, intermediate and high LIBRA index. Line indicates incidence, shaded area indicates 95% CI. Numbers of participants at risk at 6-year follow-up were 791 in low (408 intervention; 383 control), 756 in intermediate (400 intervention; 356 control) and 738 in high (406 intervention, 332 control) LIBRA groups. LIBRA LIfestyle for BRAin Health

comparable when including non-modifiable risk factors in the LIBRA index.

The concept of selecting people at increased risk of dementia for preventive interventions to magnify the intervention effect is widely supported among experts in the field and has been incorporated in the design of recent multi-domain prevention trials [6, 7]. Our results do not support this strategy, and are even in contrast with this concept, at least in later life, suggesting a more favourable effect of the intervention in those with a low

Table 3 Intervention effect on incident all-cause dementia across the models, by LIBRA group

	LIBRA group	Intervention, n/N (%)	Control, n/N (%)	Hazard ratio (95% CI)	p value for interaction
Model 1: LIBRA index	Low	33/567 (5.8%)	43/524 (8.2%)	0.71 (0.45–1.12)	Ref.
	Intermediate	39/576 (6.8%)	32/505 (6.3%)	1.06 (0.66–1.69)	0.23
	High	41/606 (6.8%)	32/496 (6.5%)	1.02 (0.64–1.62)	0.27
Model 2: LIBRA index including education	Low	28/555 (5.0%)	39/498 (7.8%)	0.64 (0.40–1.05)	Ref.
	Intermediate	38/525 (7.2%)	31/482 (6.4%)	1.11 (0.69–1.79)	0.12
	High	46/660 (7.0%)	35/525 (6.7%)	1.03 (0.66–1.59)	0.17
Model 3: LIBRA index including age, sex and education	Low	32/564 (5.7%)	33/515 (6.4%)	0.88 (0.54–1.43)	Ref.
	Intermediate	35/568 (6.2%)	34/510 (6.7%)	0.91 (0.57–1.47)	0.94
	High	45/608 (7.4%)	38/480 (7.9%)	0.92 (0.59–1.41)	0.92
Model 4: LIBRA index excluding coronary heart disease	Low	36/559 (6.0%)	45/559 (8.1%)	0.75 (0.48–1.16)	Ref.
	Intermediate	35/570 (6.1%)	28/477 (5.9%)	1.05 (0.64–1.72)	0.32
	High	42/580 (7.2%)	34/489 (7.0%)	1.01 (0.64–1.59)	0.34

LIBRA LIfestyle for BRAin Health, *CI* confidence interval, *Ref.* reference category

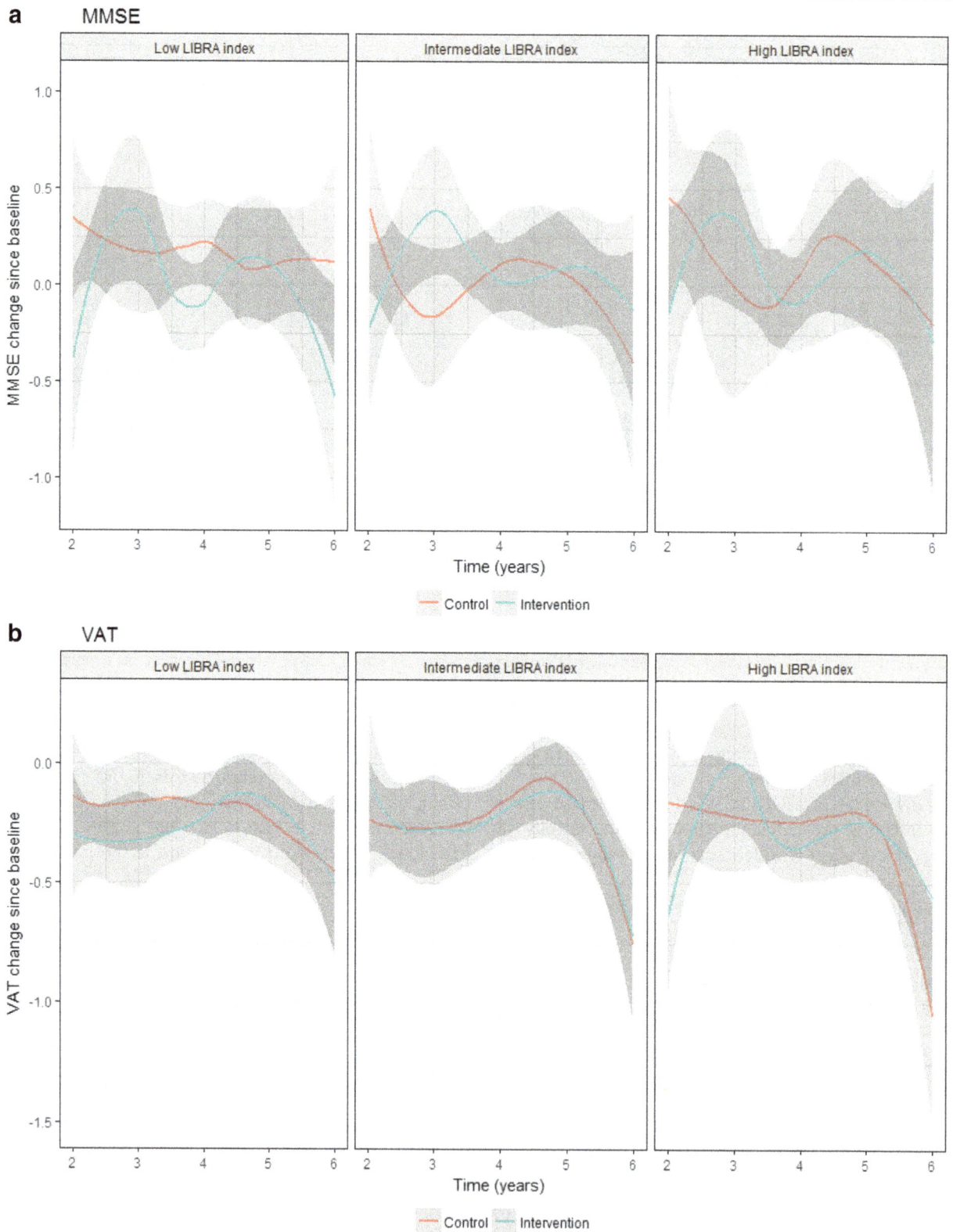

Fig. 2 Effect of intervention on MMSE (**a**) and VAT (**b**) change since baseline in LIBRA groups. Trajectories of change in MMSE and VAT since baseline comparing control group (red line) to intervention group (blue line) in each LIBRA group, as predicted with multilevel growth model. Positive value indicates increase in MMSE/VAT since baseline, negative value indicates decrease. LIBRA LIfestyle for BRAin Health, MMSE Mini-Mental State Examination, VAT Visual Association Test

LIBRA index. A potential explanation for this is that the contrast between the intervention and control conditions was too small, partly due to Hawthorne effects and improvements in the standard care for cardiovascular risk management during the trial [5]. Although a greater reduction in systolic BP could be achieved in participants with a higher LIBRA index, this was the case in both the intervention and control groups and the difference between the treatment groups was smallest in the high LIBRA group. Another potential explanation for our results is that the LIBRA index does not successfully classify dementia risk in this older population aged 70–78 years. Indeed, our analyses did not show an association between a high LIBRA index and increased risk of dementia. Since preDIVA is an RCT, this could potentially (partly) be due to the fact that the dementia risk was influenced during the trial by the intervention and/or Hawthorne effects [5]. For example, systolic BP decreased by approximately 8 mmHg in the intervention group and 4 mmHg in the control group, and the decline was steepest in participants with hypertension at baseline [5]. In one of the LIBRA validation studies, a higher LIBRA index was associated (at group level) with an increased risk of dementia in people aged 70–79 years [11]. The individual predictive accuracy in late life was poor, however, with a C statistic of 0.50, and seemed to decrease with increasing age. Investigating the utility of the LIBRA index as a selection tool for prevention trials at a younger age (55–70 years) may yield different results. A third potential explanation is that the factors in the LIBRA index and in other dementia risk scores are dichotomous and not designed to precisely quantify the magnitude of the risk/protective factor or the room for improvement. For example, the potential for improvement is different for someone with a systolic BP of 125 mmHg on antihypertensive medication compared to a person with a systolic BP of 155 mmHg without medication, although both are weighted equally in the LIBRA index with the dichotomous score for hypertension (including both high BP and/or antihypertensive medication use). In order for a risk estimation tool to be useful for selection of high-risk populations for dementia prevention trials, the potential for improvement should be taken into account (e.g. by distinguishing treated or untreated hypertension).

Regardless of the LIBRA index performance in high-age populations, the concept of selecting people at high risk of dementia may only be appropriate for younger people (i.e. age < 70 years). In older people at high risk of dementia, cerebrovascular and neurodegenerative damage may already be irreversible, while those with a low risk could still benefit from risk factor improvement in order to maintain cognitive function. Also, several observational studies have shown a diminishing or even inverting association between risk factors and incident dementia in older people, as for example the J-shaped relation with BP [25]. Therefore, future trials should perhaps either focus on people with lowest dementia risk in old age or highest dementia risk in midlife. This would, however, imply that substantially larger sample sizes or longer follow-up will be required, as incidence rates in these groups are lower.

A strength of this analysis is that preDIVA is, up until now, the only multi-domain prevention trial with dementia as the primary outcome. The population-based approach with few exclusion criteria renders preDIVA a suitable study to test whether the LIBRA index is a promising tool to select high-risk groups from the general population. A limitation is the overall neutral result of the preDIVA trial, perhaps limiting the possibility to detect high-risk groups who benefit most. However, a significant effect of the intervention was found in the per-protocol analysis among participants with untreated hypertension at baseline (HR 0.54, 95% CI 0.32–0.92) [5], while the results of the present analyses do not show a trend towards improved treatment effects in higher LIBRA groups. Another limitation is that no other neuropsychological tests were performed besides the MMSE and VAT to detect more subtle cognitive changes. We did not have information on two of the 12 LIBRA items, including cognitive activity which is the strongest-weighted item in the LIBRA index [9]. These factors were, however, already identified as risk factors that need further validation in the systematic review and Delphi consensus used to design the LIBRA index, and were also not included in the validation study among people in late life (70–79 years) [11, 12]. Furthermore, it may be argued that cognitive activity at this age is not as much a modifiable risk factor but rather an early indicator of developing cognitive decline and dementia [26].

Conclusions

Within our study population of community-dwelling people aged 70–78 years, a modifiable dementia risk score does not identify heterogeneity in the treatment effect of a multi-domain intervention to prevent dementia or cognitive decline. This suggests that in older adults a high LIBRA index may not be a suitable parameter to select participants for a dementia prevention trial. Specific characteristics of the preDIVA study, including the overall neutral effect of the intervention and relatively high age group, may have contributed to the lack of discriminating capacity of the LIBRA index.

medication, history of cardiovascular disease and diabetes. **Table S5.** Treatment effect on vascular risk factors in LIBRA groups. **Table S6.** Baseline characteristics of participants included in and excluded from cognitive analyses. **Table S7.** Treatment effect on cognition in LIBRA groups (DOCX 533 kb)

Abbreviations

BMI: Body mass index; BP: Blood pressure; CI: Confidence interval; CVD: Cardiovascular disease; HR: Hazard ratio; ISRCTN: International Standard Randomised Controlled Trial Number; LIBRA: LIfestyle for BRAin Health; MD: Mean difference; MMSE: Mini-Mental State Examination; preDIVA: Prevention of Dementia by Intensive Vascular Care; RCT: Randomised controlled trial; VAT: Visual Association Test

Acknowledgements

The authors would like to thank all participants, general practitioners and practice nurses involved in the preDIVA study. They also would like to thank Lisa S.M. Eurelings, Suzanne A. Ligthart and Carin E. Miedema for their hard work for the preDIVA study.

Funding

The preDIVA trial was supported by the Dutch Ministry of Health, Welfare and Sports (50–50110–98-020), the Innovatiefonds Zorgverzekeraars (Innovation Fund of Collaborative Health Insurances, 05–234) and ZonMw (The Netherlands Organisation for Health Research and Development, 62000015).
The analyses presented here are based on funding from the European Union Seventh Framework Programme (FP7/2007–2013) under grant agreement n° 305374 and an EU Joint Programme—Neurodegenerative Disease Research (JPND) project. The JPND project is supported through the following funding organisations under the aegis of the JPND (www.jpnd.eu): Finland, Suomen Akatemia (Academy of Finland,291803); France, L'Agence Nationale de la Recherche (The French National Research Agency, ANR-14-JPPS-0001-02); Germany, Bundesministerium für Bildung und Forschung (BMBF) (The Federal Ministry of Education and Research, FKZ01ED1509); Sweden, Vetenskapsrådet (VR) (Swedish Research Council, 529–2014-7503); the Netherlands, ZonMw (The Netherlands Organisation for Health Research and Development, 733051041).

Authors' contributions

SK and ER were responsible for the conception of the study. TvM, MPH-B, EPMvC, WAvG, KD, SK and ER contributed to the design of the study. The preDIVA trial was supervised by EPMvC, WAvG and ER. J-WvD helped in data management and outcome adjudication. Data analysis and drafting of the manuscript was performed by TvM. All authors contributed to data interpretation and approved the final manuscript.

Competing interests

The authors declare that they have no competing interests.

Author details

[1]Department of Neurology, Academic Medical Center (AMC), Meibergdreef 9, 1105, AZ, Amsterdam, the Netherlands. [2]Department of Neurology, Donders Institute for Brain, Cognition and Behaviour, Radboud University Medical Center, Nijmegen, the Netherlands. [3]Department of General Practice, Amsterdam Public Health Research Institute, Academic Medical Center (AMC), Amsterdam, the Netherlands. [4]Department of Psychiatry and Neuropsychology, Alzheimer Center Limburg, Maastricht University, Maastricht, the Netherlands.

References

1. World Health Organisation: World report on ageing and health. World Health Organisation: Luxembourg; 2015.
2. Scheltens P, Blennow K, Breteler MMB, de Strooper B, Frisoni GB, Salloway S, Van der Flier WM. Alzheimer's disease. Lancet. 2016;388:505–17.
3. Norton S, Matthews FE, Barnes DE, Yaffe K, Brayne C. Potential for primary prevention of Alzheimer's disease: an analysis of population-based data. Lancet Neurol. 2014;13:788–94.
4. Richard E, Andrieu S, Solomon A, Mangialasche F, Ahtiluoto S, Moll van Charante EP, Coley N, Fratiglioni L, Neely AS, Vellas B, et al. Methodological challenges in designing dementia prevention trials—the European Dementia Prevention Initiative (EDPI). J Neurol Sci. 2012;322:64–70.
5. Moll van Charante EP, Richard E, Eurelings LS, van Dalen JW, Ligthart SA, van Bussel EF, Hoevenaar-Blom MP, Vermeulen M, van Gool WA. Effectiveness of a 6-year multidomain vascular care intervention to prevent dementia (preDIVA): a cluster-randomised controlled trial. Lancet. 2016; 388(10046):797–805.
6. Ngandu T, Lehtisalo J, Solomon A, Levalahti E, Ahtiluoto S, Antikainen R, Backman L, Hanninen T, Jula A, Laatikainen T, et al. A 2 year multidomain intervention of diet, exercise, cognitive training, and vascular risk monitoring versus control to prevent cognitive decline in at-risk elderly people (FINGER): a randomised controlled trial. Lancet. 2015;385:2255–63.
7. Andrieu S, Guyonnet S, Coley N, Cantet C, Bonnefoy M, Bordes S, Bories L, Cufi MN, Dantoine T, Dartigues JF, et al. Effect of long-term omega 3 polyunsaturated fatty acid supplementation with or without multidomain intervention on cognitive function in elderly adults with memory complaints (MAPT): a randomised, placebo-controlled trial. Lancet Neurol. 2017;16:377–89.
8. Imtiaz B, Tolppanen AM, Kivipelto M, Soininen H. Future directions in Alzheimer's disease from risk factors to prevention. Biochem Pharmacol. 2014;88:661–70.
9. Schiepers OJ, Kohler S, Deckers K, Irving K, O'Donnell CA, van den Akker M, Verhey FR, Vos SJ, de Vugt ME, van Boxtel MP. Lifestyle for Brain Health (LIBRA): a new model for dementia prevention. Int J Geriatr Psychiatry. 2018; 33(1):167–75.
10. Wiersma T, Smulders YM, Stehouwer CD, Konings KT, Lanphen J. Summary of the multidisciplinary guideline on cardiovascular risk management (revision 2011). Ned Tijdschr Geneeskd. 2012;156:A5104.
11. Vos SJB, van Boxtel MPJ, Schiepers OJG, Deckers K, de Vugt M, Carriere I, Dartigues JF, Peres K, Artero S, Ritchie K, et al. Modifiable risk factors for prevention of dementia in midlife, late life and the oldest-old: validation of the LIBRA index. J Alzheimers Dis. 2017;58:537–47.
12. Deckers K, van Boxtel MP, Schiepers OJ, de Vugt M, Munoz Sanchez JL, Anstey KJ, Brayne C, Dartigues JF, Engedal K, Kivipelto M, et al. Target risk factors for dementia prevention: a systematic review and Delphi consensus study on the evidence from observational studies. Int J Geriatr Psychiatry. 2015;30:234–46.
13. Pocklington C, Gilbody S, Manea L, McMillan D. The diagnostic accuracy of brief versions of the Geriatric Depression Scale: a systematic review and meta-analysis. Int J Geriatr Psychiatry. 2016;31:837–57.
14. Stel VS, Smit JH, Pluijm SM, Visser M, Deeg DJ, Lips P. Comparison of the LASA Physical Activity Questionnaire with a 7-day diary and pedometer. J Clin Epidemiol. 2004;57:252–8.
15. Kivipelto M, Ngandu T, Laatikainen T, Winblad B, Soininen H, Tuomilehto J. Risk score for the prediction of dementia risk in 20 years among middle aged people: a longitudinal, population-based study. Lancet Neurol. 2006;5:735–41.
16. American Psychiatric Association. Diagnostic and Statistical Manual of Mental Disorders. 4th ed. Washington, DC: American Psychiatric Association; 2000.
17. Folstein MF, Folstein SE, McHugh PR. "Mini-mental state". A practical method for grading the cognitive state of patients for the clinician. J Psychiatr Res. 1975;12:189–98.
18. Lindeboom J, Schmand B, Tulner L, Walstra G, Jonker C. Visual association test to detect early dementia of the Alzheimer type. J Neurol Neurosurg Psychiatry. 2002;73:126–33.
19. Bellera CA, MacGrogan G, Debled M, de Lara CT, Brouste V, Mathoulin-Pelissier S. Variables with time-varying effects and the cox model: some statistical concepts illustrated with a prognostic factor study in breast cancer. BMC Med Res Methodol. 2010;10:20.

20. Hinchliffe SR, Lambert PC. Flexible parametric modelling of cause-specific hazards to estimate cumulative incidence functions. BMC Med Res Methodol. 2013;13:13.

21. Piepoli MF, Hoes AW, Agewall S, Albus C, Brotons C, Catapano AL, Cooney MT, Corra U, Cosyns B, Deaton C, et al. European guidelines on cardiovascular disease prevention in clinical practice: the sixth joint task force of the European Society of Cardiology and Other Societies on cardiovascular disease prevention in clinical practice (constituted by representatives of 10 societies and by invited experts)developed with the special contribution of the European Association for Cardiovascular Prevention & rehabilitation (EACPR). Eur Heart J. 2016;2016(37):2315–81.

22. Voogdt-Pruis HR, Van Ree JW, Gorgels AP, Beusmans GH. Adherence to a guideline on cardiovascular prevention: a comparison between general practitioners and practice nurses. Int J Nurs Stud. 2011;48:798–807.

23. Gee KA. Multilevel growth modeling:an introductory approach to analyzing longitudinal data for evaluators. Am J Eval. 2014;35:543–61.

24. R Core Team. R: a language and environment for statistical computing. Vienna: R Foundation for Statistical Computing; 2017.

25. Ruitenberg A, Skoog I, Ott A, Aevarsson O, Witteman JC, Lernfelt B, van Harskamp F, Hofman A, Breteler MM. Blood pressure and risk of dementia: results from the Rotterdam study and the Gothenburg H-70 study. Dement Geriatr Cogn Disord. 2001;12:33–9.

26. Wilson RS, Barnes LL, Aggarwal NT, Boyle PA, Hebert LE, Mendes de Leon CF, Evans DA. Cognitive activity and the cognitive morbidity of Alzheimer disease. Neurology. 2010;75:990–6.

27. Kilbride HS, Stevens PE, Eaglestone G, Knight S, Carter JL, Delaney MP, Farmer CK, Irving J, O'Riordan SE, Dalton RN, Lamb EJ. Accuracy of the MDRD (Modification of Diet in Renal Disease) study and CKD-EPI (CKD Epidemiology Collaboration) equations for estimation of GFR in the elderly. Am J Kidney Dis. 2013;61:57–66.

7

Does taking statins affect the pathological burden in autopsy-confirmed Alzheimer's dementia?

Jana Crum[1], Jeffrey Wilson[1] and Marwan Sabbagh[2,3]*

Abstract

Background: The efficacy of cholesterol lowering agents, specifically statins, in slowing the rate of decline of cognitive function in Alzheimer's disease (AD) patients is not yet fully understood. Our team's previously published paper showed that patients who used statins demonstrated no increase in cognitive decline in mild cognitive impairment when compared with nonusers. Further, AD patients on statins demonstrated a slight decreasing trend in cognitive decline. The purpose of this study is therefore to investigate the association between stain use in AD confirmed by clinical diagnosis and autopsy and the pathological burden (plaques, tangles, Braak stage). The hypothesis leading this investigation is that prolonged statin use associates with lower AD pathology at autopsy.

Methods: We queried the National Alzheimer's Coordinating Center (NACC) database for autopsy-confirmed AD cases. Of the Uniform Data Set (UDS) participants who are deceased, 16,163 were diagnosed with dementia at their last UDS visit prior to death, and autopsy data are available for 3945 patients. These patients were then stratified into two groups based upon statin use. The two groups were then analyzed for their pathological AD burden, including total plaques, total tangles, age at death, age of onset, and Braak stage.

Results: NACC data were available for 1816 subjects with clinically and pathologically confirmed AD; 1558 were not on statins and 258 were on statins. No significant differences in age at death, age at onset, Braak stages, mean total tau, and mean total amyloid were found between the two subject groups. When statin use was analyzed by apolipoprotein E (ApoE) genotype carrier statins, the presence of ApoE4 did not influence the effects (or lack thereof) of statin use.

Conclusions: Prolonged statin use in pathologically confirmed AD dementia does not appear to influence the amount of burden of plaques and tangles or Braak stage. These observations were not altered by the presence of absence of ApoE4.

Keywords: Statins, Alzheimer's disease, Dementia, Post mortem, Senile plaques, Neurofibrillary tangles, Braak stages

Background

Alzheimer's disease (AD) is the sixth leading cause of death in the United States. In 2017, Alzheimer's dementia or related dementias were the primary cause of death for 33% of seniors who expired [1]. It is projected that by 2050, 14 million Americans will have dementia due to Alzheimer's disease [1]. Due to the increasing burden Alzheimer's disease adds to the American healthcare system, more than $2.9 billion of the NIH's research budget has been allocated to AD and AD-related research in 2017 [2].

Numerous studies have investigated the role that cholesterol and lipoproteins play in AD. The direct effects of plasma cholesterol and related lipoproteins on the incidence and severity of dementia and cognitive decline remain a controversial topic deserving of deeper exploration. Recent discoveries have opened up new lines of inquiry to help the neuroscience community more accurately understand and depict the connection between these two variables. Increasing evidence links brain cholesterol with both

* Correspondence: sabbagm@ccf.org
[2]Department of Neurology, Barrow Neurological Institute, Phoenix, AZ, USA
[3]Cleveland Clinic Lou Ruvo Center for Brain Health, 888 W. Bonneville Ave, Las Vegas, NV 89106, USA
Full list of author information is available at the end of the article

plaques and tangles [3]. A positive correlation has been shown between HDL levels and MMSE performance and a negative correlation between LDL levels and immediate and delayed recall [4]. Several epidemiological studies also showed that elevated total serum cholesterol was a significant risk factor for Alzheimer's disease, regardless of ApoE status [5]. Lowering cholesterol levels via statins is associated with reducing Aβ [6]. Subjects with incident dementia have demonstrated higher total cholesterol at their first visit [7]. Cholesterol levels and atherosclerosis have also been found to associate with Alzheimer's disease [8]. Because lipoproteins appear to adversely affect cognitive functioning, statins have long been purported to play a role in cognitive decline; however, some within the neuroscience community disagree with the notion that the role between statins and dementia is worthy of further exploration. Our study set out to provide compelling evidence that, rather, the relationship between the two is one which we can no longer afford to overlook in our battle against AD and other related forms of dementia.

Evidence that statins decrease the risk of incident dementia is convincing from an epidemiological standpoint. Some studies show that statin users have a fivefold lower risk of incident Alzheimer's disease and a threefold lower risk of MCI [7]. Three major clinical trials have investigated the role of statins in cognitive decline. The CLASP study in 2011 assessed the use of simvastatin in probable Alzheimer's disease. No significant difference in cognitive decline was found between simvastatin and a placebo when measured by the ADAS-Cog [9]. The LEADe trial in 2010 studied atorvastatin therapy in mild to moderate Alzheimer's disease. Again, no net benefit was found resulting from statin therapy compared with placebo over 72 weeks [10] as measured by the ADAS-Cog and ADAS-CGIC. These two clinical trials contradict the initial findings in 2005 by Sparks et al. [11] that displayed a significantly decreased rate of cognitive decline by atorvastatin on the ADAS-cog and MMSE over 6 months. These values approached those which would have suggested compelling significance at the 12 month mark as well [11]. All three of these trials focused on subjects with Alzheimer's dementia.

Our team's previously published study explained that patients who used statins showed no negative effects of statins on cognitive decline in amnestic MCI. Further, MCI subjects on statins demonstrated a slight decrease in cognitive decline [12]. This study builds on these results to pose the question asking whether or not statin use decreases the amount of AD pathology at the time of autopsy.

The connection between statins and AD and other forms of dementia warrants exploration. Many studies have investigated the efficacy of statins in reducing AD diagnosis and progression. The purpose of the study is to determine whether statin use in clinically and autopsy confirmed AD is associated with a lower pathological burden (plaques, tangles, Braak stage). This study was carried out to confirm the hypothesis that chronic statin use associates with less AD pathology at autopsy.

Methods

Study sample

All data were obtained from the Uniform Data Set (UDS), the Neuropathology Data Set, and the Researcher's Data Dictionary—Genetic Data from the National Alzheimer's Coordinating Center (NACC), a database funded by the National Institute on Aging (NIA); compilation of the data began in September 2015. The dataset includes subjects with a range of cognitive characteristics spanning normal cognition, mild cognitive impairment, and dementia. The demographic, clinical, and specimen data from 39 past and present Alzheimer's Disease Centers were also analyzed, which enroll and follow subjects with their own various protocols. The UDS was collected via a standardized evaluation of subjects during either an office visit, a home visit, or over telephone conversations with a trained clinician or clinic personnel. The information needed was provided by either the subjects themselves or their informants during annual assessment. Written informed consent was obtained from all subjects and informants. Research using the NACC database was approved by the Institutional Review Board at the University of Washington.

This investigation analyzed data gathered by the NACC, established in 1999 in response to a call for a permanent Alzheimer's disease data-coordinating center and database. Through making this information available to researchers, the NACC aims to maintain and increase the research capability of the NACC database, facilitate and conduct research using NACC data, collaborate with national or international efforts on AD and other dementias, and maintain the NIA-required administrative coordination of ADC meetings and ADC communications [13].

The NACC's data request website provided all of the data necessary for this study. The data were compiled by the NACC in a dataset. The proposal posed in the query questioned the effect of statins on the neuropathology of dementia due to Alzheimer's disease. To facilitate acquisition of pertinent variables, the following keywords were used: "Alzheimer's disease/LOAD", "Neuropathology", "Braak stage", "APOE", "Cross-sectional", and "Statin". The start date of the UDS (September 2005) was used, and the data freeze includes data through December 2016.

AD participants who came to autopsy were assessed based upon their use of statins (+ or −). Participants were placed in either the statin positive or statin negative group. All statin types were grouped together, and no other medications designed to lower lipids were considered. First, the demographical configuration of the subject was determined by categorizing each subject into groups, such as age at onset, age at death, duration of AD, gender, and education level. Subjects were further stratified by the volume of statin users vs nonusers for each demographical factor. Each subject's Braak stage, overall amyloid load, and overall tau load were analyzed. These subgroups were then cross-analyzed based upon the internal number of statin users vs nonstatin users.

Linear models were fitted to investigate the effects of group difference on NACC age, duration of AD, age at onset, Braak stage, total amyloid, and tau overall. The predictor in these models was statin use or nonuse, and significance was declared based on a probability of type I error level as 0.05 ($\alpha = 0.05$). The assumptions of normality and independence of outcomes among patients were satisfied. Homogeneity was checked, and no evidence concluded otherwise.

Results

Overall demographics

The demographic composition of the subjects analyzed is presented in Table 1. For both statin user and nonuser populations, the median age at time of autopsy was 83 years. In addition, males comprised most of both subject groups, representing 60.47% and 53.98% of statin users and nonusers respectively. A total of 532 (29.5%) subjects obtained a graduate or professional degree (mean 19.7 years of education). Of the 1801 subjects with educational background information available, only 256 (14.8%) took statins as recorded in the NACC database. At each level of educational achievement, nonstatin users vastly outnumbered statin users. Duration of AD and gender illustrated a statistically significant difference, with p values of 0.015 and 0.030 respectively, with regards to the amount of statin users vs nonusers.

Pathological impact

Pathological load differences between statin users and nonstatin users are presented in Table 2. Braak stage showed no statistically significant difference between

Table 1 Demographics of gender and education by statin

	Nonstatin	Statin
Gender		
Male	841 (54%)	156 (54%)
Female	717 (46%)	102 (39.5%)
Education		
Primary school	129 (8.3%)	19 (7.4%)
High school diploma	310 (20.1%)	54 (21.1%)
Some college	263 (17.0%)	42 (16.4%)
Bachelor degree	382 (24.7%)	70 (27.3%)
Graduate/professional school	461 (29.8%)	71 (27.7%)

Table 2 Parameter estimates and significance values for responses by statin regardless of Apo E status

	N	Mean	Standard error of the mean	p value
Age at death				
Non statin	1558	81.72	0.274	0.324
Statin	258	81.07	0.530	
Duration of AD				
Nonstatin	1520	8.8053	0.11082	0.015
Statin	256	8.0938	0.27669	
Age at onset of AD				
Nonstatin	1520	72.0526	0.29309	0.846
Statin	256	72.1992	v.57622	
Braak stage				
Nonstatin	1552	4.8853	0.03685	0.292
Statin	258	4.7829	0.08682	
Total amyloid load				
Nonstatin	1557	2.3378	0.02420	0.635
Statin	258	2.3682	0.05838	
Total tau load				
Nonstatin	1155	1.9957	0.01036	0.683
Statin	193	1.9845	0.02595	

AD Alzheimer's disease

statin groups, $p = 0.292$. Neither overall tau nor amyloid load demonstrated a statistically significant difference in subject clusters, p = 0.683 and 0.635 respectively.

Table 3 shows how the effect of statins on the parameters explored are influenced by ApoE genotype. In nonstatin users, there were significant differences. Age at death and age of onset were significantly younger for ApoE4 carriers. ApoE4 carriers also had significantly higher CERAD neuritic plaque scores, tau scores, and Braak stages.

In statin users, there were also significant differences. Age at death and age of onset were significantly younger in ApoE4 carriers. Tau scores were significantly higher in ApoE4 carriers, but neuritic plaque scores and Braak stages did not differ in the statin group between ApoE4 and non-ApoE4 carriers (Table 4).

Discussion

This study was carried out to confirm the hypothesis that chronic statin use associates with less AD pathology at autopsy. Based upon the analysis of the NACC dataset and assessment of the AD pathological load by subject statin use, several key findings were identified. Statin users demonstrated no statistically significant differences in any pathological load than nonstatin users. No differences for Braak stages, overall tau, and overall amyloid load were found. Upon further analysis, in each level of overall amyloid level,

Table 3 Parameter estimates and significance values for responses by statin inclusive of ApoE status

Statin use	APOE4	Mean	p value	Mean difference	Standard error of the difference	95% confidence interval of the difference		
						Lower	Upper	
0								
Age at death	1.00	79.64						
	0.00	81.86	0.014	−2.228	0.895	−3.999	−0.457	Significant
Education level	1.00	15.59	0.879	−0.132	0.868	−1.835	1.570	Not significant
	0.00	15.72						
Estimated onset age	1.00	69.13						
	0.00	72.25	0.002	−3.118	0.992	−5.083	−1.153	Significant
Tauopathy	1.00	2.01						
	0.00	0.34	0.000	1.672	0.076	1.523	1.820	Significant
Density of neocortical neuritic plaques (amyloid CERAD score)	1.00	2.60						
	0.00	2.32	0.000	0.271	0.075	0.123	0.419	Significant
Braak stage	1.00	5.29						
	0.00	4.87	0.000	0.420	0.112	0.199	0.642	Significant
1								
Age at death	1.00	76.81	0.036	−4.543	2.159	−8.795	−0.291	Significant
	0.00	81.36						
Education level	1.00	14.13	0.444	−1.598	2.085	−5.704	2.508	Not significant
	0.00	15.72						
Estimated onset age	1.00	67.19	0.001	−5.346	1.335	−8.104	−2.587	Significant
	0.00	72.53						
Tauopathy	1.00	2.06						
	0.00	0.37	0.000	1.691	0.183	1.330	2.051	Significant
Density of neocortical neuritic plaques (amyloid CERAD score)	1.00	2.56	0.393	0.207	0.242	−0.270	0.684	Not significant
	0.00	2.36						
Braak stage	1.00	5.25	0.167	0.498	0.359	−0.210	1.206	Not significant
	0.00	4.75						

APO apolipoprotein, *CERAD* Consortium to Establish a Registry for Alzheimer's Disease
0 means ApoE 4 NON carrier
1 means ApoE 4 Carrier

nonstatin users drastically outnumbered statin users suggesting that statin use in AD is relatively small. Further, we find that the effect of statin use is not confounded or impacted by ApoE carrier status. These data suggest that statin use did not protect against AD pathology in autopsy-confirmed AD dementia cases. Additionally, these data suggest that statins do not negatively impact AD.

An additional finding is that ApoE4 carriers had increases in Braak stages, tau pathology, and amyloid CERAD plaque counts. This is in line with previously published reports [14, 15].

Limitations on generalization of this study are many. First, because it is a case–control study, we rely on what is captured in the database. It is possible that many participants were on statins in the past but are no longer. Second, with our stratification, we could not include the amount of and time for which subjects used statins and the type of statin used. The length of time the statin therapy is employed may contribute to the macroscale impact statins seem to have on the duration of subjects' AD battle. Also, no comorbidities were taken into consideration. For example, hypercholesterolemia is a risk factor for AD and would alter selection of statin use in that population. The subjects in this study may have had no use for statin intake, therefore the low statin use levels. Another limitation is that neuropathological measures of plaques, tangles, and Braak staging are somewhat limited, the plaque measures in particular as they only tell part of the amyloid story—they represent the insoluble amyloid but not the soluble species, wherein

Table 4 Group statistics

Statin use		APOE4	N	Mean	Standard deviation	Standard error of the mean
0						
	Age at death	1.00	99	78.96	8.415	0.846
		0.00	1459	81.16	10.957	0.287
	Education level	1.00	99	15.59	2.966	0.298
		0.00	1459	15.72	8.601	0.225
	Estimated onset age	1.00	99	111.61	185.605	18.654
		0.00	1459	91.61	128.096	3.354
	Tauopathy	1.00	99	2.01	0.267	0.027
		0.00	1459	.34	2.698	0.071
	Density of neocortical neuritic plaques (amyloid CERAD score)	1.00	99	2.60	0.699	0.070
		0.00	1459	2.32	0.983	0.026
	Braak stage	1.00	99	5.29	1.042	0.105
		0.00	1459	4.87	1.488	0.039
1						
	Age at death	1.00	16	76.19	6.036	1.509
		0.00	242	80.60	8.591	0.552
	Education level	1.00	16	14.13	3.074	0.769
		0.00	242	15.72	8.290	0.533
	Estimated onset age	1.00	16	67.19	4.764	1.191
		0.00	242	80.19	84.564	5.436
	Tauopathy	1.00	16	2.06	0.250	0.063
		0.00	242	0.37	2.673	0.172
	Density of neocortical neuritic plaques (amyloid CERAD score)	1.00	16	2.56	0.727	0.182
		0.00	242	2.36	0.950	0.061
	Braak stage	1.00	16	5.25	0.856	0.214
		0.00	242	4.75	1.419	0.091

APO apolipoprotein, *CERAD* Consortium to Establish a Registry for Alzheimer's Disease
0 means ApoE 4 NON carrier
1 means ApoE 4 Carrier

the highly aggregative and arguably more toxic oligo-meric forms exist. As such, it is possible that statin exposure is protective against levels of soluble amyl-oid, wherein amyloid trafficking supported by choles-terol/lipoproteins and some of their receptors (e.g., LRP1 and others thought to be important receptors in active amyloid clearance from the brain) are thought to be important, but these are not variables assessed. Yet another limitation is that statins might exert protective benefits beyond plaques and tangles. Hypoxia and inflammation are two mechanisms that can adversely contribute to cognitive decline and which statins have been claimed to be protective, sug-gesting that these are also factors that could have ex-plained their associations with clinical data but cannot be excluded from this study.

Future studies should investigate whether the amount of time of statin use impacts on the AD pathological load of subjects.

Conclusions

Prolonged statin use in pathologically confirmed AD dementia does not appear to influence the amount of burden of plaques and tangles or Braak stage and the effect is not altered by the presence or absence of ApoE4. Our hypothesis that chronic statin use might be associated with lower AD pathological burden was not confirmed despite the large body of evidence that statin use might protect against AD changes. The dif-ference here is that our study was focused on autopsy-confirmed AD and not longitudinal cohorts. This postmortem study indicates that chronic statins do not alter AD pathology at the end of life. Statins might exert beneficial effects earlier in the disease but appear not to impact the pathology when investigated post mortem.

Acknowledgements
Laura Cordes MS was retained to assist in drafting the rebuttal, address reviewer concerns, and perform substantive revising and editing of the manuscript.

Funding
Supported by the National Institute on Aging (NIA) (P30 AG19610), the Barrow Neurological Foundation, and the Keep Memory Alive Foundation. The National Alzheimer's Coordinating Center (NACC) database is funded by NIA/National Institutes of Health Grant U01 AG016976. NACC data are contributed by the NIA-funded Alzheimer Disease Centers: P30 AG019610 (PI Eric Reiman, MD), P30 AG013846 (PI Neil Kowall, MD), P50 AG008702 (PI Scott Small, MD), P50 AG025688 (PI Allan Levey, MD, PhD), P50 AG047266 (PI Todd Golde, MD, PhD), P30 AG010133 (PI Andrew Saykin, PsyD), P50 AG005146 (PI Marilyn Albert, PhD), P50 AG005134 (PI Bradley Hyman, MD, PhD), P50 AG016574 (PI Ronald Petersen, MD, PhD), P50 AG005138 (PI Mary Sano, PhD), P30 AG008051 (PI Thomas Wisniewski, MD), P30 AG013854 (PI M. Marsel Mesulam, MD), P30 AG008017 (PI Jeffrey Kaye, MD), P30 AG010161 (PI David Bennett, MD), P50 AG047366 (PI Victor Henderson, MD, MS), P30 AG010129 (PI Charles DeCarli, MD), P50 AG016573 (PI Frank LaFerla, PhD), P50 AG005131 (PI James Brewer, MD, PhD), P50 AG023501 (PI Bruce Miller, MD), P30 AG035982 (PI Russell Swerdlow, MD), P30 AG028383 (PI Linda Van Eldik, PhD), P30 AG053760 (PI Henry Paulson, MD, PhD), P30 AG010124 (PI John Trojanowski, MD, PhD), P50 AG005133 (PI Oscar Lopez, MD), P50 AG005142 (PI Helena Chui, MD), P30 AG012300 (PI Roger Rosenberg, MD), P30 AG049638 (PI Suzanne Craft, PhD), P50 AG005136 (PI Thomas Grabowski, MD), P50 AG033514 (PI Sanjay Asthana, MD, FRCP), P50 AG005681 (PI John Morris, MD), and P50 AG047270 (PI Stephen Strittmatter, MD, PhD).

Authors' contributions
JC performed the data requisition and initial draft of the manuscript. JW performed the statistical analysis. MS conceived of the project and completed the draft of the manuscript. All authors read and approved the final manuscript.

Consent for publication
Provided by the NACC after prior review.

Competing interests
JC declares no competing interests. JW and MS declare no competing financial interests.

Author details
[1] Arizona State University, Tempe, AZ, USA. [2] Department of Neurology, Barrow Neurological Institute, Phoenix, AZ, USA. [3] Cleveland Clinic Lou Ruvo Center for Brain Health, 888 W. Bonneville Ave, Las Vegas, NV 89106, USA.

References
1. Alzheimer's Association 2018 Alzheimer's and Disease Facts and Figures. www.alz.org/media/HomeOffice/facts%20and%20figures/facts-and-figures.pdf.
2. National Institutes of Health Estimates of Funding for Various Research, Condition, and Disease Categories (RCDC). https://report.nih.gov/rcdc.
3. Kandiah N, Feldman HH. Therapeutic potential of statins in Alzheimer's disease. J Neurol Sci. 2009;283(1–2):230–4.
4. Sparks DL, Kryscio RJ, Connor DJ, et al. Cholesterol and cognitive performance in normal controls and the influence of elective statin use after conversion to mild cognitive impairment: results in a clinical trial cohort. Neurodegener Dis. 2010;7(1–3):183–6.
5. McGuinness B, Craig D, Bullock R, Malouf R, Passmore P. Statins for the treatment of dementia. Cochrane Database Syst Rev. 2014;7:CD007514.
6. Chuang C, Lin C, Lin M, Sung F, Kao C. Decreased prevalence of dementia associated with statins: a national population-based study. Eur J Neurol. 2015;22(6):912–8.
7. Beydoun MA, Beason-Held LL, Kitner-Triolo MH, et al. Statins and serum cholesterol's associations with incident dementia and mild cognitive impairment. J Epidemiol Community Health. 2011;65(11):949–57.
8. Malfitano AM, Marasco G, Proto MC, Laezza C, Gazzerro P, Bifulco M. Statins in neurological disorders: an overview and update. Pharmacol Res. 2014; 88(0):74–83.
9. Sano M, Bell K, Galasko D, et al. A randomized, double-blind, placebo-controlled trial of simvastatin to treat Alzheimer disease. Neurology. 2011; 77(6):556–63.
10. Feldman HH, Doody RS, Kivipelto M, et al. Randomized controlled trial of atorvastatin in mild to moderate Alzheimer disease: LEADe. Neurology. 2010;74(12):956–64.
11. Sparks DL, Sabbagh MN, Connor DJ, et al. Atorvastatin therapy lowers circulating cholesterol but not free radical activity in advance of identifiable clinical benefit in the treatment of mild-to-moderate AD. Curr Alzheimer Res. 2005;2(3):343–53.
12. Smith KB, Kang P, Sabbagh MN, Initiative A's DN. The effect of statins on rate of cognitive decline in mild cognitive impairment. Alzheimers Dement. 2017;3(2):149–56. https://doi.org/10.1016/j.trci.2017.01.001.
13. Beekly DL, Ramos EM, Lee WW, Deitrich WD, Jacka ME, Wu J, Hubbard JL, Koepsell TD, Morris JC, Kukull WA, NIA Alzheimer's Disease Centers. The National Alzheimer's Coordinating Center (NACC) database: the Uniform Data Set. Alzheimer Dis Assoc Disord. 2007;21(3):249–58.
14. Ogm TG, Scharmagl H, März W, Bohl J. Apolipoprotein E isoforms and the development of low and high Braak stages of Alzheimer's disease-related lesions. Acta Neuropathol. 1999;98(3):273–80.
15. Ghebremedhin E, Schultz C, Braak E, Braak H. High frequency of apolipoprotein E epsilon4 allele in young individuals with very mild Alzheimer's disease-related neurofibrillary changes. Exp Neurol. 1998;153(1):152–5.

8

Patterns of cognitive function in middle-aged and elderly Chinese adults—findings from the EMCOA study

Yu An[1†], Lingli Feng[1,2†], Xiaona Zhang[1], Ying Wang[1], Yushan Wang[1], Lingwei Tao[1], Yanhui Lu[1,3], Zhongsheng Qin[4] and Rong Xiao[1*] (ID)

Abstract

Background: The principal aim of this study was to demonstrate the gender-specific cognitive patterns among middle-aged and elderly Chinese adults, investigate the risk factors on global and domain-specific cognitive performance in men and women, respectively, and report demographically adjusted norms for cognitive tests.

Methods: The Effects and Mechanism of Cholesterol and Oxysterol on Alzheimer's disease (EMCOA) study enrolled 4573 participants aged 50–70 years in three Chinese cities. All participants underwent an extensive neuropsychological test battery. Composite scores for specific domains were derived from principal component analysis (PCA). Multivariate linear regression models were used to determine gender-specific risk factors and demographically adjusted normative data.

Results: Three cognitive domains of verbal memory, attention/processing speed/executive function, and cognitive flexibility were extracted. A female advantage in verbal memory was observed regardless of age, whereas men tended to outperform women in global cognition and attention/processing speed/executive function. The effects of education on women were more substantial than men for general cognition and attention/processing speed/executive function. For all the cognitive tests, regression-based and demographically adjusted normative data were calculated.

Conclusions: There is a need for gender-specific intervention strategies for operationalizing cognitive impairment.

Keywords: Cognitive pattern, Gender-specific, Global and domain-specific, Normative data, Cross-sectional, Middle-aged and elderly

Background

According to the World Alzheimer Report 2015 released by Alzheimer's Disease International (ADI), 900 million people aged 60 years or above are now living worldwide, with this number expected to increase by 138–239% in middle-income countries such as China between 2015 and 2050 [1]. This is a noteworthy estimation given that normal aging is accompanied by deterioration across a spectrum of cognitive functions related to memory, attention, executive function, processing speed, and so on

[2]. As a chronic and progressive neurodegenerative disorder that is strongly age-associated, dementia involves a severe loss of cognitive function beyond the normal aging process [3]. It can impede independent living and impose considerable personal, social, and economic burdens. Age-related cognitive impairment and the global impact of dementia has become a priority public health issue considering that the aging population constitutes a rapidly increasing proportion of the total population [4]. In the absence of an effective treatment, there is a responsibility for researchers to develop strategies to reduce the risk and slow the progression associated with mental aging.

Research on age-related cognitive impairment has shown that assessment of cognitive performance over

* Correspondence: xiaor22@ccmu.edu.cn
†Yu An and Lingli Feng contributed equally to this work.
[1]School of Public Health, Capital Medical University, No.10 Xitoutiao, You An Men Wai, Beijing 100069, China
Full list of author information is available at the end of the article

the lifespan is a heterogeneous process [5]. On one hand, advanced age conveys positive influences on verbal abilities and production, and implicit and autobiographical memory due to growing knowledge and life experience. On the other hand, advanced age also conveys negative influences on processing speed, explicit memory, and verbal fluency due to age-related deterioration of the brain [6]. Diversity in cognitive performance and different rates of cognitive decline have been reported to be altered with regard to demographic characteristics, education, lifestyle, physical conditions, social engagement, and economic resources [7–9]. In fact, the influence of these sociodemographic characteristics on cognitive function is not homogeneous and they may interact with each other to yield distinctive patterns of cognitive performance. In particular, our previous studies have found that numerous cognitive scores were significantly different between men and women [10]. Lifestyle risk factors for mild cognitive impairment (MCI) are also gender-specific, in which smoking was only significant in men [11]. However, the gender-specific cognitive patterns and related risk factors are still under debate with respect to discrepant results across countries and are thus in need of further investigation. The elucidation of these different effects is crucial for understanding what determines healthy cognitive aging.

Including an estimated 218 million older people and 9.5 million people living with dementia, China has become a region with the most people living with dementia in 2015 [1]. Given this, many studies focused on older individuals in different stages of dementia, such as MCI [12–14]. Nevertheless, cognitive aging may begin in mid-life and has also been extensively investigated outside the context of dementia. Therefore, detection of cognitive decline in at-risk middle-aged and elderly groups has become a research priority [15]. Making firm identification and diagnosis between normal aging, MCI, and different subtypes of dementia requires the use of normative standards. Unbiased identification and diagnosis requires an individual's cognitive performance to be compared to a normal sample from a comparable cognitively healthy population [16]. However, most commonly used neuropsychological tests only have norms for elderly populations aged 60 years or above. The norms for cognitive function are relatively under-researched among Chinese middle-aged and elderly adults owing to the lack of large-scale community-based studies. It can be problematic to draw clinical inferences from normative studies only for elderly populations aged 60 years or above.

A large-scale community-based study in China, the Effects and Mechanisms of Cholesterol and Oxysterol on Alzheimer's disease (EMCOA) study, offers an opportunity to explore normal cognitive performance across the age spectrum of 50–70 years. This epidemiological investigation, begun in 2014, was primarily designed to prospectively determine the effects of dietary cholesterol and oxysterols on the incidence of Alzheimer's disease (AD)/MCI in the middle-aged and elderly population. The present study emerged to investigate gender-specific cognitive patterns, explore risk factors for global or domain-specific cognitive performance in men and women, respectively, and to establish reliable normative information in Chinese middle-aged and elderly adults.

Methods

Setting

The present study was within the framework of the EMCOA study, an ongoing community-based cohort study of Chinese adults aged 50–70 years living in three Chinese cities of Beijing, Linyi, and Jincheng, and was registered on the Chinese Clinical Trial Registry as ChiCTR-OOC-17011882. The baseline examination took place between January 2014 and December 2015 and follow-up examinations take place every 2 years. The project was conducted by a synergistic collaboration among the Capital Medical University, Linyi Health Examination Center affiliated with Linyi People's Hospital, Jincheng Health Examination Center affiliated with Jincheng People's Hospital, and several community-based health centers affiliated with Beijing Chaoyang District Center for Disease Control and Prevention. Eligibility criteria for the EMCOA study included adults aged 50–70 years with no history of neuropsychiatric disorders or neoplastic diseases (malignant and benign tumor growths, e.g. head-neck tumors, metastatic lung, or upper digestive tumors) [17] and who simultaneously agreed to participate in the study. Exclusion criteria were as follows: 1) diagnosed with any neurodegenerative disease by neurologists (e.g., MCI or dementia); 2) suffering from cognitive impairment caused by depression, stroke, traumatic brain injury, or other severe organ dysfunction; 3) declined to participate in the study; 4) currently taking medication or dietary supplement to improve cognitive function; and 5) uncorrected visual or hearing impairment. The study protocols of the EMCOA study were reviewed and approved by the Ethics Committee of the Capital Medical University (2013SY35) and participants provided written informed consent.

Study population

The present analysis is based on the information obtained at the baseline examination. A total of 5805 individuals responded to the invitation and agreed to participate in this study. After checking the participants, 1232 participants were excluded for the following reasons: 531 due to neuropsychiatric problems (e.g., dementia, depression, or cerebral aneurysm), 680 due to the participant's failure to complete the whole examination, and 21 due to other reasons. Finally, large cross-sectional data from 4573 middle-aged and elderly participants entered the study and were used for this analysis (Fig. 1). Of the 4573 participants, 2247 (49.1%) were men and 2326 (50.9%) were women.

Cognitive test battery

Participants underwent neuropsychological evaluation in a private and quiet room carried out by technicians with formal training. A battery of well-validated Chinese version tests that possess high inter- and intra-rater reliability were administered to assess cognitive performance. Audio tape recordings of standardized testing procedures were reviewed across study sites to ensure consistency. We included the following cognitive tests: the Mini-Mental State Examination (MMSE) [18]; the Montreal Cognitive Assessment Test (MoCA) [19]; the Auditory Verbal Learning Test (AVLT) [20] using summarized scores of immediate recall (AVLT-IR), short recall (AVLT-SR), and long recall (AVLT-LR); the Symbol Digit Modalities Test (SDMT) [21]; the Wechsler Memory Scale Revised for China (WMS-RC) subtests Logical Memory Test—immediate recall (LMT-IR) [22], Digit Span Forwards (DSF), and Digit Span Backwards (DSB) [23]; the Trail Making Test (TMT) A and B [24]; and the Stroop Color-Word Test-Interference Trial (SCWT-IT) [25]. A detailed description of the procedure and modifications made to these measures can be found in Additional file 1: Supplementary methods and results.

Covariates

At enrollment, a questionnaire on sociodemographics (gender, date of birth, years of formal education, employment, monthly household income, etc.), lifestyle (residence status, reading habits, physical activity, smoking, drinking, etc.), and clinical data (past and family medical history) was used to obtain information from the participants and/or their family member. Details of covariates are shown in Additional file 1.

Data analysis

Principal component analysis (PCA) with varimax rotation was employed as a data-reduction technique to obtain composite scores for specific cognitive domains. The analysis of covariance was used to compare cognitive patterns between men and women. Sociodemographic characteristics, lifestyle, and medical variables, as well as cognitive performance between men and women, are reported as mean (standard deviation (SD)), median (interquartile range), or frequency (percentage). Reported p values refer to the Student t test, Mann Whitney U test, Kruskal-Wallis test, or chi-square test as appropriate. We used multivariate linear regression analysis for global and domain-specific cognitive performance as continuous outcomes. All models were adjusted for potential risk factors (sociodemographic characteristics, lifestyle, and medical variables) and stratified by gender. Heterogeneity of risk factors between men and women was assessed as gender × risk factor interactions which were included in overall models with the main effect terms. For interactions in multiple testing, an adjusted p value < 0.05, taking into

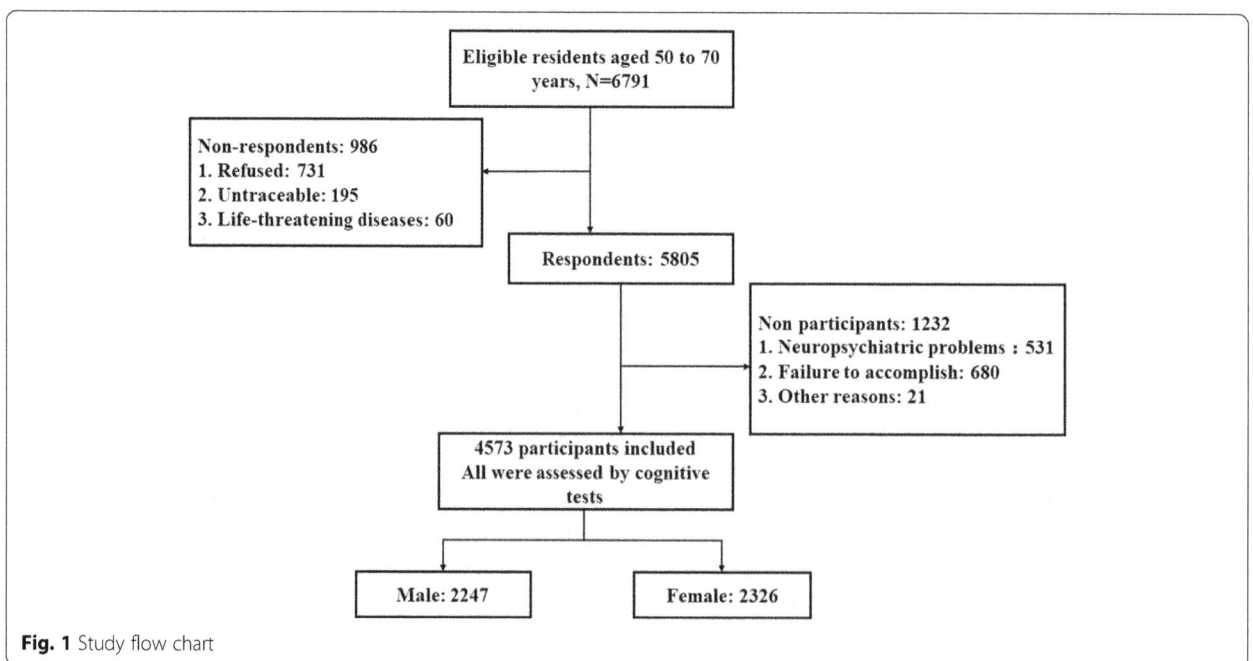

Fig. 1 Study flow chart

Table 1 Cognitive tests of participants

Cognitive test	Total number	Mean	SD	Skew
MMSE	4494	28.11	2.137	−2.217
MoCA	4514	24.79	3.568	−1.242
AVLT-IR	4495	15.2209	4.98377	0.265
AVLT-SR	4483	5.23	2.522	0.040
AVLT-LR	4452	4.57	2.759	0.127
SDMT	4492	33.63	11.453	0.158
DSF	3923	7.72	1.448	−0.735
DSB	3920	4.03	1.292	−0.302
TMT-A	4486	69.75	27.295	1.029
TMT-B	4452	168.16	70.199	1.013
LMT-IR	4427	10.7408	5.10170	−0.067
SCWT-IT	4410	40.2502472	23.16964651	10.304

Skew > 0, positive skewed distribution; skew < 0, negative skewed distribution
AVLT-IR Auditory Verbal Learning Test—immediate recall, *AVLT-LR* Auditory Verbal Learning Test—long recall, *AVLT-SR* Auditory Verbal Learning Test—short recall, *DSB* digit span backwards, *DSF* digit span forwards, *MMSE* Mini-Mental State Examination, *MoCA* Montreal Cognitive Assessment, *SCWT-IT* Stroop Color-Word Test Interference Trial, *SDMT* Symbol Digit Modalities Test, *TMT* Trail Making Test, *LMT-IR* Logical Memory Test—immediate recall

account the false discovery rate (FDR) [26], was considered as statistically significant. The norms of these cognitive tests were also established and stratified according to variables that most associated with cognitive performance, and the details are shown in Additional file 1. All analyses were carried out using SPSS for Windows, version 23.0 (SPSS, Chicago, IL USA) and statistical significance was set at $p < 0.05$.

Table 2 Principal components analysis for the cognitive subtests

Cognitive subtest	Components		
	Verbal memory	Attention/processing speed/executive function	Cognitive flexibility
AVLT-IR	**0.859348**	0.1786355	−0.02420138
AVLT-SR	**0.925347**	0.1656561	0.013152043
AVLT-LR	**0.919844**	0.1586545	0.007458428
SDMT	0.268641	**0.6900593**	0.107590145
DSF	0.056095	**0.5391598**	−0.48831854
DSB	0.256134	**0.5315925**	−0.36294081
TMT-A	0.09689	**0.7970535**	0.091785669
TMT-B	0.110346	**0.7881209**	0.142030366
LMT-IR	0.427479	**0.5010345**	−0.13808383
SCWT-IT	0.042578	0.2260081	**0.759748898**

Bold entries indicate measures with high loadings on each factor
AVLT-IR Auditory Verbal Learning Test—immediate recall, *AVLT-LR* Auditory Verbal Learning Test—long recall, *AVLT-SR* Auditory Verbal Learning Test—short recall, *DSB* digit span backwards, *DSF* digit span forwards, *SCWT-IT* Stroop Color-Word Test Interference Trial, *SDMT* Symbol Digit Modalities Test, *TMT* Trail Making Test, *LMT-IR* Logical Memory Test—immediate recall

Table 3 Characteristics of cognitive domains in participants

Cognitive domain	Total number	Mean	SD	Skew
Memory performance	3696	0.000	1.000	0.188
Attention/processing speed/executive function	3696	0.000	1.000	−0.624
Cognitive flexibility	3696	0.000	1.000	3.871

Each cognitive domain is the mean of the composite scores
Skew > 0, positive skewed distribution; skew < 0, negative skewed distribution

Results
Global and domain-specific cognitive performance

The means and SDs of all the cognitive tests are presented in Table 1. The PCA generated three principal components from 10 subtests with eigen values > 1 which accounted for 64.83% of the total initial variance in cognitive test performance (Table 2). The compound scores were calculated subsequently for: 1) verbal memory; 2) attention/processing speed/executive function; and 3) cognitive flexibility. The first component, primarily comprised of immediate, short, and long recall of AVLT, was interpreted to reflect verbal memory. The second component was interpreted to reflect attention/

Table 4 Age group, education level, and cognitive performance between men and women

	Men (n = 2247)	Women (n = 2326)	p value
Age group (years), n (%)			0.086
50–54	550 (24.5%)	576 (24.8%)	
55–59	693 (30.8%)	767 (33.0%)	
60–64	671 (29.9%)	684 (29.4%)	
65–70	293 (13.0%)	251 (10.8%)	
Education level, n (%)			< 0.001**
Elementary school	218 (9.7%)	551 (23.7%)	
Junior middle school	666 (29.6%)	818 (35.2%)	
Senior middle school	678 (30.2%)	619 (26.6%)	
college and above	650 (28.9%)	293 (12.6%)	
Global cognitive function, mean (IQR)			
MMSE	29 (28, 30)	26 (24, 28)	< 0.001**
MoCA	28 (27, 30)	25 (22, 27)	< 0.001**
Domain-specific cognitive function, mean (IQR)			
Verbal memory	−0.10 (−0.73, 0.64)	0.03 (−0.68, 0.73)	0.003*
Attention/processing speed/ executive function	0.29 (−0.38, 0.77)	−0.03 (−0.83, 0.59)	< 0.001**
Cognitive flexibility	−0.08 (−0.63, 0.39)	0.12 (−0.39, 0.67)	< 0.001**

Data shown as *n* (%) were compared between two groups using the chi-square test
Data with skewed distribution shown as median (interquartile range (IQR)) were compared between two groups using the Mann Whitney *U* test
MMSE Mini-Mental State Examination, *MoCA* Montreal Cognitive Assessment
*$P < 0.05$; **$P < 0.001$

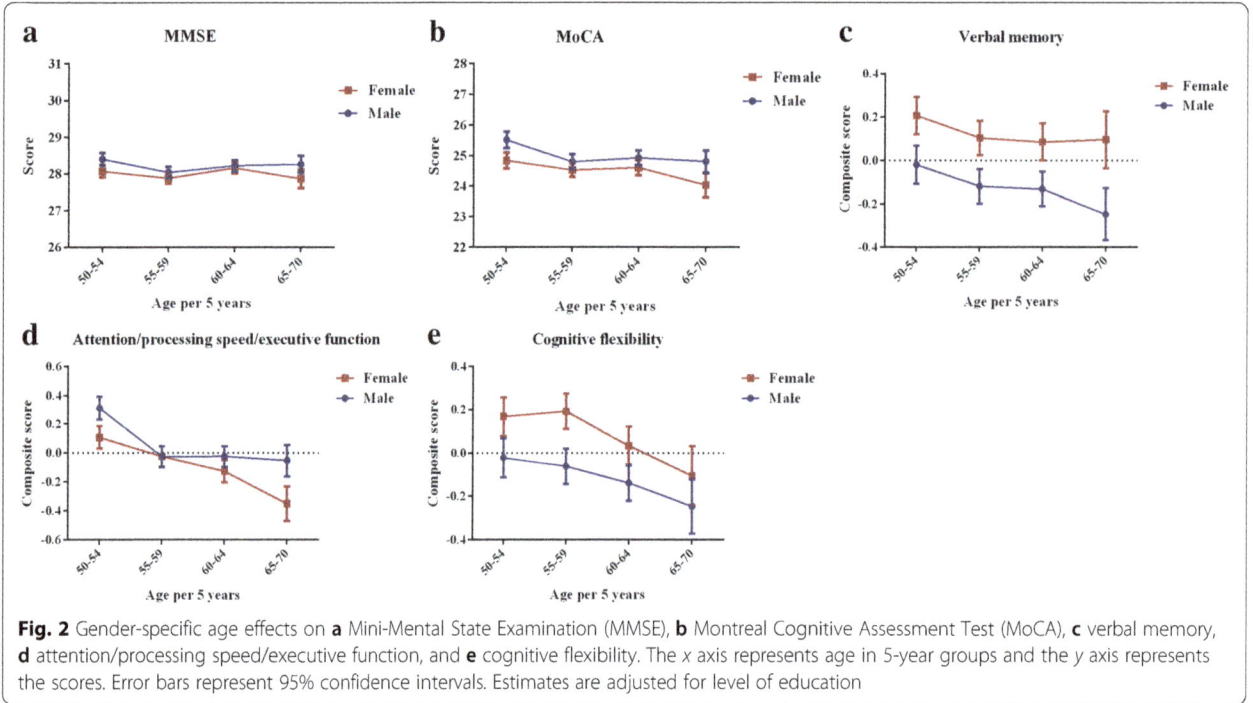

Fig. 2 Gender-specific age effects on **a** Mini-Mental State Examination (MMSE), **b** Montreal Cognitive Assessment Test (MoCA), **c** verbal memory, **d** attention/processing speed/executive function, and **e** cognitive flexibility. The x axis represents age in 5-year groups and the y axis represents the scores. Error bars represent 95% confidence intervals. Estimates are adjusted for level of education

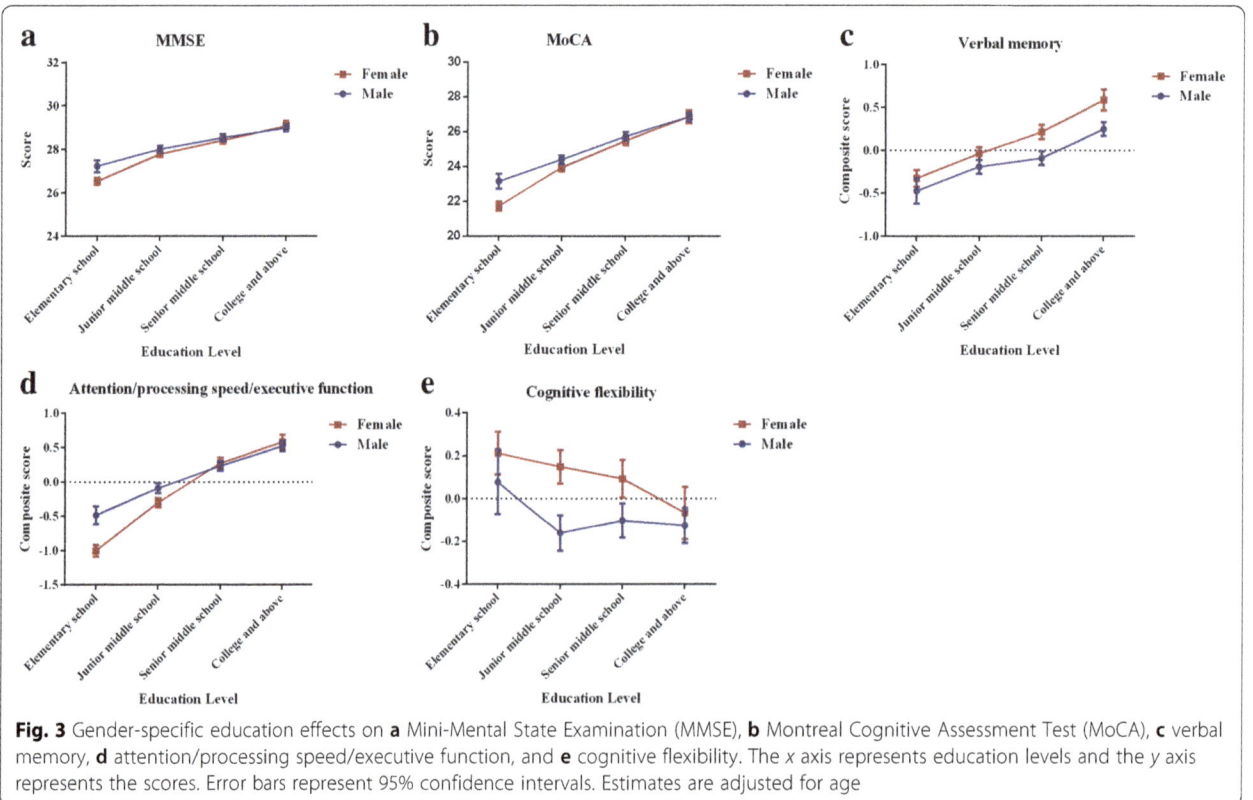

Fig. 3 Gender-specific education effects on **a** Mini-Mental State Examination (MMSE), **b** Montreal Cognitive Assessment Test (MoCA), **c** verbal memory, **d** attention/processing speed/executive function, and **e** cognitive flexibility. The x axis represents education levels and the y axis represents the scores. Error bars represent 95% confidence intervals. Estimates are adjusted for age

Table 5 General characteristics of the participants

	Men	Women	p value
Number, n (%)	2247 (49.1%)	2326 (50.9%)	–
Sociodemographic characteristics			
Age (years), median (IQR)	59 (55, 62)	58 (54, 62)	0.045*
Education (years), median (IQR)	12 (9, 15)	9 (9, 12)	< 0.001**
Occupation, n (%)			< 0.001**
Manual work	452 (20.1%)	723 (31.1%)	
White-collar work	921 (41.0%)	453 (19.5%)	
Monthly income, n (%)			< 0.001**
Low	607 (27.0%)	868 (37.3%)	
Medium	734 (32.7%)	722 (31.1%)	
High	906 (40.3%)	736 (31.6%)	
BMI (kg/m^2), mean ± SD	25.38 ± 3.12	24.59 ± 3.16	< 0.001**
BMI group, n (%)			< 0.001**
Underweight	19 (0.8%)	27 (1.16%)	
Normal weight	992 (44.1%)	1268 (54.5%)	
Overweight	1018 (45.3%)	805 (34.6%)	
Obese	218 (9.7%)	226 (9.7%)	
Lifestyle, n (%)			
Solitude	42 (1.9%)	45 (1.9%)	0.871
Reading habits	1450 (64.5%)	1125 (48.4%)	< 0.001**
Physically active	1612 (71.7%)	1712 (73.6%)	0.158
Current smoker	973 (43.3%)	62 (2.7%)	< 0.001**
Current drinker	1123 (50.0%)	127 (5.5%)	< 0.001**
Medical history, n (%)			
Diabetes	372 (16.6%)	281 (12.1%)	< 0.001**
Hypertension	784 (34.9%)	664 (28.5%)	< 0.001**
Hyperlipidemia	476 (21.2%)	494 (21.2%)	0.964
Stroke	32 (1.4%)	26 (1.1%)	0.355
Coronary heart disease	203 (9.0%)	140 (6.0%)	< 0.001**
Family history of dementia	160 (7.1%)	204 (8.8%)	0.039*

Data shown as median (interquartile range (IQR)) were compared between two groups using the Mann Whitney U test
Data shown as mean ± standard deviation (SD) were compared between two groups using the Student t test
Data shown as n (%) were compared between two groups using the chi-square test
BMI body mass index
*P < 0.05; **P < 0.001

processing speed/executive function, with SDMT, LMT-IR, TMT A and B, DSF, and DSB contributing substantially. The third component was interpreted with SCWT-IT to reflect cognitive flexibility. The means and SDs of the composite scores of the three specific domains used in the analyses are presented in Table 3. All the cognitive tests had skewed distribution and the specific domains were symmetric.

Gender-specific cognitive patterns

Women scored better than men on verbal memory and cognitive flexibility, whereas men scored better on the

MMSE, MoCA, and attention/processing speed/executive function (Table 4).

The gender-specific cognitive patterns are presented in Figs. 2 and 3, which show mean levels and 95% confidence intervals (CIs) of cognitive performance stratified by age or education. On one hand, the female cognitive advantage across all ages was significant for verbal memory performance. Age was significantly associated with each cognitive measure in both men and women. On the other hand, a significant gender discrepancy existed for education level, and women tended to be less educated. In the elementary school educated group, women

Table 6 Gender-specific associations of sociodemographic characteristics, lifestyle, and medical history with cognitive performance

	MMSE			MoCA			Verbal memory			Attention/processing speed/executive function			Cognitive flexibility		
	Men	Women	p^a	Men	Women	p	Men	Women	p	Men	Women	p	Men	Women	p
Sociodemographic characteristics															
Age	-0.038	-0.031	0.446	-0.078*	-0.063	0.327	-0.054	-0.114*	0.187	-0.185**	-0.110*	0.923	-0.096*	-0.042	0.311
Education years	0.163**	0.308**	<0.001#	0.225**	0.369**	<0.001#	0.087	0.196**	0.226	0.253**	0.403**	<0.001#	-0.08	-0.037	0.128
Occupation															
Manual work	Ref	Ref	Ref	Ref	Ref	Ref	Ref	Ref	Ref	Ref	Ref	Ref	Ref	Ref	Ref
White-collar work	0.01	0.067	0.069	0.110*	0.066	0.118	0.100*	0.081	0.954	0.104*	0.155**	0.006	-0.007	0.004	0.114
Monthly income															
Low	Ref	Ref	Ref	Ref	Ref	Ref	Ref	Ref	Ref	Ref	Ref	Ref	Ref	Ref	Ref
Medium	0.133*	0.069	0.656	0.083*	0.058	0.557	0.026	0.043	0.401	0.055	-0.004	0.995	0.107*	-0.008	0.933
High	0.179**	0.058	0.96	0.137*	0.056	0.888	0.133*	0.063	0.306	0.069	-0.023	0.589	0.157*	-0.064	0.059
Body mass index															
Healthy	Ref	Ref	Ref	Ref	Ref	Ref	Ref	Ref	Ref	Ref	Ref	Ref	Ref	Ref	Ref
Underweight	0.008	-0.003	0.939	-0.001	-0.004	0.807	-0.021	-0.101*	0.222	-0.012	0.034	0.198	0.002	0.09	0.133
Overweight	0.041	-0.036	0.426	0.042	-0.063	0.034	0.092	-0.015	0.316	-0.029	-0.049	0.778	0.021	0.02	0.295
Obesity	0.076	-0.039	0.111	0.073	0.011	0.93	0.085	-0.023	0.271	-0.038	-0.073*	0.243	-0.038	0.052	0.078
Lifestyle															
Solitude	-0.043	0.051	0.045	-0.095*	0.005	0.045	-0.013	0.028	0.415	0.007	0.007	0.929	-0.009	0.026	0.271
Reading habits	0.079*	0.097*	0.113	0.169**	0.185**	0.051	0.143**	0.123*	0.729	-0.002	0.056	0.022	0.031	-0.118	0.057
Physically active	0.015	-0.063	0.295	-0.046	-0.07	0.726	-0.038	-0.053	0.892	0.100*	0.046	0.917	0.029	-0.019	0.343
Current smoker	-0.074*	-0.023	0.984	-0.058*	-0.001	0.467	-0.102*	-0.001	0.2	-0.016	-0.002	0.894	-0.057	0.019	0.277
Current drinker	0.055	0.012	0.922	0.059	0.042	0.4	0.063	0.064	0.281	0.014	-0.001	0.996	0.015	-0.015	0.61
Medical history															
Diabetes	-0.009	-0.01	0.961	0.002	-0.002	0.967	-0.071*	-0.021	0.487	-0.008	-0.031	0.559	0.002	-0.037	0.548
Hypertension	-0.007	-0.047	0.343	-0.048	-0.074*	0.343	-0.036	-0.036	0.852	0.014	-0.048	0.08	-0.053	-0.002	0.245
Hyperlipidemia	-0.004	0.021	0.285	0.015	0.021	0.463	0.032	0.007	0.997	0.017	0.067	0.282	0.01	0.074	0.257
Stroke	-0.106*	-0.006	0.063	-0.035	0.001	0.475	-0.014	0.042	0.234	-0.002	-0.043	0.284	0.031	-0.100*	0.061
Coronary heart disease	-0.056	0.05	0.023	-0.053	0.03	0.081	-0.142**	-0.027	0.069	0.082	0.043	0.602	0.018	0.011	0.79
Family history of dementia	-0.041	0.013	0.207	-0.01	0.017	0.446	0.013	0.041	0.612	-0.026	0.022	0.309	-0.056	-0.056	0.989

Multivariate linear regression analysis with the enter method was performed on all variables and standardized regression coefficients are presented

MMSE Mini-Mental State Examination, MoCA Montreal Cognitive Assessment

^a p for interactions

*P < 0.05, **P < 0.001; false discovery rate adjusted #P < 0.05

Table 7 Proportion of variance accounted for cognitive performance in linear regression analyses for 12 cognitive tests

Cognitive tests	Model 1	Model 2	ΔR^2
MMSE	0.150	0.176	0.026
MoCA	0.255	0.314	0.059
AVLT-IR	0.124	0.161	0.037
AVLT-SR	0.118	0.16	0.042
AVLT-LR	0.118	0.168	0.050
SDMT	0.279	0.304	0.025
DSF	0.084	0.108	0.024
DSB	0.140	0.159	0.019
TMT-A	0.214	0.232	0.018
TMT-B	0.172	0.193	0.021
LMT-IR	0.201	0.242	0.041
SCWT-IT	0.016	0.018	0.002

The values represent the proportion of variance (R^2) in the regression model
In model 1, the linear regression analysis was performed only on age, gender, and education
In model 2, the linear regression analysis was performed on all the sociodemographic, lifestyle, and medical variables
Both models used the enter method
AVLT-IR Auditory Verbal Learning Test—immediate recall, *AVLT-LR* Auditory Verbal Learning Test—long recall, *AVLT-SR* Auditory Verbal Learning Test—short recall, *DSB* digit span backwards, *DSF* digit span forwards, *MMSE* Mini-Mental State Examination, *MoCA* Montreal Cognitive Assessment, *SCWT-IT* Stroop Color-Word Test Interference Trial, *SDMT* Symbol Digit Modalities Test, *TMT* Trail Making Test, *LMT-IR* Logical Memory Test—immediate recall

performed significantly worse than men in MMSE, MoCA, and attention/processing speed/executive function. However, this difference was eliminated in those with a higher education. In the senior middle school and college and above educated group, women performed the same as men in the aforementioned cognitive performance and even better than men for verbal memory. With respect to cognitive flexibility, women achieved significantly higher scores than men only for junior and senior middle school education.

Gender-specific risk factors for cognitive performance
The comparison of sociodemographic characteristics, lifestyle, and medical variables between men and women are provided in Table 5. Compared with men, women included in our analysis were slightly younger ($p = 0.04$) and less likely to be engaged in white-collar work ($p < 0.001$). Women also reported lower education ($p < 0.001$) and income ($p < 0.001$). Meanwhile, a higher prevalence of being overweight and a lower prevalence of underweight body mass index (BMI) was observed in men compared with women ($p < 0.001$). With regard to lifestyle, men were more likely than women to be current smokers ($p < 0.001$) and to report current alcohol use and reading habits ($p < 0.001$). Differences in disease

prevalence were such that men were more likely than women to report diabetes ($p < 0.001$), hypertension ($p < 0.001$), and coronary heart disease ($p < 0.001$), whereas women were more likely to have a family history of dementia ($p = 0.039$).

We examined the gender-specific risk factors on cognitive performance using multivariate analysis (Table 6) and found that sociodemographic, lifestyle, and medical variables had different effects on cognitive performance in men and women. For sociodemographic characteristics, male global and domain-specific cognitive performance was positively associated with education, intellectual occupation, and higher monthly income, whereas it was negatively associated with age. Similarly, female cognitive performance was also positively associated with education and a white-collar occupation and negatively associated with age. Furthermore, being underweight and obesity also negatively impacted female verbal memory and attention/processing speed/executive function. For lifestyle, both male and female global cognitive performance and verbal memory benefited from reading habits. Meanwhile, solitude and smoking were negatively associated with male global cognitive score and verbal memory while being physically active had a positive influence on male attention/processing speed/executive function. For medical variables, diabetes and coronary heart disease were associated with lower verbal memory score in men, hypertension was associated with lower MoCA scores in women, and stroke was associated with a lower MMSE score in men and cognitive flexibility score in women. Significant differences between men and women were observed for an association of years of education with MMSE, MoCA, and attention/processing speed/executive function. The effects of increased education years on general cognition and attention/processing speed/executive function were significantly greater in women than men ($p < 0.001$ for interaction, and $p < 0.05$ after FDR adjustment).

Development of normative data for 12 cognitive tests and related z score
The predictive scores and normative data were developed based on three variables of age, gender, and education from multivariate regression models (Table 7). The equations are shown in Additional file 1 and the regression coefficients are presented in Table 8. Next, the predictive scores were used to generate demographically adjusted z scores which can be converted to a percentile that indicates the individual's cognitive performance among peers of comparable age, gender, and education. The normative data of 12 cognitive tests were determined and stratified by age, gender, and education (Table 9, Fig. 4a-l). Furthermore, the reference

Table 8 Regression coefficients of the normative data equations

Cognitive tests	Gender	Age	Education	Gender × age	Gender × education	Age × education	Age^2	Education^2	Constant
MMSE	−1.041	–	0.084	–	0.078	–	–	–	27.599
MoCA	0.127	–	0.233	−0.031	0.127	–	–	–	23.136
AVLT-IR	–	–	0.282	–	0.11	–	−0.001	–	12.727
AVLT-SR	–	–	–	–	0.06	–	−0.001	0.006	5.028
AVLT-LR	–	–	–	–	0.057	–	−0.001	0.007	4.505
SDMT	−5.477	−0.323	0.461	–	0.681	–	–	–	45.41
DSF	–	–	0.186	–	–	−0.001	–	–	6.502
DSB	−0.391	−0.019	–	–	0.026	–	–	0.004	4.864
TMT-A	24.601	5.309	–	–	−1.877	–	−0.039	–	−114.999
TMT-B	–	–	–	0.969	−4.493	–	–	–	152.416
LMT-IR	−1.751	–	–	–	0.129	–	–	0.019	9.071
SCWT-IT	−0.277	–	–	–	0.005	0.001	–	−0.004	3.686

The values represented unstandardized regression coefficient
AVLT-IR Auditory Verbal Learning Test—immediate recall, *AVLT-LR* Auditory Verbal Learning Test—long recall, *AVLT-SR* Auditory Verbal Learning Test—short recall, *DSB* digit span backwards, *DSF* digit span forwards, *MMSE* Mini-Mental State Examination, *MoCA* Montreal Cognitive Assessment, *SCWT-IT* Stroop Color-Word Test Interference Trial, *SDMT* Symbol Digit Modalities Test, *TMT* Trail Making Test, *LMT-IR* Logical Memory Test—immediate recall

Table 9 Regression-based normative data of cognitive performance stratified by age, gender, and education as appropriate

		Education level							
		Elementary school		Junior middle school		Senior middle school		College and above	
	Age	Male	Female	Male	Female	Male	Female	Male	Female
MMSE	50–54	27.19 ± 0.47	26.74 ± 0.51	28.01 ± 0.00	27.67 ± 0.00	28.49 ± 0.00	28.38 ± 0.00	29.06 ± 0.08	29.21 ± 0.12
	55–59	27.38 ± 0.35	26.66 ± 0.58	28.01 ± 0.00	27.67 ± 0.00	28.49 ± 0.00	28.38 ± 0.00	29.04 ± 0.08	29.21 ± 0.12
	60–64	27.42 ± 0.30	26.76 ± 0.48	28.01 ± 0.00	27.67 ± 0.00	28.49 ± 0.00	28.38 ± 0.00	29.03 ± 0.08	29.19 ± 0.12
	65–70	27.45 ± 0.26	26.72 ± 0.53	28.01 ± 0.00	27.67 ± 0.00	28.49 ± 0.00	28.38 ± 0.00	29.02 ± 0.07	29.20 ± 0.12
MoCA	50–54	22.91 ± 1.06	22.32 ± 1.04	24.75 ± 0.04	24.25 ± 0.08	25.81 ± 0.04	25.69 ± 0.08	27.10 ± 0.19	27.40 ± 0.25
	55–59	23.18 ± 0.77	21.88 ± 1.18	24.58 ± 0.04	23.94 ± 0.08	25.67 ± 0.04	25.42 ± 0.09	26.89 ± 0.18	27.12 ± 0.27
	60–64	23.12 ± 0.68	21.79 ± 1.00	24.43 ± 0.04	23.65 ± 0.09	25.53 ± 0.05	25.13 ± 0.09	26.74 ± 0.18	26.78 ± 0.24
	65–70	23.05 ± 0.58	21.42 ± 1.07	24.29 ± 0.05	23.35 ± 0.10	25.37 ± 0.05	24.84 ± 0.09	26.54 ± 0.17	26.47 ± 0.27
AVLT-IR	50–54	12.54 ± 1.15	13.52 ± 1.07	14.53 ± 0.09	15.50 ± 0.08	15.67 ± 0.08	16.99 ± 0.08	17.08 ± 0.23	18.75 ± 0.26
	55–59	12.63 ± 0.83	13.05 ± 1.21	14.16 ± 0.10	15.17 ± 0.10	15.36 ± 0.10	16.70 ± 0.10	16.67 ± 0.22	18.44 ± 0.29
	60–64	12.28 ± 0.75	12.90 ± 1.03	13.79 ± 0.11	14.82 ± 0.11	15.02 ± 0.11	16.35 ± 0.11	16.33 ± 0.22	18.04 ± 0.25
	65–70	12.09 ± 0.64	12.44 ± 1.10	13.43 ± 0.15	14.43 ± 0.13	14.61 ± 0.13	15.97 ± 0.12	15.87 ± 0.24	17.63 ± 0.28
AVLT-SR	50–54	4.25 ± 0.28	4.64 ± 0.33	4.91 ± 0.06	5.44 ± 0.06	5.45 ± 0.05	6.17 ± 0.05	6.28 ± 0.15	7.18 ± 0.16
	55–59	4.11 ± 0.21	4.38 ± 0.38	4.66 ± 0.07	5.21 ± 0.07	5.24 ± 0.07	5.97 ± 0.07	6.01 ± 0.14	6.97 ± 0.18
	60–64	3.91 ± 0.20	4.21 ± 0.33	4.42 ± 0.07	4.97 ± 0.07	5.02 ± 0.08	5.74 ± 0.07	5.78 ± 0.15	6.71 ± 0.15
	65–70	3.68 ± 0.19	3.93 ± 0.34	4.17 ± 0.10	4.71 ± 0.09	4.74 ± 0.09	5.48 ± 0.08	5.47 ± 0.16	6.43 ± 0.19
AVLT-LR	50–54	3.57 ± 0.30	3.94 ± 0.34	4.27 ± 0.07	4.77 ± 0.06	4.86 ± 0.06	5.55 ± 0.06	5.78 ± 0.16	6.65 ± 0.18
	55–59	3.39 ± 0.22	3.65 ± 0.38	3.99 ± 0.08	4.51 ± 0.08	4.62 ± 0.08	5.32 ± 0.08	5.47 ± 0.16	6.40 ± 0.20
	60–64	3.15 ± 0.21	3.44 ± 0.33	3.70 ± 0.09	4.24 ± 0.08	4.36 ± 0.09	5.05 ± 0.08	5.21 ± 0.16	6.10 ± 0.17
	65–70	2.89 ± 0.20	3.12 ± 0.35	3.42 ± 0.11	3.94 ± 0.10	4.04 ± 0.10	4.76 ± 0.10	4.85 ± 0.18	5.78 ± 0.21
SDMT	50–54	27.67 ± 3.34	26.70 ± 3.88	33.38 ± 0.46	33.95 ± 0.40	36.64 ± 0.39	39.35 ± 0.39	40.81 ± 0.76	45.76 ± 0.97
	55–59	27.18 ± 2.43	24.68 ± 4.40	31.68 ± 0.44	32.38 ± 0.44	35.20 ± 0.46	37.96 ± 0.45	39.02 ± 0.74	44.27 ± 1.09
	60–64	26.00 ± 2.22	23.91 ± 3.74	30.10 ± 0.46	30.88 ± 0.45	33.74 ± 0.47	36.46 ± 0.45	37.57 ± 0.73	42.62 ± 0.91
	65–70	24.76 ± 1.92	22.11 ± 4.00	28.66 ± 0.56	29.34 ± 0.50	32.12 ± 0.49	34.95 ± 0.48	35.76 ± 0.80	40.98 ± 1.09
DSF	50–54	6.98 ± 0.36	7.12 ± 0.26	7.61 ± 0.02	7.60 ± 0.01	7.97 ± 0.02	7.97 ± 0.02	8.41 ± 0.07	8.40 ± 0.06
	55–59	7.10 ± 0.25	7.06 ± 0.28	7.55 ± 0.01	7.55 ± 0.01	7.90 ± 0.02	7.90 ± 0.02	8.29 ± 0.06	8.31 ± 0.07
	60–64	7.09 ± 0.21	7.08 ± 0.22	7.49 ± 0.02	7.50 ± 0.02	7.84 ± 0.02	7.84 ± 0.02	8.21 ± 0.06	8.21 ± 0.06
	65–70	7.09 ± 0.17	7.03 ± 0.23	7.45 ± 0.02	7.45 ± 0.02	7.76 ± 0.02	7.77 ± 0.02	8.01 ± 0.06	8.12 ± 0.06
DSB	50–54	3.68 ± 0.14	3.46 ± 0.16	4.01 ± 0.03	3.85 ± 0.02	4.31 ± 0.02	4.23 ± 0.02	4.75 ± 0.08	4.76 ± 0.08
	55–59	3.63 ± 0.10	3.35 ± 0.18	3.91 ± 0.03	3.76 ± 0.03	4.22 ± 0.03	4.15 ± 0.03	4.64 ± 0.07	4.67 ± 0.09
	60–64	3.56 ± 0.10	3.29 ± 0.15	3.82 ± 0.03	3.67 ± 0.03	4.14 ± 0.03	4.06 ± 0.03	4.55 ± 0.07	4.57 ± 0.08

Table 9 Regression-based normative data of cognitive performance stratified by age, gender, and education as appropriate (Continued)

| | Age | Education level | | | | | | | |
| | | Elementary school | | Junior middle school | | Senior middle school | | College and above | |
		Male	Female	Male	Female	Male	Female	Male	Female
	65–70	3.48 ± 0.08	3.19 ± 0.16	3.74 ± 0.03	3.58 ± 0.03	4.04 ± 0.03	3.97 ± 0.03	4.44 ± 0.07	4.48 ± 0.09
TMT-A	50–54	73.20 ± 5.61	86.91 ± 8.02	63.65 ± 1.79	71.67 ± 1.58	58.69 ± 1.51	60.69 ± 1.50	51.49 ± 1.99	47.32 ± 2.34
	55–59	76.71 ± 4.03	92.67 ± 9.07	69.24 ± 1.18	76.81 ± 1.18	63.34 ± 1.26	65.24 ± 1.23	57.11 ± 1.58	52.26 ± 2.40
	60–64	79.22 ± 3.63	93.31 ± 7.67	72.48 ± 0.69	79.99 ± 0.69	66.51 ± 0.73	68.55 ± 0.70	60.23 ± 1.18	55.86 ± 1.82
	65–70	80.25 ± 2.98	96.41 ± 8.30	73.80 ± 0.18	81.52 ± 0.17	68.18 ± 0.16	70.20 ± 0.18	62.06 ± 0.87	57.45 ± 1.93
TMT-B	50–54	185.28 ± 13.15	208.77 ± 19.14	162.40 ± 1.37	172.83 ± 2.43	149.42 ± 1.17	146.31 ± 2.32	133.17 ± 2.74	114.61 ± 4.93
	55–59	185.13 ± 9.54	220.24 ± 21.71	167.50 ± 1.31	182.26 ± 2.61	153.73 ± 1.38	154.64 ± 2.68	138.67 ± 2.64	123.53 ± 5.62
	60–64	188.41 ± 8.62	225.69 ± 18.55	172.22 ± 1.37	191.23 ± 2.68	158.10 ± 1.39	163.61 ± 2.70	143.05 ± 2.63	133.24 ± 4.67
	65–70	191.91 ± 7.39	236.12 ± 19.69	176.56 ± 1.69	200.48 ± 2.97	162.97 ± 1.47	172.66 ± 2.85	148.55 ± 2.74	143.10 ± 5.74
LMT-IR	50–54	8.26 ± 0.71	7.28 ± 0.97	9.99 ± 0.00	9.40 ± 0.00	11.56 ± 0.00	11.35 ± 0.00	13.83 ± 0.35	13.64 ± 0.00
	55–59	8.56 ± 0.52	7.46 ± 0.79	9.99 ± 0.00	9.40 ± 0.00	11.56 ± 0.00	11.35 ± 0.00	13.73 ± 0.34	14.03 ± 0.42
	60–64	8.61 ± 0.45	7.34 ± 0.89	9.99 ± 0.00	9.40 ± 0.00	11.56 ± 0.00	11.35 ± 0.00	13.70 ± 0.34	14.04 ± 0.42
	65–70	8.66 ± 0.38	7.50 ± 0.75	9.99 ± 0.00	9.40 ± 0.00	11.56 ± 0.00	11.35 ± 0.00	13.64 ± 0.31	13.96 ± 0.41
SCWT-IT	50–54	35.18 ± 3.74	30.32 ± 3.10	38.31 ± 0.41	33.42 ± 0.32	36.47 ± 0.45	33.24 ± 0.41	31.26 ± 1.08	30.20 ± 0.74
	55–59	37.66 ± 3.11	30.43 ± 3.79	39.89 ± 0.41	34.69 ± 0.36	38.16 ± 0.56	34.73 ± 0.49	33.65 ± 1.06	32.10 ± 0.88
	60–64	38.78 ± 3.00	31.78 ± 3.45	41.40 ± 0.45	35.94 ± 0.38	39.96 ± 0.59	36.41 ± 0.52	35.67 ± 1.07	34.19 ± 0.74
	65–70	39.97 ± 2.80	32.13 ± 4.07	42.85 ± 0.57	37.28 ± 0.44	42.07 ± 0.66	38.19 ± 0.58	38.37 ± 1.19	36.58 ± 1.00

Predictors in final multivariate linear regression analysis were age, gender and level of education

AVLT-IR Auditory Verbal Learning Test—immediate recall, AVLT-LR Auditory Verbal Learning Test—long recall, AVLT-SR Auditory Verbal Learning Test—short recall, DSB digit span backwards, DSF digit span forwards, MMSE Mini-Mental State Examination, MoCA Montreal Cognitive Assessment, SCWT-IT Stroop Color-Word Test Interference Trial, SDMT Symbol Digit Modalities Test, TMT Trail Making Test, LMT-IR Logical Memory Test—immediate recall

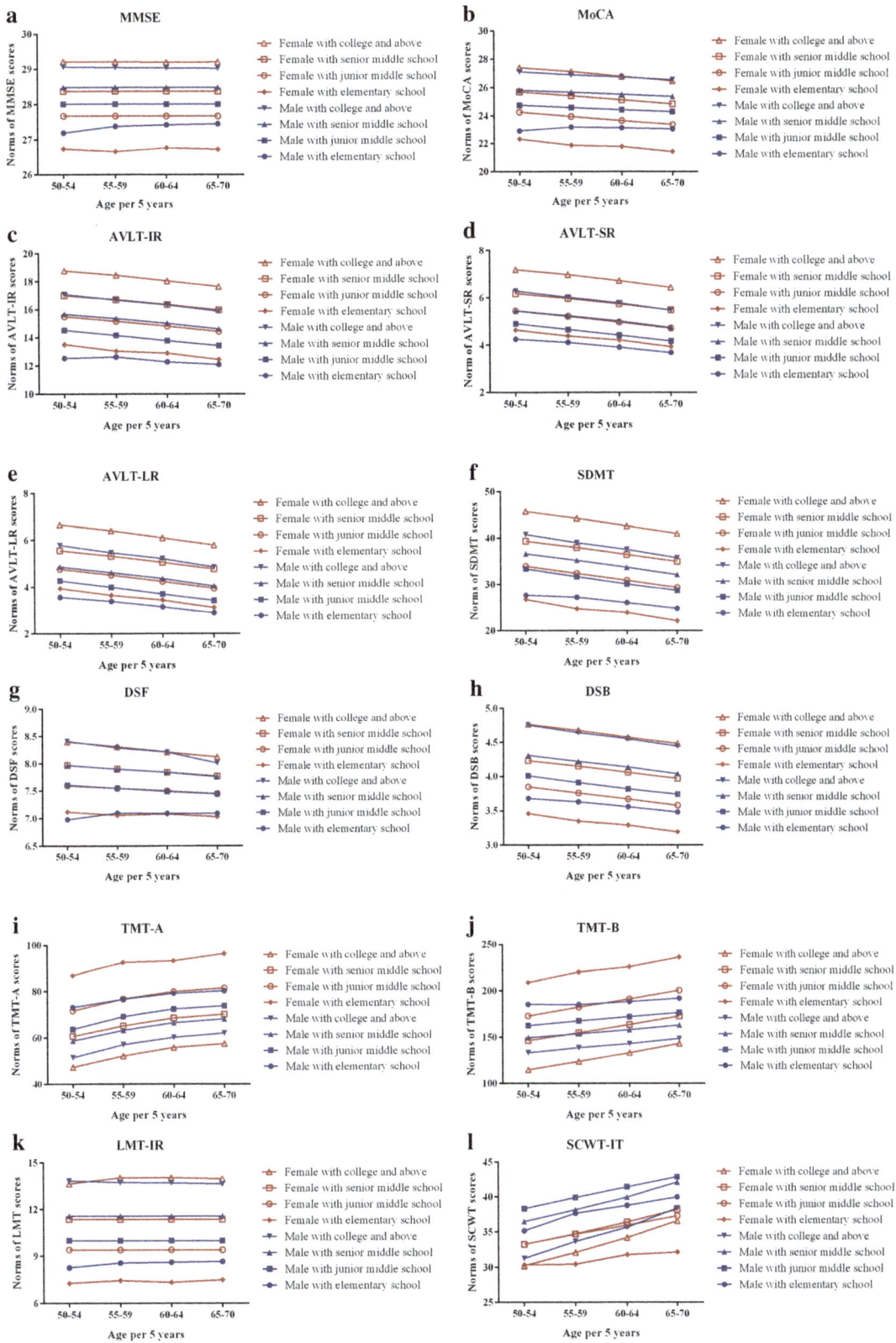

Fig. 4 (See legend on next page.)

cut-off values are also shown (Table 10) to define cognitive impairment.

Discussion

This large community-based study in three Chinese areas is among the first to: 1) examine gender-specific cognitive patterns; 2) explore the gender-specific risk and protective factors; and 3) establish age-, gender-, and education-specific normative data for 12 cognitive tests among a Chinese middle-aged and elderly population. Prior studies mostly employed single or limited cognitive measures and smaller samples to establish restricted normative data [27–29]. Consequently, they may not capture the wide range of cognitive function needed to reflect early changes in mid-life with gender-specific initial ability levels. Thus, encompassing and comparing a wide spectrum of cognitive function may be particularly valuable in identifying modifiable risk factors and critical periods of cognitive impairment following mid-life.

Gender-specific cognitive patterns

An increasing number of studies carried out in Chinese populations have shown gender-specific cognitive patterns both in China and abroad [30–33]. The rate of global cognitive decline was faster among females than males according to MMSE [30]. In agreement with the Rotterdam Study [34], our study also did not find a rapid change in MMSE score until the age of 70 years which suggests an increased need to pay more attention to a wider range of cognitive domains since the global cognition may be stable before the age of 70 years.

Significant gender disparities were observed in three cognitive domains across different age and education groups. With respect to verbal memory, our results were partially congruent with a growing literature that suggest women perform better than men [35–38]. Interestingly, it has been reported that a female advantage in verbal memory remains consistent throughout the lifespan. Furthermore, a 10-year cohort study found that women outperformed men not only on verbal memory, but also on verbal recognition and semantic fluency tasks [39], suggesting that the female advantage for verbal memory tasks is possibly because women are inclined to use semantic clustering in recall. Contrary to verbal memory, men tended to score higher than women for attention/

processing speed/executive function, which is an important cognitive capacity to attend to or to "stay on" a task [40] to complete a task quickly and accurately under the cognitive control of behavior. However, the results only showed the male advantage in the 50–54 and 65–70 years age groups, consistent with previous reports that age-related associations for processing speed were stronger than other domains [41]. The SCWT-IT was interpreted to reflect cognitive flexibility. Van der Elst et al. [42] found clear gender differences on the Stroop interference scores. Nevertheless, the results of regression analyses showed that the influence of age, gender, and education was less profound, which indicated that deficits in Stroop tests may be influenced by intricate factors with concurrent effects.

Gender-specific risk factors for cognitive performance

Studying gender differences in cognitive function is a complex and controversial topic. Furthermore, the relevance of biological and environmental factors is not yet clear. Given the gaps in our knowledge of the gender-specific associations between these factors and cognition in previous studies, our results may be of special importance.

The effects of education on women were more substantial than in men for general cognition and attention/processing speed/executive function. As we can see from Fig. 3, education could reverse the inferiority in women and even lead to superiority in performance of global and domain-specific cognitive performance. Education may explain most of the gender disparity in cognitive pattern, which was also indicated by Lei et al. from China [31] and Lee et al. from India [43]. With respect to verbal memory, we may presume that education could strengthen the semantic clustering in recall. For attention/processing speed/executive function, the Chinese have a larger male advantage in this domain than Americans, with a potential reason being the relatively equivalent access to formal education in developed countries [40]. In former low-income environments, such as traditional rural China, families may favor sons and large gender gaps in schooling exist in low-income settings. Such long-term educational attainment disparities that Chinese women experience through their life course may affect their cognitive trajectory.

Asides from education, a large range of potentially reversible risk factors for cognitive performance were identified and show gender differences, notably white-collar

Table 10 Age-, gender-, and education-specific reference values for cognitive tests

| | | Education level | | | | | | | |
| | | Elementary school | | Junior middle school | | Senior middle school | | College and above | |
	Age	Men	Women	Men	Women	Men	Women	Men	Women
MMSE	50–54	24	24	25	25	25	25	26	26
	55–59	24	24	25	25	25	25	26	26
	60–64	24	24	25	25	25	25	26	26
	65–70	24	24	25	25	25	25	26	26
MoCA	50–54	18	18	20	20	21	21	22	23
	55–59	18	17	20	19	21	21	22	22
	60–64	18	17	20	19	21	20	22	22
	65–70	18	17	20	19	21	20	22	22
AVLT-IR	50–54	6	7	8	8	9	10	10	12
	55–59	6	6	7	8	8	10	10	11
	60–64	5	6	7	8	8	9	9	11
	65–70	5	5	6	7	8	9	9	11
AVLT-SR	50–54	1	1	1	2	2	3	3	4
	55–59	1	1	1	2	2	2	2	3
	60–64	0	1	1	1	1	2	2	3
	65–70	0	0	1	1	1	2	2	3
AVLT-LR	50–54	0	0	0	1	1	2	2	3
	55–59	0	0	0	1	1	1	2	2
	60–64	0	0	0	0	0	1	1	2
	65–70	0	0	0	0	0	1	1	2
SDMT	50–54	13	12	19	19	22	25	26	31
	55–59	12	10	17	18	20	23	24	30
	60–64	11	9	15	16	19	22	23	28
	65–70	10	7	14	15	17	20	21	26
DSF	50–54	5	5	6	6	6	6	6	6
	55–59	5	5	5	5	6	6	6	6
	60–64	5	5	5	5	6	6	6	6
	65–70	5	5	5	5	6	6	6	6
DSB	50–54	2	2	2	2	2	2	3	3
	55–59	2	2	2	2	2	2	3	3
	60–64	2	1	2	2	2	2	3	3
	65–70	2	1	2	2	2	2	3	3
TMT-A	50–54	110	123	100	108	95	97	88	84
	55–59	113	129	106	113	100	102	93	89
	60–64	116	130	109	116	103	105	97	92
	65–70	117	133	110	118	105	107	98	94
TMT-B	50–54	281	305	258	269	245	242	229	210
	55–59	281	316	263	278	250	251	235	219
	60–64	284	321	268	287	254	259	239	229
	65–70	288	332	213	296	259	269	244	239
LMT-IR	50–54	1	0	3	2	5	4	7	7
	55–59	2	0.5	3	2	5	4	7	7

Table 10 Age-, gender-, and education-specific reference values for cognitive tests *(Continued)*

| | | Education level | | | | | | | |
| | | Elementary school | | Junior middle school | | Senior middle school | | College and above | |
	Age	Men	Women	Men	Women	Men	Women	Men	Women
	60–64	2	0	3	2	5	4	7	7
	65–70	2	0.5	3	2	5	4	7	7
SCWT-IT	50–54	78	67	86	75	82	74	69	67
	55–59	83	67	89	78	85	78	75	72
	60–64	86	70	92	80	89	81	79	76
	65–70	89	71	96	83	94	85	86	82

Age-, gender-, and education-specific reference values were defined as 1.5 times root mean square error (RMSE) under the mean of normative score for MMSE, MoCA, AVLT-IR, AVLT-SR, AVLT-LR, SDMT, DSF, DSB, and LMT-IR, and 1.5 times RMSE above the mean of normative score for TMT-A, TMT-B, and SCWT-IT
AVLT-IR Auditory Verbal Learning Test—immediate recall, *AVLT-LR* Auditory Verbal Learning Test—long recall, *AVLT-SR* Auditory Verbal Learning Test—short recall, *DSB* digit span backwards, *DSF* digit span forwards, *MMSE* Mini-Mental State Examination, *MoCA* Montreal Cognitive Assessment, *SCWT-IT* Stroop Color-Word Test Interference Trial, *SDMT* Symbol Digit Modalities Test, *TMT* Trail Making Test, *LMT-IR* Logical Memory Test—immediate recall

work, a higher income level, smoking, diabetes, and coronary heart disease for men, and underweight and obesity as well as hypertension for women. Although no significant between-gender differences were observed, the subgroup analysis also indicated that these risk factors should be taken into consideration in the development of gender-specific preventive intervention programs for cognition.

The need for normative data and a comparison with normative scores

Finally in this study, we provided demographically adjusted and regression-based normative data for 12 cognitive tests. The overall sample size in our study was large and excluded cognitive disorders. The normative data and reference values are finely stratified by the most relevant demographic factors. A quick, efficient, and straightforward method to obtain z scores and percentile rank estimates for specific participants is also provided for clinical researchers.

Normative data have been shown to be indispensable for distinguishing normal aging from early transition to cognitive impairment. Undoubtedly, it would be better to endorse age-, gender-, or education-specific cut-off scores based on demographically adjusted normative data in research. As a result, researchers have tried to yield better screening accuracy instead of uniform cut-off scores [44, 45]. Differences are noted when compared with prior studies for normative scores in the Chinese [46, 47]. These differences are likely attributed to distinction in reporting of the normative data. The present study employed a regression-based approach instead of typical methods (e.g., means and SDs calculated from raw scores). The problem intrinsically related to the latter is the need for a relatively smaller size of subgroups [48]. In the regression-based approach, norms are derived from equations by using the data for all the

samples and the abovementioned problem disappears with no need for a subdivided sample. Also, the unbalanced data will not affect the norms in the regression-based approach because the estimation of the regression weights cannot be biased by any imbalance in the sample but only results in some loss of statistical power [49]. Furthermore, normative data and an estimated z score (and ultimately percentile rank) can even be obtained for particular participants with certain demographic characteristics out of the sample [50].

Certain limitations of this study are noted. First, the present cross-sectional study reported "conventional" norms based on exclusion of participants with evident clinical neurodegenerative diseases instead of "robust" norms that follow individuals longitudinally. It further excludes individuals with subclinical/latent neurological diseases, which may provide less appropriate norms and decreased sensitivity to mild deficits [51], although some research has suggested similarities between two norms in identifying early cognitive impairment [52]. Second, the present study did not take the residential area into consideration, such as a differentiation between urban and rural regions, which may contribute to local differences in education, occupational experiences, income, and lifestyle over the lifespan. Third, since all the medical variables were self-reported, participants may underestimate their symptoms or hesitate to report their real medical status to avoid being perceived as complainers.

Conclusions

In summary, this study holds significance as it contributes to the ongoing investigation of gender-specific cognitive patterns and predictors of cognitive performance among middle-aged and elderly Chinese. Males were inclined to outperform females in global cognition and attention/processing speed/executive function, while females tended to do better on verbal memory as well as cognitive flexibility. These cognitive disparities were considerably mitigated or even reversed but not fully explained by education. Meanwhile, the regression-based and demographically adjusted normative score was provided for 12 cognitive tests to serve as an additional resource and guidance for clinical researchers. Taken together, our findings call for future longitudinal follow-up to improve our knowledge of cognitive patterns and related risk factors. We believe that better understanding the biology of gender differences in cognitive patterns will not only be conducive to advocating a healthy lifestyle and promoting gender-specific interventions to prevent or minimize cognitive impairment but will also be integral to the investigation of personalized, gender-specific new therapies.

Abbreviations
AD: Alzheimer's disease; ADI: Alzheimer's Disease International; AVLT: Auditory Verbal Learning Test; AVLT-IR: Auditory Verbal Learning Test—immediate recall; AVLT-LR: Auditory Verbal Learning Test—long recall; AVLT-SR: Auditory Verbal Learning Test—short recall; BMI: Body mass index; DSB: Digit span backwards; DSF: Digit span forwards; EMCOA: Effects and Mechanism of Cholesterol and Oxysterol on Alzheimer's disease; FDR: False discovery rate; LMT-IR: Logical Memory Test—immediate recall; MCI: Mild cognitive impairment; MMSE: Mini-Mental State Examination; MoCA: Montreal Cognitive Assessment Test; PCA: Principal component analysis; SCWT-IT: Stroop Color-Word Test Interference Trial; SD: Standard deviation; SDMT: Symbol Digit Modalities Test; TMT: Trail Making Test; WMS-RC: Wechsler Memory Scale Revised for China

Acknowledgements
The authors are indebted to Deqiang Zheng, Dian He, and Yanxia Luo from the Department of Epidemiology and Health Statistics of Capital Medical University for their statistical advice. The authors also thank Hongguo Rong, Junfang Zhao, and the medical and ancillary staff of the Health Examination Center in Linyi and Jincheng and Beijing Chaoyang District Center for Disease Control and Prevention for assistance in the field survey. They also thank all participants for their time.

Funding
This work was supported by the State Key Program of the National Natural Science Foundation of China (grant no. 81330065) and National Natural Science Foundation of China (grant no. 81673149).

Authors' contributions
RX conceptualized and designed the study, obtained funding, and supervised data collection. YA and LF conducted the data analysis, and drafted and critically revised the manuscript. XZ, YiW, YuW, LT, YL, and ZQ made substantial contributions to the acquisition of data, and analysis and interpretation of data. All authors read and approved the final manuscript.

Consent for publication
All the co-authors and participants have given their consent for publication.

Competing interests
The authors declare that they have no competing interests.

Author details
[1]School of Public Health, Capital Medical University, No.10 Xitoutiao, You An Men Wai, Beijing 100069, China. [2]Peking university First Hospital, Beijing, China. [3]Linyi Mental Health Center, Linyi, Shandong, China. [4]Jincheng People's Hospital, Jincheng, Shanxi, China.

References
1. Prince M, Wimo A, Guerchet M, Ali G, Wu Y, Prina M. World Alzheimer Report 2015. The global impact of dementia. An analysis of prevalence, incidence, cost & trends. London: Alzheimer's Disease International (ADI); 2015.
2. Albert MS. Changes in cognition. Neurobiol Aging. 2011;32(Suppl 1):S58–63.
3. Tariq S, Barber PA. Dementia risk and prevention by targeting modifiable vascular risk factors. J Neurochem. 2017;144(5):565–81.
4. Prince M, Bryce R, Albanese E, Wimo A, Ribeiro W, Ferri CP. The global prevalence of dementia: a systematic review and metaanalysis. Alzheimers Dement. 2013;9(1):63–75.
5. Paulo AC, Sampaio A, Santos NC, Costa PS, Cunha P, Zihl J, Cerqueira J, Palha JA, Sousa N. Patterns of cognitive performance in healthy ageing in northern Portugal: a cross-sectional analysis. PLoS One. 2011;6(9):e24553.
6. Bergman I, Almkvist O. Neuropsychological test norms controlled for physical health: does it matter? Scand J Psychol. 2015;56(2):140–50.
7. Xu W, Tan L, Wang HF, Jiang T, Tan MS, Tan L, Zhao QF, Li JQ, Wang J, Yu JT. Meta-analysis of modifiable risk factors for Alzheimer's disease. J Neurol Neurosurg Psychiatry. 2015;86(12):1299–306.
8. Kesse-Guyot E, Andreeva VA, Lassale C, Hercberg S, Galan P. Clustering of midlife lifestyle behaviors and subsequent cognitive function: a longitudinal study. Am J Public Health. 2014;104(11):e170–7.
9. Bennett DA, Arnold SE, Valenzuela MJ, Brayne C, Schneider JA. Cognitive and social lifestyle: links with neuropathology and cognition in late life. Acta Neuropathol. 2014;127(1):137–50.
10. Lu Y, An Y, Yu H, Che F, Zhang X, Rong H, Xi Y, Xiao R. Sex-specific nonlinear associations between serum lipids and different domains of cognitive function in middle to older age individuals. Metab Brain Dis. 2017; 32(4):1089–97.
11. Lu Y, An Y, Guo J, Zhang X, Wang H, Rong H, Xiao R. Dietary intake of nutrients and lifestyle affect the risk of mild cognitive impairment in the Chinese elderly population: a cross-sectional study. Front Behav Neurosci. 2016;10:229.
12. Johnson DK, Storandt M, Morris JC, Galvin JE. Longitudinal study of the transition from healthy aging to Alzheimer disease. Arch Neurol. 2009; 66(10):1254–9.
13. Hedden T, Oh H, Younger AP, Patel TA. Meta-analysis of amyloid-cognition relations in cognitively normal older adults. NEUROLOGY. 2013;80(14): 1341–8.
14. Bennett DA, Wilson RS, Schneider JA, Evans DA, Beckett LA, Aggarwal NT, Barnes LL, Fox JH, Bach J. Natural history of mild cognitive impairment in older persons. Neurology. 2002;59(2):198–205.
15. Larouche E, Tremblay MP, Potvin O, Laforest S, Bergeron D, Laforce R, Monetta L, Boucher L, Tremblay P, Belleville S, et al. Normative data for the Montreal cognitive assessment in middle-aged and elderly Quebec-French people. Arch Clin Neuropsychol. 2016; https://doi.org/10.1093/arclin/acw076.
16. Schneider AL, Sharrett AR, Gottesman RF, Coresh J, Coker L, Wruck L, Selnes OA, Deal J, Knopman D, Mosley TH. Normative data for 8 neuropsychological tests in older blacks and whites from the atherosclerosis risk in communities (ARIC) study. Alzheimer Dis Assoc Disord. 2015;29(1):32–44.
17. Migdanis I, Gioulbasanis I, Lianou E, Migdanis A, Kanaki M, Kiriakou GI, Sgantzos M, Kapsoritakis A, Kontogianni M. Nutritional status and

objective assessment of functional status in patients with neoplastic diseases receiving antineoplastic therapy: preliminary results. Clin Nutr ESPEN. 2018;24:186.

18. Folstein MF, Folstein SE, McHugh PR. "Mini-mental state". A practical method for grading the cognitive state of patients for the clinician. J Psychiatr Res. 1975;12(3):189–98.

19. Nasreddine ZS, Phillips NA, Bedirian V, Charbonneau S, Whitehead V, Collin I, Cummings JL, Chertkow H. The Montreal cognitive assessment, MoCA: a brief screening tool for mild cognitive impairment. J Am Geriatr Soc. 2005; 53(4):695–9.

20. Ma J, Zhang Y, Guo Q. Comparison of vascular cognitive impairment—no dementia by multiple classification methods. Int J Neurosci. 2015;125(11): 823–30.

21. Price KL, DeSantis SM, Simpson AN, Tolliver BK, McRae-Clark AL, Saladin ME, Baker NL, Wagner MT, Brady KT. The impact of clinical and demographic variables on cognitive performance in methamphetamine-dependent individuals in rural South Carolina. Am J Addict. 2011;20(5):447–55.

22. Wang C, An Y, Yu H, Feng L, Liu Q, Lu Y, Wang H, Xiao R. Association between exposure to the Chinese famine in different stages of early life and decline in cognitive functioning in adulthood. Front Behav Neurosci. 2016;10:146.

23. Miu J, Negin J, Salinas-Rodriguez A, Manrique-Espinoza B, Sosa-Ortiz AL, Cumming R, Kowal P. Factors associated with cognitive function in older adults in Mexico. Glob Health Action. 2016;9:30747.

24. Wei M, Shi J, Li T, Ni J, Zhang X, Li Y, Kang S, Ma F, Xie H, Qin B, et al. Diagnostic accuracy of the Chinese version of the trail-making test for screening cognitive impairment. J Am Geriatr Soc. 2017;66(1):92–9.

25. Chan RC, Hoosain R, Lee TM, Fan YW, Fong D. Are there sub-types of attentional deficits in patients with persisting post-concussive symptoms? A cluster analytical study. Brain Inj. 2003;17(2):131–48.

26. BENJAMINI Y, HOCHBERG Y. Controlling the false discovery rate—a practical and powerful approach to multiple testing. J Royal Stat Soc Series B-Methodological. 1995;57(1):289–300.

27. Malek-Ahmadi M, Powell JJ, Belden CM, O'Connor K, Evans L, Coon DW, Nieri W. Age- and education-adjusted normative data for the Montreal cognitive assessment (MoCA) in older adults age 70–99. Neuropsychol Dev Cogn B Aging Neuropsychol Cogn. 2015;22(6):755–61.

28. Yancar DE, Ozcan T. Evaluating the relationship between education level and cognitive impairment with the Montreal cognitive assessment test. PSYCHOGERIATRICS. 2015;15(3):186–90.

29. Amaral-Carvalho V, Caramelli P. Normative data for healthy middle-aged and elderly performance on the Addenbrooke cognitive examination-revised. Cogn Behav Neurol. 2012;25(2):72–6.

30. Wu Y, Zhang D, Pang Z, Oksuzyan A, Jiang W, Wang S, Li S, Kruse T, Christensen K, Tan Q. Gender-specific patterns in age-related decline in general health among Danish and Chinese: a cross-national comparative study. Geriatr Gerontol Int. 2012;12(3):431–9.

31. Lei X, Smith JP, Sun X, Zhao Y. Gender differences in cognition in China and reasons for change over time: evidence from CHARLS. J Econ Ageing. 2014; 4:46–55.

32. Lei X, Hu Y, McArdle JJ, Smith JP, Zhao Y. Gender differences in cognition among older adults in China. J Hum Resour. 2012;47(4):951–71.

33. Chang ES, Dong X. A battery of tests for assessing cognitive function in U.S. Chinese older adults—findings from the PINE study. J Gerontol A Biol Sci Med Sci. 2014;69(Suppl 2):S23–30.

34. Hoogendam YY, Hofman A, van der Geest JN, van der Lugt A, Ikram MA. Patterns of cognitive function in aging: the Rotterdam study. Eur J Epidemiol. 2014;29(2):133–40.

35. Proust-Lima C, Amieva H, Letenneur L, Orgogozo JM, Jacqmin-Gadda H, Dartigues JF. Gender and education impact on brain aging: a general cognitive factor approach. Psychol Aging. 2008;23(3):608–20.

36. Matos GM, Pinho MS, Rodrigues SM. Effects of socio-demographic variables on performance on the Cambridge neuropsychological automated tests for the assessment of dementia and Portuguese norms for older adults living in retirement homes. Clin Neuropsychol. 2016; 30(2):284–317.

37. Li R. Why women see differently from the way men see? A review of sex differences in cognition and sports. J Sport Health Sci. 2014;3(3):155–62.

38. Laws KR, Irvine K, Gale TM. Sex differences in cognitive impairment in Alzheimer's disease. World J Psychiatry. 2016;6(1):54–65.

39. Li R, Singh M. Sex differences in cognitive impairment and Alzheimer's disease. Front Neuroendocrinol. 2014;35(3):385–403.

40. Weir D, Lay M, Langa K. Economic development and gender inequality in cognition: a comparison of China and India, and of SAGE and the HRS sister studies. J Econ Ageing. 2014;4:114–25.

41. Lipnicki DM, Crawford JD, Dutta R, Thalamuthu A, Kochan NA, Andrews G, Lima-Costa MF, Castro-Costa E, Brayne C, Matthews FE, et al. Age-related cognitive decline and associations with sex, education and apolipoprotein E genotype across ethnocultural groups and geographic regions: a collaborative cohort study. PLoS Med. 2017;14(3):e1002261.

42. Van der Elst W, Van Boxtel MP, Van Breukelen GJ, Jolles J. The Stroop color-word test: influence of age, sex, and education; and normative data for a large sample across the adult age range. Assessment. 2006;13(1):62–79.

43. Lee J, Shih R, Feeney K, Langa KM. Gender disparity in late-life cognitive functioning in India: findings from the longitudinal aging study in India. J Gerontol B Psychol Sci Soc Sci. 2014;69(4):603–11.

44. Lu J, Li D, Li F, Zhou A, Wang F, Zuo X, Jia XF, Song H, Jia J. Montreal cognitive assessment in detecting cognitive impairment in Chinese elderly individuals: a population-based study. J Geriatr Psychiatry Neurol. 2011;24(4):184–90.

45. Tan JP, Li N, Gao J, Wang LN, Zhao YM, Yu BC, Du W, Zhang WJ, Cui LQ, Wang QS, et al. Optimal cutoff scores for dementia and mild cognitive impairment of the Montreal cognitive assessment among elderly and oldest-old Chinese population. J Alzheimers Dis. 2015;43(4):1403–12.

46. Wang Q, Sun J, Ma X, Wang Y, Yao J, Deng W, Liu X, Collier DA, Li T. Normative data on a battery of neuropsychological tests in the Han Chinese population. J Neuropsychol. 2011;5(Pt 1):126–42.

47. Collinson SL, Fang SH, Lim ML, Feng L, Ng TP. Normative data for the repeatable battery for the assessment of neuropsychological status in elderly Chinese. Arch Clin Neuropsychol. 2014;29(5):442–55.

48. Van Breukelen GJ, Vlaeyen JW. Norming clinical questionnaires with multiple regression: the pain cognition list. Psychol Assess. 2005;17(3):336–44.

49. Zachary RA, Gorsuch RL. Continuous norming: implications for the WAIS-R. J Clin Psychol. 1985;41(1):86–94.

50. Shirk SD, Mitchell MB, Shaughnessy LW, Sherman JC, Locascio JJ, Weintraub S, Atri A. A web-based normative calculator for the uniform data set (UDS) neuropsychological test battery. Alzheimers Res Ther. 2011;3(6):32.

51. Clark LR, Koscik RL, Nicholas CR, Okonkwo OC, Engelman CD, Bratzke LC, Hogan KJ, Mueller KD, Bendlin BB, Carlsson CM, et al. Mild cognitive impairment in late middle age in the Wisconsin registry for Alzheimer's prevention study: prevalence and characteristics using robust and standard neuropsychological normative data. Arch Clin Neuropsychol. 2016; https://doi.org/10.1093/arclin/acw024.

52. Ritchie LJ, Frerichs RJ, Tuokko H. Effective normative samples for the detection of cognitive impairment in older adults. Clin Neuropsychol. 2007;21(6):863–74.

Functional connectivity in cognitive control networks mitigates the impact of white matter lesions in the elderly

Gloria Benson[1][*] ⓘ, Andrea Hildebrandt[2,3], Catharina Lange[4], Claudia Schwarz[1], Theresa Köbe[1,5,6], Werner Sommer[3], Agnes Flöel[7] and Miranka Wirth[1,8*]

Abstract

Background: Cerebrovascular pathology, quantified by white matter lesions (WML), is known to affect cognition in aging, and is associated with an increased risk of dementia. The present study aimed to investigate whether higher functional connectivity in cognitive control networks mitigates the detrimental effect of WML on cognition.

Methods: Nondemented older participants (≥ 50 years; $n = 230$) underwent cognitive evaluation, fluid-attenuated inversion recovery (FLAIR) magnetic resonance imaging (MRI), and resting state functional magnetic resonance imaging (fMRI). Total WML volumes were quantified algorithmically. Functional connectivity was assessed in preselected higher-order resting state networks, namely the fronto-parietal, the salience, and the default mode network, using global and local measures. Latent moderated structural equations modeling examined direct and interactive relationships between WML volumes, functional connectivity, and cognition.

Results: Larger WML volumes were associated with worse cognition, having a greater impact on executive functions ($\beta = -0.37$, $p < 0.01$) than on memory ($\beta = -0.22$, $p < 0.01$). Higher global functional connectivity in the fronto-parietal network and higher local connectivity between the salience network and medial frontal cortex significantly mitigated the impact of WML on executive functions, (unstandardized coefficients: $b = 2.39$, $p = 0.01$; $b = 3.92$, $p = 0.01$) but not on memory ($b = -5.01$, $p = 0.51$, $b = 2.01$, $p = 0.07$, respectively). No such effects were detected for the default mode network.

Conclusion: Higher functional connectivity in fronto-parietal and salience networks may protect against detrimental effects of WML on executive functions, the cognitive domain that was predominantly affected by cerebrovascular pathology. These results highlight the crucial role of cognitive control networks as a neural substrate of cognitive reserve in older individuals.

Keywords: White matter lesions, Functional connectivity, Reserve, Protective factors, Cognitive control networks

Background

Cerebrovascular pathology, as quantified through white matter lesions (WML), is present in more than 50% of the elderly population [1]. WML are known to affect brain structure [2, 3] and cognitive performance [4–7], and have been associated with an increased risk of stroke and dementia [8]. Identifying beneficial lifestyle factors and brain mechanisms that protect against the negative effects of

* Correspondence: Gloria.benson@charite.de; miranka.wirth@charite.de
[1]NeuroCure Clinical Research Center, Department of Neurology, Charité – Universitätsmedizin Berlin, Freie Universität Berlin, Humboldt-Universität zu Berlin, Berlin Institute of Health, Berlin, Germany
Full list of author information is available at the end of the article

cerebrovascular pathology may be beneficial in preventing cognitive failure.

Cognitive dysfunction related to WML has been shown to be attenuated by protective lifestyle factors, such as educational attainment, cognitive enrichment, and physical activity [3, 9, 10], adding to the growing body of evidence for the concept of cognitive reserve (CR) [11]. Neuroimaging studies have extended the concept of CR to the level of functional brain mechanisms [12, 13]. It is suggested that those individuals with high CR have brain activation patterns that reflect higher neural efficiency, which may help maintain cognitive functions in the face of brain pathology [14]. While the reserve hypothesis has been well established in the context of WML with behavioral measures of CR [9, 15–17], the functional mechanisms within neural networks that may convey reserve in cerebrovascular pathology remain to be understood.

Some neuroimaging studies have provided an indication of active neuronal compensation in the context of WML. For example, in a working memory task, older individuals with higher WML volumes showed higher task-related brain activation across different levels of task complexity in anterior cingulate and middle frontal regions [18]. Fernández-Cabello et al. [19] found that older individuals with a high CR and a high WML load over-recruited fronto-parietal areas during task performance when compared with young individuals. These findings imply that higher neural capacity in brain regions subserving cognitive control could buffer the negative impacts of WML. More clarification is needed, however, on the moderating role of functional brain networks.

Recently, higher functional connectivity within major hubs of cognitive control networks have been proposed as neural correlates of CR [20]. Cognitive control networks are linked to reserve-associated protective factors [21], and have been suggested to play a compensatory role in the presence of early Alzheimer's disease (AD) pathology [22]. More specifically, it was demonstrated that higher global connectivity in the fronto-parietal network [23] and higher local connectivity from the anterior cingulate cortex (a central hub of the salience network) [24, 25] may offer protection against the detrimental effects of age-related neuropathology. All together, these results motivated us to choose cognitive control networks, the fronto-parietal and the salience network, to examine reserve mechanisms and their moderating role in cerebrovascular pathology.

In the present study, we investigate whether resting state functional connectivity in cognitive control networks, as a proxy of CR, plays a role in mitigating the negative effect of cerebrovascular pathology on cognitive performance (Fig. 1, panel A). To this end, we assessed the relationships between the extent of WML (WML load), cognition, and functional connectivity using structural equation modeling (SEM) and tested for moderation effects in a sample of 230 nondemented individuals. We hypothesized the following: 1) a detrimental effect of WML on cognitive domains, such as executive functions and memory [6]; and 2) a moderating role of global and local functional connectivity in the fronto-parietal and salience networks, with the default mode network as control. More precisely, we expected that the negative relationship between WML load and cognitive performance would be reduced in individuals with higher levels of functional connectivity.

Methods
Participants

In total, 230 nondemented older participants, healthy older individuals ($n = 140$), and individuals with mild cognitive impairment (MCI; $n = 90$) were included in this study. Participants were aged between 50 and 80 years and were native German speakers. The healthy older individuals were recruited from the general community via advertisement. The Mini-Mental State Examination (MMSE) [26] was used to exclude pre-existing cognitive impairment (a score < 26 led to exclusion). Amnestic MCI patients were recruited from the memory clinic of the Department of Neurology at the Charité University Hospital, Berlin, and a Neurology specialist practice in Berlin (Dr. J. Bohlken). Individuals with MCI were diagnosed according to the standardized Mayo Clinic criteria [27]. Exclusion criteria for both groups included severe medical, neurological, or psychiatric disease. Detailed information of the samples has been provided previously [28, 29].

Neuropsychological testing

Participants underwent a full neuropsychological test battery focused on a variety of cognitive domains. Based on their relevance for the present research questions, the following psychometric tests were selected for further analysis: learning and memory performance was evaluated by the German version of the Auditory Verbal Learning Test (VLMT) [30], providing subscores for learning ability (total immediate recall), delayed recall, and recognition. Executive functions were measured by the Trail Making Test (TMT) version A and B [31, 32] and the interference score from the Stroop Color-Word interference test [33]. In addition, working memory and language abilities, respectively, were measured using the forward and backward digit span conditions from the Wechsler Digit span task [34] and phonemic and alternating word fluency [35].

Acquisition preprocessing and analysis of the neuroimaging data
Magnetic resonance imaging (MRI) acquisition

Scans were acquired using a 3-Tesla Magnetom Trio (Tim Trio; Siemens AG, Erlangen, Germany) at two different sites using identical imaging protocols. T1-weighted images were acquired with magnetization-prepared rapid acquisition gradient-echo (MPRAGE) with the following parameters: repetition time (TR = 1900 ms; TE = 2.52 ms; 192 sagittal slices; size = $1.0 \times 1.0 \times 1.0$ mm^3; flip angle = 9°). Functional scans were obtained at rest using T2*-weighted EPI sequence (TR = 2300 ms; TE = 30 ms; 34 slices; size = $3.0 \times 3.0 \times 4.0$ mm^3; flip angle = 90°). Subjects were instructed to keep their eyes closed and not think of anything in particular. Fluid attenuated inverse

A. Hypothesized relationships

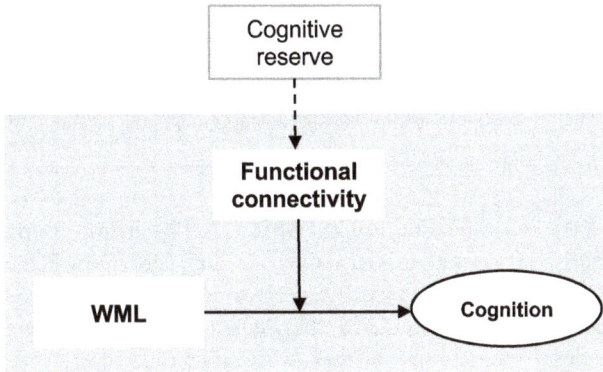

B.0. Schematic illustration of the pre-selected resting state networks (RSNs)

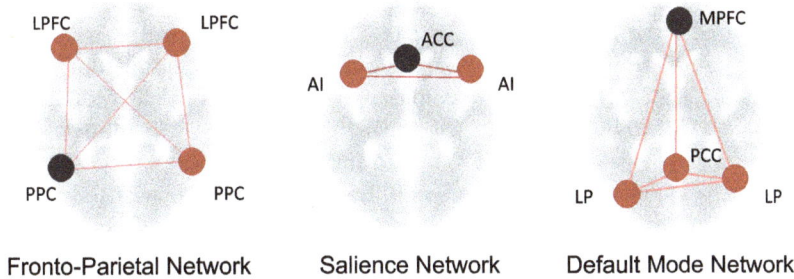

Fronto-Parietal Network   Salience Network   Default Mode Network

B.1. Assessment of global connectivity measures

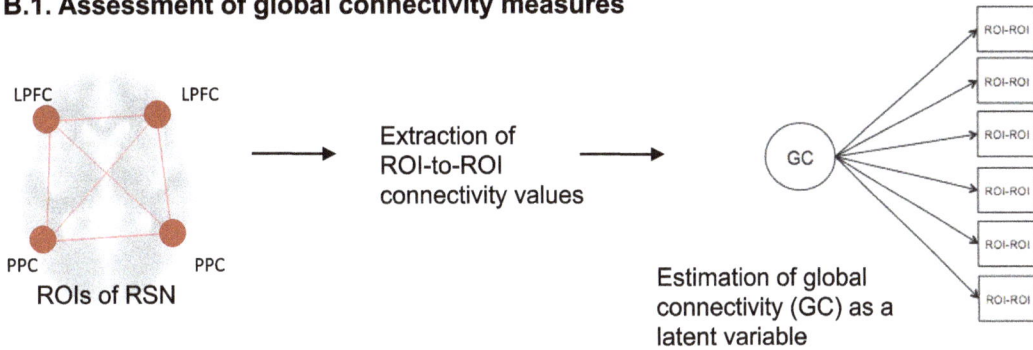

ROIs of RSN   Extraction of ROI-to-ROI connectivity values   Estimation of global connectivity (GC) as a latent variable

B.2. Assessment of local connectivity measures

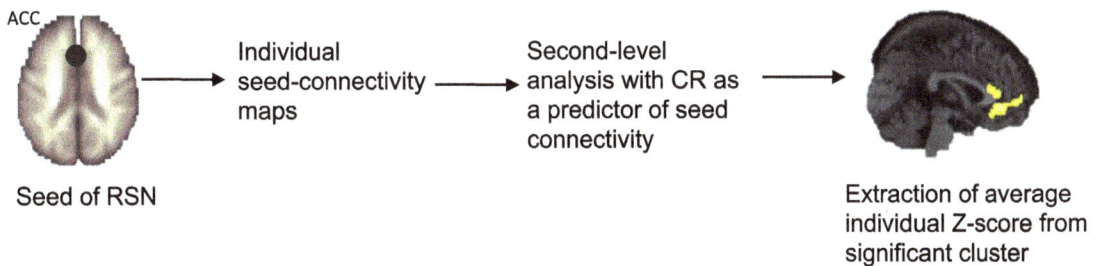

Seed of RSN   Individual seed-connectivity maps   Second-level analysis with CR as a predictor of seed connectivity   Extraction of average individual Z-score from significant cluster

Fig. 1 (See legend on next page.)

(See figure on previous page.)
Fig. 1 Panel A: Hypothesized relationships. The relationships analyzed in this study are shaded in gray. Functional connectivity, as a proxy of cognitive reserve (CR), may act as a moderator between white matter lesions and cognition. Panel B.0: Regions of interest (ROIs) for each resting state network as provided by CONN atlas. ROIs selected as seeds in the local connectivity measure are presented in grey. Panel B.1: Schematic representation of the assessment of global connectivity measures. Panel B.2: Assessment of local connectivity measure with our behavioral measure of CR indicated by years of education, premorbid intelligence, and lifestyle index. ACC anterior cingulate cortex, AI anterior insula, LP lateral parietal, LPFC lateral prefrontal cortex, MPFC medial prefrontal cortex, PCC posterior cingulate cortex, PPC posterior parietal cortex, WML white matter lesions

recovery (FLAIR) T2-weighted images (TR = 8000 ms; TE = 100 ms; 2370 inversion time; 232 × 256 matrix size = 0.86 × 0.86 × 5.0 mm³; flip angle = 130°; slice gap = 5.0 mm) were acquired to measure WML. Neuroimaging measurements and neuropsychological test sessions were obtained in close proximity (mean time delay, 12.9 days; range, 1–40 days).

Assessment of WML and vascular risk

Total WML volumes were segmented automatically using the FLAIR images and the "lesion growth algorithm" of the lesion segmentation toolbox (LST) under the freely available Statistical Parametric Mapping (SPM) software package (version SPM8, Wellcome Trust Centre for Neuroimaging, Institute of Neurology, UCL, London, UK; [36]). Processing and parameter settings (kappa = 0.30, binarization threshold = 0.50) were exactly as described previously [37]. The total WML volume was obtained by multiplying the number of WML voxels according to the binary WML map by the voxel volume. For each subject, WML volume ratio was computed as the volume of WML divided by the total intracranial (TIV) volume. Individual TIV was assessed with the Tissue Volumes utility in SPM 12 (Wellcome Trust Centre for Neuroimaging, London, UK; www.fil.ion.ucl.ac.uk/spm). It computes the total by summing the volumes of grey matter, white matter, and cerebrospinal fluid (CSF) from the corresponding segmented images [38]. Frequency maps were calculated for each group, both separately and for the entire sample. To this aim, the frequency (i.e., number of participants with WML in specific voxels relative to total number of participants) was computed voxel-wise based on binarized WML segmentation maps previously warped to the anatomic Montreal Neurologic Institute reference space.

In addition, we computed the validated Framingham risk index of cardiovascular disease (CVD) as a combined measure of vascular risk to validate the WML measure based on the present sample [39]. This measure involves age, sex, total cholesterol, high-density lipoprotein (HDL) cholesterol, systolic blood pressure, medical history of diabetes, treatment for hypertension, and smoking status.

Preprocessing and analysis of resting state functional MRI

The publicly available CONN Functional Connectivity Toolbox version 17C (www.nitrc.org/projects/conn), in conjunction with SPM 12 (Wellcome Department of Cognitive Neurology, London, UK; www.fil.ion.ucl.ac.uk/spm), was used to perform all preprocessing steps [40]. In detail, we used the default preprocessing pipeline: raw functional images were slice-time corrected, realigned (motion corrected), and coregistered to each participant's MPRAGE image. Images were then normalized to the Montreal Neurological Institute (MNI) standard space and spatially smoothed with an 8-mm Gaussian filter. Identification of outlier scans was performed using Artifact Detection Tools (http://www.nitrc.org/projects/artifact_detect; [40]). Specifically, this regresses out scans as nuisance covariates in the first-level analysis exceeding 3 standard deviations (SD) in mean global intensity and frame-to-frame differences exceeding 0.5 mm (combination of translational and rotational displacements). There were no significant differences between the two groups in the number of outlier scans ($p = 0.6$) or mean motion ($p = 0.2$); details in Additional file 1 (Table S2). Resting state images were band-pass filtered (0.008–0.09 Hz) and corrected with the implemented component correction (CompCor) strategy [41], including the removal of white/CSF time series, motion, and artifact-outlier regressors, to reduce the influence of blood oxygen level-dependent (BOLD) signals unrelated to neural activity. This approach limits the influence of confounds such as head motion, peripheral physiology, and other imaging artifacts.

Functional connectivity assessment

Functional connectivity was assessed within preselected cognitive control networks, namely the fronto-parietal network and the salience network, using global and local connectivity measures (Fig. 1, panel B.0). The default mode network was added for comparison reasons. Global network connectivity was estimated within each resting state network, using the atlas network region(s) of interest (ROI) (8-mm radius spheres) provided by CONN. ROI-to-ROI connectivity values (Fisher-transformed correlation coefficients) at false discovery rate (FDR)-corrected level were extracted for each ROI pair within each network [40] The ROI-to-ROI connectivity values were used as indicators of latent variables (one for each network) in SEM (see below) for estimating global functional connectivity within each resting state network (Fig. 1, panel B.1).

Local network connectivity was assessed within each resting state network by extracting those brain regions that significantly correlated with our behavioral measure of CR (explained in detail below), similar to previous approaches [24]. Individual connectivity maps were derived using seed-to-voxel analyses from CONN (Fig. 1, panel B.2). Whole brain correlational maps were generated by extracting the mean resting state BOLD time course for each seed ROI and calculating the Fisher-transformed correlation coefficients with the BOLD time course throughout the whole brain. For each network the following ROIs (Fig. 1, Panel B.0) were used as seeds: fronto-parietal network (left posterior parietal cortex (LPPC): −46,−58,49), salience network (anterior cingulate cortex (ACC): 0,22,35), and default mode network (medial prefrontal cortex (MPFC): 1,55,−3). We chose these seeds as they are characterized as core network hubs [42, 43] and are areas involved in reserve-related functional connectivity findings [20, 24, 44]. Individual connectivity maps were then subjected to voxel-wise second-level analysis with our behavioral measure of CR as a predictor of local connectivity related to reserve. Significant clusters were extracted at a cluster-level threshold of $p < 0.05$, FDR-corrected for multiple comparison, and a voxel-level threshold of $p < 0.005$. Finally, the average Z scores across each individual cluster for each subject were used as a local connectivity measure.

Modeling procedure and measurement models

The SEM builds upon multiple observed variables to estimate latent variables. We used the software Mplus for the purpose of modeling [45]. Structural equational modeling allows estimation of the relationship between observed variables and the latent variable they intend to measure (measurement models), and relationships between multiple latent variables (structural models). The advantage of latent variables is that they represent the shared variance among multiple observed variables that are conceivable realizations of cognitive ability as a construct. Thus, latent variables are adjusted for measurement error and for the specificity of applied assessment methods in a given study. Due to this adjustment, results based on latent variables are generalized above measurement methods.

To that end, we established the best fitting measurement models, separately for cognition, CR, and each resting state network, aiming to estimate the number and structure of latent variables that are necessary to explain the relationships across all these measured variables at the levels of brain and behavior.

Cognition, connectivity, and cognitive reserve estimate models

The cognitive model included a latent variable of global cognition (G), indicated by all selected psychometric tests.

Above G, executive functions and memory were modeled as nested latent variables under G. As mentioned previously, executive functions were indicated by TMT versions A and B, and Stroop interference, while memory was indicated by VLMT total immediate recall, delayed recall, and recognition. The first model postulated G with the specific nested variables added in a stepwise fashion and testing for model fit improvement through latent variable addition. For subsequent analyses of specific relationships within a given cognitive domain, the latent variables memory and executive functions were assessed as separate latent factors. Additional file 1 (Table S1) provides the fit of all estimated measurement models.

For each resting state network, global network connectivity was estimated as a latent variable, as indicated by the functional ROI-to-ROI connectivity among the major network nodes. To account for the shared variance of pairs of ROI-to-ROI connectivity values, some residual covariance between connectivity indicators was introduced (i.e., MPFC-right lateral parietal (LP) with MPFC-left LP). The model fit for each resting state network is provided in Additional file 1 (Table S1).

Finally, we estimated a behavioral measure of CR as a latent variable based on the following observed measures: years of education, premorbid intelligence, and a combined measure of self-reported healthy lifestyle behaviors (referred to as lifestyle index). Premorbid verbal intelligence was assessed by the German multiple vocabulary test [46]. The lifestyle index included a sum score of body mass index, dietary habits, physical exercise, smoking, and alcohol consumption, described in detail elsewhere [47, 48]. A high lifestyle index score indicated normal weight, never smoking, intense physical activity, moderate alcohol consumption, and a dietary pattern rich in fruits, vegetables, and whole-grain products, as well as unsaturated fatty acids.

Several statistical test and fit indices were used for assessing model fit: the ratio between χ^2 and degrees of freedom (χ^2/df ratio < 2), root-mean square error of approximation (RMSEA) ≤ 0.08, standard root mean square residual (SRMR) ≤ 0.05, and comparative fit index (CFI) ≥ 0.95 [49]. Competing models were compared by evaluating the difference of their likelihoods, using the χ^2-difference test. Missing data were dealt with by the full information maximum likelihood (FIML) algorithm, as implemented in Mplus (details of missing data provided in Table 1).

Additional statistical analyses were conducted with SPSS (version 24) to evaluate the reproducibility of our results when simplified modeling is applied. Restricted regression models were computed to control for covariates such as age and total grey matter volume. Cook distance (> 1) was used to detect potential influential cases [50].

Table 1 Characteristics of the study group showing means, standard deviation, and range of the total sample and dichotomized by group

	Total sample	HO	MCI	
N (n women)	230 (115)	140 (71)	90 (44)	
Age (years)	65.2 ± 7.6 (50–80)	63 ± 6.9 (50–79)	68.6 ± 7.5 (50–80)	**
APOE4 carrier (%)	71 (30%) (n = 228)	27 (19%)	44 (49%)	**
WML/TIV	0.17 ± 0.37 (0–2.8) (n = 229)	0.11 ± 0.25 (0–1.5)	0.28 ± 0.48 (0–2.8)	**
Cognitive reserve				
Education	15.8 ± 3.3 (6–29)	16 ± 3.1 (10–25)	15 ± 3.7 (6–29)	
MWT	31.9 ± 2.7 (21–37)	32.4 ± 2 (24–37)	31.1 ± 3 (21–37)	
Lifestyle index	16.2 ± 2.6 (7–22) (n = 139)	16.3 ± 2.5 (7–20)	16.1 ± 2.7 (9–22)	
Cognition				
MMSE	28.7 ± 1.2 (24–30)	29.0 ± 1.1 (26–30)	28.3 ± 1.4 (24–30)	**
G factor score	–	0.35 ± 0.8 (−1.6 to 1.8)	−0.55 ± 0.9 (−1.3 to 2.6)	**
Executive function factor score	–	0.25 ± 0.6 (−1.2 to 2.7)	−0.39 ± 1.1 (−1.1 to 4.7)	**
Memory factor score	–	0.33 ± 0.8 (−1.9 to 1.7)	−0.52 ± 0.9 (−2.5 to 1.3)	**

Numbers are expressed as mean ± standard deviation, the ranges shown in parenthesis
Cognition variables are the factor scores estimated in the latent variable models. Because the latent variables of cognition were scaled by standardization (M = 0; σ = 0), they are not displayed for the whole group. Group-specific average factor score can be thus interpreted as deviations from the whole sample average
White matter lesions (WML) data were missing in one participant (mild cognitive impairment (MCI): n = 1), and lifestyle index was missing in 91 participants (healthy older (HO): n = 61, MCI: n = 12)
APOE4 apolipoprotein E, MMSE Mini-Mental State Examination, MWT German multiple vocabulary test, TIV transcranial intracranial volume
**p < 0.01, independent sample test for continuous variables and chi-square test for categorical variables

Statistical analysis

The analysis objectives of this study can be summarized as follows. First, the direct effect of WML on cognitive performance (G, memory, and executive function in the overall cognitive model) was estimated. Next, we tested whether functional connectivity (global and local measures) within each resting state network moderated the relationship between WML and executive function and memory, respectively (Fig. 1, panel A). To this aim, we estimated latent moderated structures implemented in Mplus [51]. The moderation was assessed through an interactive term, modeled by the product of WML and functional connectivity values, respectively. Latent variables of executive functions and memory were then regressed onto WML volumes, functional connectivity measures, and their interactive term.

All models were estimated based on the whole sample of nondemented individuals, which includes healthy older individuals and individuals with MCI. This was done to include a larger spectrum of individuals in whom there is sufficient pathology to cause cognitive impairment. We furthermore conducted sensitivity analysis using multigroup structural equation modeling to explore, post hoc, the significant moderation effects within each group (healthy older individuals vs. MCI). Thus, latent interactions for testing moderation effects of functional connectivity on the relationship between WML and cognition were estimated separately, but simultaneously for healthy older individuals vs MCI. Because the model included a latent interaction between functional connectivity and the relationship between WML and cognition, such a model can be established as a latent interaction model using the mixture modeling framework of Mplus. In this framework the groups (healthy older individuals and MCI) are treated as known latent classes whereas the latent interaction is estimated simultaneously, but separately for the two classes (participant groups).

Factor scores, extracted from each latent variable, were used to visualize selected interactive relationships from regression models to better understand their directionality using the R package Jtool (available at: https://cran.r-project.org/web/packages/jtools/). Centered mean predicted scores were estimated for executive function and memory on two levels of low and high (−1 SD and +1 SD) functional connectivity measures. Finally, a mediation model was included to further validate our WML measure with CVD risk score and cognition [51].

Results

Sample characteristics

Descriptive information on the total sample of nonde-mented older participants as well as participants dichot-omized by group is provided in Table 1. The MCI group had a higher frequency of APOE4 carriers, was signifi-cantly older, and performed significantly worse on the cognitive measures (cognitive scores for each test are provided in Additional file 1: Table S3). The groups did not otherwise differ demographically. The lesion fre-quency maps of participants for the total sample and for each group category are provided in Fig. 2. The figure shows lesions situated predominately in periventricular areas with more pronounced lesions in the frontal regions.

Relationships between WML and cognition

Structural equational modeling confirmed negative rela-tionships between WML volumes and cognitive per-formance (Model fit: $\chi^2 = 73.06$, df = 36, $\chi^2/\text{df} = 2.02$, RMSEA = 0.06, SRMR = 0.04, CFI = 0.96). Larger WML volumes were significantly related to lower G ($\beta_1 = -0.27$, $p < 0.01$), having an even higher impact on execu-tive functions ($\beta_2 = -0.37$, $p < 0.01$) compared with mem-ory ($\beta_3 = -0.22$, $p < 0.01$) (Fig. 3). These effects remained significant when controlling for age and grey matter volume.

In a follow-up analysis, we added CVD risk to the model defined as a predictor of WML volumes and cog-nition to further validate our WML measure (model fit: $\chi^2 = 74$, df = 43, $\chi^{2/}\text{df} = 1.72$ RMSEA = 0.05, SRMR = 0.04, CFI = 0.97). CVD risk was related to worse cogni-tion (executive functions $\beta = -0.30$, $p < 0.01$ and memory $\beta = -0.26$ $p < 0.01$). This relationship was mediated by WML load, as indicated by a significant indirect effect ($\beta = -0.12$, confidence interval (CI) −0.244 to −0.001, and $\beta = -0.08$, CI −0.154 to −0.002) for executive func-tions and memory, respectively. Finally, there was no significant relationship between CVD risk factor and our behavioral measure of CR ($r = -0.046$, $p = 0.49$).

Relationships between WML, connectivity, and cognition

Global connectivity

First, we modeled global functional connectivity as a latent variable for each resting state network. The model fit for each resting state network is provided in Additional file 1 (Table S1). All standardized factor loadings were statisti-cally significant. Next, we tested whether global connectiv-ity measures moderated the relationship between WML and cognition. Global connectivity of the fronto-parietal network showed a significant moderating effect on the re-lationship between WML and executive function (non-standardized coefficient: $b = 2.39$, $p = 0.01$), but not for memory (nonstandardized coefficient: $b = -5.01$, $p = 0.51$).

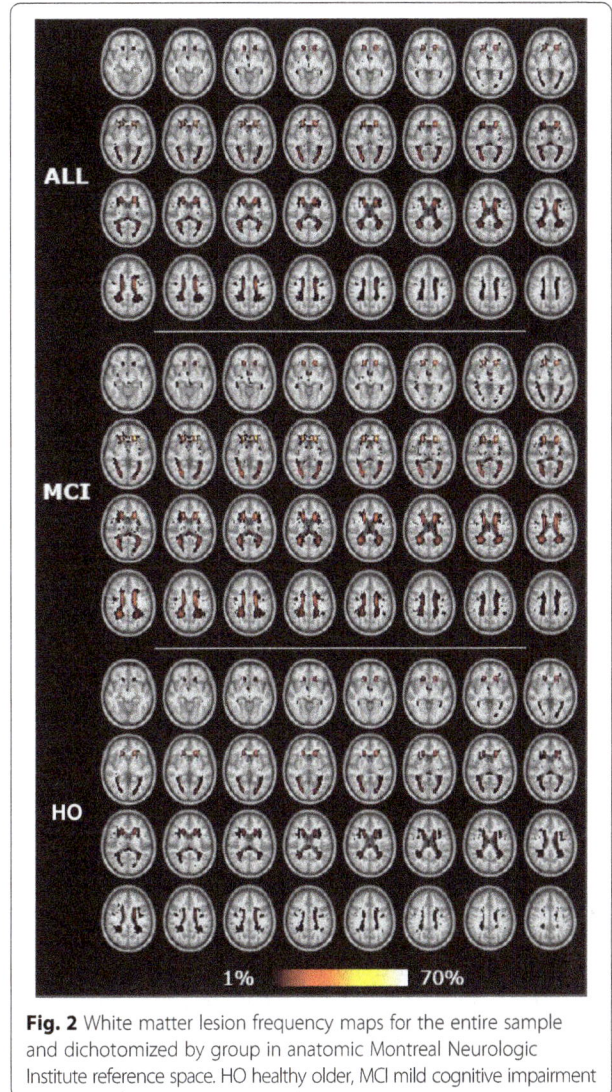

Fig. 2 White matter lesion frequency maps for the entire sample and dichotomized by group in anatomic Montreal Neurologic Institute reference space. HO healthy older, MCI mild cognitive impairment

Specifically, the negative impact of WML on executive functions was reduced in individuals with higher levels of global connectivity in the fronto-parietal network (Fig. 4a). No significant interactions between WML and global con-nectivity were found for the salience network (nonstan-dardized coefficients: $b = 0.24$, $p = 0.89$; $b = 0.15$, $p = 0.64$) and the default mode network (nonstandardized coeffi-cients: $b = 0.19$, $p = 0.55$; $b = 0.05$, $p = 0.80$) for executive functions and memory, respectively.

Local connectivity

For our local connectivity measure, we first used the behavioral measure of CR (modeled as a latent variable) as a predictor of local connectivity. Specific regions within the fronto-parietal network, the salience network, and the default mode network were positively related with CR at the given statistical threshold (with clusters in Additional file 1: Table S4). When testing for moderation effects, local

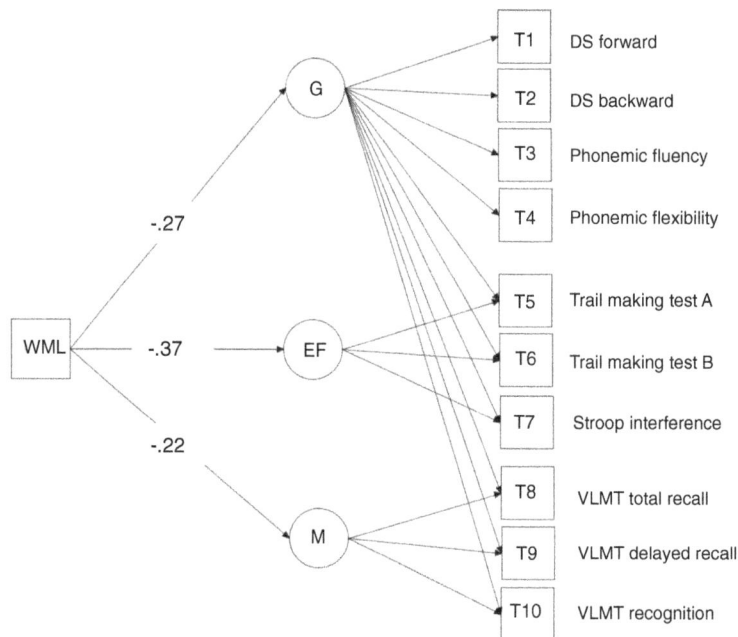

Fig. 3 Schematic representation of the structural equation model with path coefficients showing the direct effect of white matter lesions (WML) on the latent variables of global cognition (G), executive functions (EF), and memory (M). Note that the executive function tests were inverted to indicate better performance with higher scores. DS digit span, VLMT Auditory Verbal Learning Test

connectivity in the salience network (cluster shown in Fig. 4b, medial frontal cortex, cingulate gyrus; peak voxel MNI: $-12 + 38-4$, $p < 0.01$) showed a significant moderation effect on the relationship between WML volumes and executive functions (nonstandardized coefficient: $b = 3.92$, $p = 0.01$) and a trend for memory (nonstandardized coefficient: $b = 2.01$, $p = 0.07$). The negative impact of WML on executive functions was reduced in individuals with higher local connectivity in the ACC (Fig. 4b). No significant interactions between WML and local connectivity in the fronto-parietal network (nonstandardized coefficient: $b = -0.41$, $p = 0.85$; $b = -1.10$, $p = 0.31$) and the default mode network (non-standardized coefficient: $b = -0.82$, $p = 0.52$; $b = 0.38$, $p = 0.70$) were found for executive functions and memory, respectively (data not shown). All the effects reported above remained significant after controlling for age and grey matter volume.

Post-hoc multigroup analysis
Multigroup SEM examined the associations (moderations) across each diagnostic group, where the groups are handled as a higher-order moderator variable and interaction effects of functional connectivity on the relationship between WML and cognition are estimated within groups (see the explanation in the methods section). In the MCI sample, the moderating effect for global connectivity of the fronto-parietal network between WML and cognition remained significant for executive function (nonstandardized coefficient: $b = 3.10$,

$p < 0.01$). Likewise, the moderating effect of local connectivity within the salience network remained significant for both executive function and memory (nonstandardized coefficient: $b = 8.97$, $p < 0.01$; $b = 5.65$, $p < 0.01$, respectively). However, these moderating effects were not statistically substantial in the sample of healthy older individuals, for either the global fronto-parietal connectivity on executive function (nonstandardized coefficient: $b = 0.96$, $p = 0.31$), or for the local connectivity of the salience network (nonstandardized coefficient: $b = 1.28$, $p = 0.35$; $b = -0.34$, $p = 0.78$) executive functions and memory, respectively.

Discussion
The present study evaluated the moderating impact of functional connectivity on the relationship between WML and cognitive performance in nondemented older individuals. Our results indicated that higher levels of functional connectivity in the fronto-parietal network and salience network in part mitigate the negative effect of WML on executive functions, the cognitive domain most affected by cerebrovascular pathology. Analyses were performed with SEM, allowing us to abstract from measurement error and task specificity [45]. Our results support the notion that higher functional connectivity in cognitive control networks may serve as protective neural mechanism that allow better preservation of cognitive ability in the presence of cerebrovascular pathology.

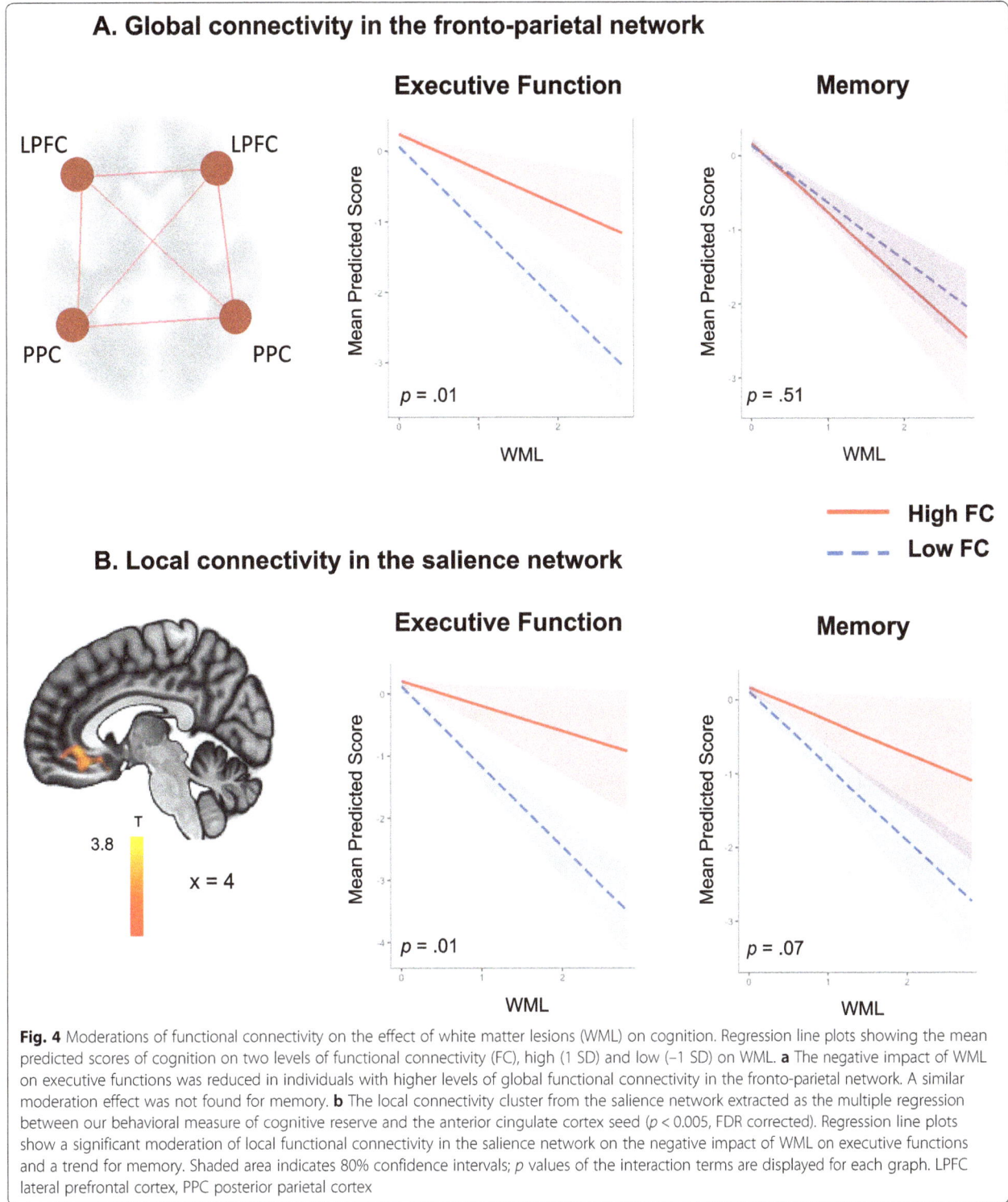

Fig. 4 Moderations of functional connectivity on the effect of white matter lesions (WML) on cognition. Regression line plots showing the mean predicted scores of cognition on two levels of functional connectivity (FC), high (1 SD) and low (–1 SD) on WML. **a** The negative impact of WML on executive functions was reduced in individuals with higher levels of global functional connectivity in the fronto-parietal network. A similar moderation effect was not found for memory. **b** The local connectivity cluster from the salience network extracted as the multiple regression between our behavioral measure of cognitive reserve and the anterior cingulate cortex seed ($p < 0.005$, FDR corrected). Regression line plots show a significant moderation of local functional connectivity in the salience network on the negative impact of WML on executive functions and a trend for memory. Shaded area indicates 80% confidence intervals; p values of the interaction terms are displayed for each graph. LPFC lateral prefrontal cortex, PPC posterior parietal cortex

Our results are consistent with the established literature, suggesting an association between higher WML load and lower cognitive performance in the domains of both memory and executive functions [1, 7]. WML tend to primarily affect processing speed and executive tasks in older participants with Alzheimer's disease, MCI, and normal cognition [5, 6, 52, 53]. Our results confirmed the stronger association with executive cognitive dysfunctions, with similar path coefficients as reported previously [17]. Although not always present [6], we found an association between lower memory performance and higher WML load, consistent with previous findings [5,

52]. The topography of WML (Fig. 2) show a higher frequency of lesions in frontal and periventricular regions, which is consistent with studies that report an association between WML frequency in these regions and decreased executive function and processing speed [6, 52]. In general, WML have been associated with a decline in cognitive domains linked to prefrontal cortex function and, to a lesser extent, with medial temporal lobe-associated memory tasks [4].

Consistent with our hypothesis, we found a significant moderating effect of the global functional connectivity in the fronto-parietal network. Thus, the negative impact of WML on executive functions was attenuated in individuals with higher global functional connectivity in this network. Our results are in line with previous findings that support the protective role of fronto-parietal network connectivity as a neural substrate of CR in both normal and pathological aging [54]. Higher functional connectivity (particularly in the left hub) has been associated with higher education and higher cognitive function in cognitively normal individuals and MCI patients [54] and has been shown to diminish the effect of Alzheimer's disease pathology on cognition [23, 55]. Our results further converge with the previous findings of Franzmeier and colleagues [23, 44]. These authors have repeatedly found evidence for a compensatory effect of the global connectivity in the fronto-parietal network in Alzheimer's disease pathology. Our results extend the evidence by demonstrating a protective role of the global fronto-parietal network against the detrimental impact of cerebrovascular pathology in the elderly.

At the local level, functional connectivity from the salience network showed a significant moderation on the impact of WML on cognition. More specifically, functional connectivity between the ACC (as seed) and the medial frontal cortex significantly mitigated the negative impact of WML on executive functions and, as a trend, this moderation effect was present for the memory domain. The regions involved in the local connectivity measure of the salience network (connectivity cluster in Fig. 4b) are in line with previous reports that show a positive correlation between connectivity from the ACC and the medial frontal cortex with higher levels of education and preserved cognitive performance in healthy elders [24]. Furthermore, a previous study [20] comparing MCI patients with low and high CR showed that the ACC was involved in regions showing connectivity changes at the local level. Our findings extend the possible beneficial effects of functional connectivity against WML to include the salience network regions.

Results from the post-hoc multigroup analysis showed the estimated interactions to be significant in the whole sample and in the MCI sample alone. There may not have been enough pathology in the healthy older group,

compared with the MCI, to yield a moderating relationship of functional connectivity on cognition. The smaller sample size of the subgroups may have also led to insufficient power to identify the effect with the healthy control group only. Our findings nevertheless support the idea that compensatory mechanisms are pronounced at the prodromal disease stage, where more neuropathology is present [56].

Both the salience and the fronto-parietal network are considered as important cognitive control networks crucial for regulation and healthy brain functioning. The fronto-parietal network is important for flexibly regulating activity to other functional networks [42], just as the salience network is crucial for integrating input from various sources [57]. Both networks support successful cognition with increased functional hub connectivity linked to better cognition [25, 58]. Higher or more efficient functional connectivity in these networks may facilitate adaptive functional connectivity to other brain regions when neurodegenerative insults occur. Our results show that, indeed, functional neural mechanisms convey reserve in the presence of cerebrovascular pathology and substantiate the notion that cognitive control networks may play an important role in resilience mechanisms.

The detection of resilient or protective mechanism are of increased recent interest given the rapidly aging population [59, 60]. Functional mechanisms underlying reserve may be suitable targets for therapeutic intervention to prevent further cognitive decline. For example, combining cognitive training and noninvasive brain stimulation over task-relevant brain areas may offer a means for cognitive enhancement in older adults, as demonstrated both in healthy older adults [61] as well as in patients with MCI [62] (see also [63] for a recent review). The present study suggests that targeting hubs specifically involved in resilient mechanisms may provide an additional approach to protect cognitive function against age-related conditions in the elderly.

There are several caveats that must be taken into consideration when interpreting our results. First, although our measure of WML is reliable, our sample was prescreened for cerebrovascular disease and included individuals with MCI. Thus, the compensatory mechanisms of functional connectivity should be replicated in a sample with higher WML load. Second, our measure of global functional connectivity as a latent variable may be specific to our SEM analysis. Our findings need to be completed by other functional connectivity measures, such as inter-network functional connectivity and degree of centrality and extended to other intrinsic brain networks [64]. A future line of work might specifically explore inter-network functional connectivity in order to elucidate the relationship of functional connectivity between networks. Third, the present study focused on functional connectivity; however, structural measures of white matter tracts through diffusion tensor imaging (DTI) should also be tested for attenuation effects underlying reserve. Recent work has explored the disruption of tract-specific WML on the default mode network [65]. However, the fronto-parietal and salience networks and their moderation effects should also be explored in this modality. Fourth, WML represent only one entity of the umbrella term of cerebrovascular disease; other pathologies (i.e. lacunes, small infarcts and microbleeds) should also be considered. More pronounced effects could be observed by the incorporation of these pathologies into the model. Finally, longitudinal studies are necessary to assess the neuroprotective trajectories of functional connectivity and whether there are nonlinear relationships with the increase in further pathology.

Conclusion
The results from the current study highlight the role of functional connectivity in cognitive control networks in attenuating the detrimental effects of cerebrovascular pathology in the elderly. Our findings shed light on neural mechanisms underlying reserve in the face of cerebrovascular pathology and suggest that the fronto-parietal network and the salience network may be suitable targets for early intervention strategies that aim to enhance CR in the elderly.

Abbreviations
ACC: Anterior cingulate cortex; CR: Cognitive reserve; CVD: Cardiovascular disease; LP: Lateral parietal; MPFC: Medial prefrontal cortex; WML: White matter lesions

Acknowledgments
We sincerely thank Dr. Daria Anthonenko, Dr. Kristin Prehn, Isabel Wrachtrup Calzado, and Andrea Dell'Orco for their support in neuroimaging analysis as well as bevioural data processing and results discussion. Additionally we would like to thank Dr. Jens Bohlken for his continued support with recruiting of participants from his practice in Berlin, Germany.

Funding
This work was supported by the Deutsche Forschungsgemeinschaft (FI 379-8/1, FI 379-10/1, FI 379-11/1, and DFG-Exc 257DFG), the Hans Gerhard Creutzfeldt scholarship (FKZ CSB II, 01EO1301 TP T2), and the NeuroCure Female Post-doctoral research fellowship.

Authors' contributions
GB, AH, and MW were responsible for the conception and design of the study and drafting the manuscript. GB, TK, and CL were responsible for the acquisition of data. GB, AH, and MW were responsible for the analysis and interpretation of data. AH, CS, AF, TK, WS, CL, and MW critically revised the manuscript. All authors read and approved the final manuscript.

Competing interests
The authors declare that they have no competing interests.

Author details
[1]NeuroCure Clinical Research Center, Department of Neurology, Charité – Universitätsmedizin Berlin, Freie Universität Berlin, Humboldt-Universität zu Berlin, Berlin Institute of Health, Berlin, Germany. [2]Department of Psychology, University Medicine Greifswald, Greifswald, Germany. [3]Department of Psychology, Humboldt-Universität zu Berlin, Berlin, Germany. [4]Department of Nuclear Medicine, Charité – Universitätsmedizin Berlin, Freie Universität Berlin, Humboldt-Universität zu Berlin, Berlin Institute of Health, Berlin, Germany. [5]Department of Psychiatry, McGill University, Montreal, Quebec, Canada. [6]Douglas Mental Health University Institute, Studies on Prevention of Alzheimer's Disease Centre, Montreal, Quebec, Canada. [7]Department of Neurology, University Medicine Greifswald, Greifswald, Germany. [8]Center for Stroke Research Berlin, Charité – Universitätsmedizin Berlin, Freie Universität Berlin, Humboldt-Universität zu Berlin, Berlin Institute of Health, Berlin, Germany.

References
1. Prins ND, Scheltens P. White matter hyperintensities, cognitive impairment and dementia: an update. Nat Rev Neurol. 2015;11:157–65.
2. Raz N, Rodrigue KM. Differential aging of the brain: patterns, cognitive correlates and modifiers. Neurosci Biobehav Rev. 2006;30:730–48.
3. Wirth M, Haase CM, Villeneuve S, Vogel J, Jagust WJ. Neuroprotective pathways: lifestyle activity, brain pathology, and cognition in cognitively normal older adults. Neurobiol Aging. 2014;35:1873–82.
4. Au R, Massaro JM, Wolf PA, Young ME, Beiser A, Seshadri S, et al. Association of white matter hyperintensity volume with decreased cognitive functioning: The Framingham Heart Study. Arch Neurol. 2006;63:246–50.
5. Tullberg M, Fletcher E, DeCarli C, Mungas D, Reed BR, Harvey DJ, et al. White matter lesions impair frontal lobe function regardless of their location. Neurology. 2004;63:246–53.
6. Birdsill AC, Koscik RL, Jonaitis EM, Johnson SC, Okonkwo OC, Hermann BP, et al. Regional white matter hyperintensities: aging, Alzheimer's disease risk, and cognitive function. Neurobiol Aging. 2014;35:769–76.
7. Wirth M, Villeneuve S, Haase CM, Madison CM, Oh H, Landau SM, et al. Associations between Alzheimer disease biomarkers, neurodegeneration, and cognition in cognitively normal older people. JAMA Neurol. 2013;70:1512–9.
8. Debette S, Markus HS. The clinical importance of white matter hyperintensities on brain magnetic resonance imaging: systematic review and meta-analysis. BMJ. 2010;341:1–9.
9. Nebes R, Meltzer C, Whyte E, Scanlon J, Halligan E, Saxton J, et al. The relation of white matter hyperintensities to cognitive performance in the normal old: education matters. Neuropsychol Dev Cogn B Aging Neuropsychol Cogn. 2006;13:326–40.
10. Saczynski JS, Jonsdottir MK, Sigurdsson S, Eiriksdottir G, Jonsson PV, Garcia ME, et al. White matter lesions and cognitive performance: the role of cognitively complex leisure activity. J Gerontol A Biol Sci Med Sci. 2008;63:848–54.
11. Stern Y. What is cognitive reserve? Theory and research application of the reserve concept. J Int Neuropsychol Soc. 2002;8:448–60.
12. Bartrés-Faz D, Arenaza-Urquijo EM. Structural and functional imaging correlates of cognitive and brain reserve hypotheses in healthy and pathological aging. Brain Topogr. 2011;24:340–57.
13. Barulli D, Stern Y. Efficiency, capacity, compensation, maintenance, plasticity: emerging concepts in cognitive reserve. Trends Cogn Sci. 2013;17:502–9.
14. Stern Y. Cognitive reserve. Neuropsychologia. 2009;47:2015–28.
15. Dufouil C, Alpérovitch A, Tzourio C. Influence of education on the relationship between white matter lesions and cognition. Neurol Int. 2003;60:831–6.
16. Zieren N, Duering M, Peters N, Reyes S, Jouvent E, Hervé D, et al. Education modifies the relation of vascular pathology to cognitive function: cognitive reserve in cerebral autosomal dominant arteriopathy with subcortical infarcts and leukoencephalopathy. Neurobiol Aging. 2013;34:400–7.

17. Brickman AM, Siedlecki KL, Muraskin J, Manly JJ, Luchsinger JA, Yeung LK, et al. White matter hyperintensities and cognition: testing the reserve hypothesis. Neurobiol Aging. 2011;32:1588–98.

18. Griebe M, Amann M, Hirsch JG, Achtnichts L, Hennerici MG, Gass A, et al. Reduced functional reserve in patients with age-related white matter changes: a preliminary fMRI study of working memory. PLoS One. 2014;9:e103359.

19. Fernández-Cabello S, Valls-Pedret C, Schurz M, Vidal-Piñeiro D, Sala-Llonch R, Bargallo N, et al. White matter hyperintensities and cognitive reserve during a working memory task: a functional magnetic resonance imaging study in cognitively normal older adults. Neurobiol Aging. 2016;48:23–33 Elsevier Inc.

20. Serra L, Mancini M, Cercignani M, Di Domenico C, Spanò B, Giulietti G, et al. Network-based substrate of cognitive reserve in Alzheimer's disease. J Alzheimers Dis. 2016;55:421–30.

21. Cole MW, Yarkoni T, Repovs G, Anticevic A, Braver TS. Global connectivity of prefrontal cortex predicts cognitive control and intelligence. J Neurosci. 2012; 32:8988–99.

22. Elman JA, Oh H, Madison CM, Baker SL, Vogel JW, Marks SM, et al. Neural compensation in older people with brain amyloid-β deposition. Nat Neurosci. 2014;17:1316–8.

23. Franzmeier N, Duering M, Weiner M, Dichgans M, Ewers M. Left frontal cortex connectivity underlies cognitive reserve in prodromal Alzheimer disease. Neurology. 2017;88:1054–61.

24. Arenaza-Urquijo EM, Landeau B, La Joie R, Mevel K, Mézenge F, Perrotin A, et al. Relationships between years of education and gray matter volume, metabolism and functional connectivity in healthy elders. Neuroimage. 2013;83C:450–7.

25. Menon V. Salience Network. Brain Mapp An Encycl Ref. 2015;2:597–611.

26. Folstein MF, Folstein SE, McHugh PR. "Mini-mental state". A practical method for grading the cognitive state of patients for the clinician. J Psychiatr Res. 1975;12:189–98.

27. Knopman DS, Petersen RC. Mild cognitive impairment and mild dementia: a clinical perspective. Mayo Clin Proc. 2014;89:1452–9.

28. Kerti L, Witte AV, Winkler A, Grittner U, Rujescu D, Flöel A. Higher glucose levels associated with lower memory and reduced hippocampal microstructure. Neurology. 2013;81:1746–52.

29. Köbe T, Witte AV, Schnelle A, Grittner U, Tesky VA, Pantel J, et al. Vitamin B-12 concentration, memory performance, and hippocampal structure in patients with mild cognitive impairment. Am J Clin Nutr. 2016;103:1045–54.

30. Lezak MD, Howieson DB, Loring DW, Hannay HJ, Fischer JS. Neuropsychological assessment. 4th ed; New York, Oxford: Oxford University Press; 2004.

31. Reitan R. Validity of the Trail Making Test as an indicator of organic brain damage. Percept Mot Skills. 1958;8:271–6.

32. Woodard JL, Axelrod BN. Wechsler Memory Scale–Revised. Psychol Assess. 1987;7:445–9.

33. Koss E, Ober BA, Delis DC, Friedland RP. The Stroop color-word test: indicator of dementia severity. Int J Neurosci. 1984;24:53–61.

34. Wechsler D. WAIS-R manual: Wechsler adult intelligence scale-revised. Psychological Corporation. 1981.

35. Harth S, Müller SV, Aschenbrenner S, Tucha O, Lange KW. Regensburger Wortflüssigkeits-Test (RWT). Z Neuropsychol. 2004;15:315–21. https://doi.org/10.1024/1016-264X.15.4.315.

36. Schmidt P, Gaser C, Arsic M, Buck D, Förschler A, Berthele A, et al. An automated tool for detection of FLAIR-hyperintense white-matter lesions in multiple sclerosis. Neuroimage. 2012;59:3774–83 Elsevier Inc.

37. Lange C, Suppa P, Maurer A, Ritter K, Pietrzyk U, Steinhagen-Thiessen E, et al. Mental speed is associated with the shape irregularity of white matter MRI hyperintensity load. Brain Imaging Behav. 2017;11:1720–730

38. Malone IB, Leung KK, Clegg S, Barnes J, Whitwell JL, Ashburner J, et al. Accurate automatic estimation of total intracranial volume: a nuisance variable with less nuisance. NeuroImage. 2015;104:366–72.

39. D'Agostino RB, Vasan RS, Pencina MJ, Wolf PA, Cobain M, Massaro JM, et al. General cardiovascular risk profile for use in primary care: The Framingham heart study. Circulation. 2008;117:743–53.

40. Whitfield-Gabrieli S, Nieto-Castanon A. Conn: A functional connectivity toolbox for correlated and anticorrelated brain networks. Brain Connect. 2012;2:125–41.

41. Behzadi Y, Restom K, Liau J, Liu TT. A component based noise correction method (CompCor) for BOLD and perfusion based fMRI. NeuroImage. 2007;37:90–101.

42. Cole MW, Repovs G, Anticevic A. The frontoparietal control system: a central role in mental health. Neuroscientist. 2014;20:652–64.

43. Bressler SL, Menon V. Large-scale brain networks in cognition: emerging methods and principles. Trends Cogn Sci. 2010;14:277–90

44. Franzmeier N, Caballero MÁA, Taylor ANW, Simon-Vermot L, Buerger K, Ertl-Wagner B, et al. Resting-state global functional connectivity as a biomarker of cognitive reserve in mild cognitive impairment. Brain Imaging Behav. 2017;11:368–82.

45. Muthén L, Muthén B. Mplus user's guide. 8th ed: Los Angeles CA: Muthén & Muthén 2017.

46. Hessler J, Jahn T, Kurz A, Bickel H. The MWT-B as an estimator of premorbid intelligence in MCI and dementia. Z Neuropsychol. 2013;24:129–37.

47. Flöel A, Witte a V, Lohmann H, Wersching H, Ringelstein EB, Berger K, et al. Lifestyle and memory in the elderly. Neuroepidemiology. 2008;31:39–47 [cited 2014 Mar 15].

48. Frey I, Berg A, Grathwohl D, Keul J. Freiburger Fragebogen zur kSrperlichen Aktivit it- Entwicklung, PriJfung und Anwendung. Soz Praventivmed. 1999;44:55–64.

49. Hu LT, Bentler PM. Cutoff criteria for fit indexes in covariance structure analysis: conventional criteria versus new alternatives. Struct Equ Model. 1999;6:1–55.

50. Cook RD. Detection of influential observation in linear regression. Technometrics. 1977;19:15–8.

51. Klein A, Moosbrugger H. Maximum likelihood estimation of latent interaction effects with the LMS method. Psychometrika. 2000;65:457–74.

52. Smith EE, Salat DH, Jeng J, McCreary CR, Fischl B, Schmahmann JD, et al. Correlations between MRI white matter lesion location and executive function and episodic memory. Neurology. 2011;76:1492–9.

53. Gunning-Dixon FM, Raz N. The cognitive correlates of white matter abnormalities in normal aging: a quantitative review. Neuropsychology. 2000;14:224–32.

54. Franzmeier N, Hartmann JC, Taylor ANW, Caballero MÁA, Simon-Vermot L, Buerger K, et al. Left frontal hub connectivity during memory performance supports reserve in aging and mild cognitive impairment. J Alzheimers Dis. 2017;59:1381–92.

55. Franzmeier N, Düzel E, Jessen F, Buerger K, Levin J, Duering M, et al. Left frontal hub connectivity delays cognitive impairment in autosomal-dominant and sporadic Alzheimer's disease. Brain. 2018;141:1186–200.

56. Arenaza-Urquijo EM, Wirth M, Chételat G. Cognitive reserve and lifestyle: moving towards preclinical Alzheimer's disease. Front Aging Neurosci. 2015;7:134.

57. Menon V, Uddin LQ. Saliency, switching, attention and control: a network model of insula function. Brain Struct Funct. 2010;214:655–67.

58. Liu J, Xia M, Dai Z, Wang X, Liao X, Bi Y, et al. Intrinsic brain hub connectivity underlies individual differences in spatial working memory. Cereb Cortex. 2017;27:5496–508.

59. Pinter D, Enzinger C, Fazekas F. Cerebral small vessel disease, cognitive reserve and cognitive dysfunction. J Neurol. 2015;262:2411–9.

60. Arenaza-Urquijo EM, Vemuri P. Resistance vs resilience to Alzheimer disease. Neurol Int. 2018;90:695–703.

61. Antonenko D, Külzow N, Sousa A, Prehn K, Grittner U, Flöel A. Neuronal and behavioral effects of multi-day brain stimulation and memory training. Neurobiol Aging. 2018;61:245–54.

62. Meinzer M, Lindenberg R, Phan MT, Ulm L, Volk C, Flöel A. Transcranial direct current stimulation in mild cognitive impairment: behavioral effects and neural mechanisms. Alzheimers Dement. 2015;11:1032–40.

63. Passow S, Thurm F, Li SC. Activating developmental reserve capacity via cognitive training or non-invasive brain stimulation: potentials for promoting fronto-parietal and hippocampal-striatal network functions in old age. Front Aging Neurosci. 2017;9:33.

64. Bullmore E, Sporns O. Complex brain networks: graph theoretical analysis of structural and functional systems. Nat Rev Neurosci. 2009;10:186–98.

65. Taylor ANW, Kambeitz-Ilankovic L, Gesierich B, Simon-Vermot L, Franzmeier N, Araque Caballero M, et al. Tract-specific white matter hyperintensities disrupt neural network function in Alzheimer's disease. Alzheimer's Dement. 2017;13:225–35.

The EMIF-AD PreclinAD study: study design and baseline cohort overview

Elles Konijnenberg[1][*] (iD), Stephen F. Carter[2], Mara ten Kate[1], Anouk den Braber[1,3], Jori Tomassen[1], Chinenye Amadi[2], Linda Wesselman[1], Hoang-Ton Nguyen[4], Jacoba A. van de Kreeke[4], Maqsood Yaqub[5], Matteo Demuru[1], Sandra D. Mulder[6], Arjan Hillebrand[7], Femke H. Bouwman[1], Charlotte E. Teunissen[6], Erik H. Serné[8], Annette C. Moll[4], Frank D. Verbraak[4], Rainer Hinz[9], Neil Pendleton[2], Adriaan A. Lammertsma[5], Bart N. M. van Berckel[5], Frederik Barkhof[5,10], Dorret I. Boomsma[3], Philip Scheltens[1], Karl Herholz[2] and Pieter Jelle Visser[1,11]

Abstract

Background: Amyloid pathology is the pathological hallmark in Alzheimer's disease (AD) and can precede clinical dementia by decades. So far it remains unclear how amyloid pathology leads to cognitive impairment and dementia. To design AD prevention trials it is key to include cognitively normal subjects at high risk for amyloid pathology and to find predictors of cognitive decline in these subjects. These goals can be accomplished by targeting twins, with additional benefits to identify genetic and environmental pathways for amyloid pathology, other AD biomarkers, and cognitive decline.

Methods: From December 2014 to October 2017 we enrolled cognitively normal participants aged 60 years and older from the ongoing Manchester and Newcastle Age and Cognitive Performance Research Cohort and the Netherlands Twins Register. In Manchester we included single individuals, and in Amsterdam monozygotic twin pairs. At baseline, participants completed neuropsychological tests and questionnaires, and underwent physical examination, blood sampling, ultrasound of the carotid arteries, structural and resting state functional brain magnetic resonance imaging, and dynamic amyloid positron emission tomography (PET) scanning with [18F]flutemetamol. In addition, the twin cohort underwent lumbar puncture for cerebrospinal fluid collection, buccal cell collection, magnetoencephalography, optical coherence tomography, and retinal imaging.

Results: We included 285 participants, who were on average 74.8 ± 9.7 years old, 64% female. Fifty-eight participants (22%) had an abnormal amyloid PET scan.

Conclusions: A rich baseline dataset of cognitively normal elderly individuals has been established to estimate risk factors and biomarkers for amyloid pathology and future cognitive decline.

Keywords: Preclinical Alzheimer's disease, Amyloid, Cognitively normal, Monozygotic twins, [18F]flutemetamol

Background

Alzheimer's disease (AD) is the most common cause of dementia and is characterized by amyloid plaques and neurofibrillary tangles with subsequently progressive neuronal loss and eventually death [1]. Aggregation of amyloid is supposed to be the first event in AD and starts years before cognitive impairment occurs [2–4].

Postmortem pathological and biomarker studies have demonstrated that 20–40% of cognitively normal elderly individuals possess abnormal amyloid levels in their brain [4–9]. These subjects are considered to be in the preclinical stage of AD [10, 11]. This presymptomatic window provides a unique opportunity for secondary prevention studies, as subjects have limited brain damage and no symptoms yet. Understanding the pathophysiological mechanisms underlying amyloid pathology in this preclinical stage of AD might also be critical to

* Correspondence: e.konijnenberg@vumc.nl
[1]Alzheimer Center, Department of Neurology, VU University Medical Center, Neuroscience Amsterdam, PO Box 7057, 1007 MB Amsterdam, The Netherlands
Full list of author information is available at the end of the article

identify possible drug targets for the development of effective treatments.

There are, however, several research challenges for the development of prevention strategies in the preclinical AD stage. First, amyloid markers are needed for the diagnosis of preclinical AD. There is an urgent need for readily applicable screening markers, such as blood or imaging markers, to identify cognitively normal subjects at increased risk for amyloid pathology so that more expensive or invasive tests such as positron emission tomography (PET) scan or cerebrospinal fluid (CSF) via lumbar puncture can be performed in more selected populations. A number of markers have already been identified for this purpose but these need to be validated in preclinical/prodromal stages of the disease [12–15]. Second, there is still an incomplete understanding of what drives the development of amyloid pathology in cognitively normal subjects. Previous studies have identified a limited number of risk factors for amyloid pathology, such as Apolipoprotein E (APOE) genotype, age, and level of education [4, 16–18]. These established risk factors, however, can only explain part of the risk for amyloid pathology. Third, amyloid pathology has been associated with an increased risk for cognitive decline, but the rate of decline varies greatly [19]. A few possible prognostic factors in preclinical AD have been identified but they await replication [20, 21]. Fourth, current normative data for biomarkers and cognitive markers may be suboptimal as many cognitively normal subjects already have amyloid pathology. Finally, CSF and PET biomarkers for amyloid pathology do not match in about 15% of cases [22–24], in particular in cognitively normal subjects. It has been suggested that amyloid changes can be detected earlier in CSF than by PET but this requires further investigation [25].

In this paper, we describe the study design of the multisite PreclinAD study, which aims to address these clinical research challenges. Within this study, cognitively normal elderly individuals are recruited from the Manchester and Newcastle Age and Cognitive Performance Research Cohort (ACPRC) in Manchester [26] and the Netherlands Twin Register (NTR) in Amsterdam [27]. From the NTR we recruited monozygotic (MZ) twins. When a relation is observed between two markers, studying MZ twins enables exploring the nature of the observed relation: the MZ twin differences approach gives the possibility to study the relation excluding confounding by genetic factors (the twins are genetically identical); and the cross-twin cross-trait design, studying whether marker 1 in one twin can predict marker 2 in their co-twin, gives the opportunity to study the contribution of shared familial factors (genes and common environment) to the relation. Previous studies using AD-type dementia as an outcome estimated the amount of variance explained by genetic factors to be around 80% [28], suggesting a major genetic role in the development of AD. However, there is a lack of studies estimating the contribution of genetic and environmental influences on AD biomarkers in nondemented individuals and the role of environmental risk and protective factors for AD remains unclear [18].

The PreclinAD study aimed to: validate existing and discover new markers for amyloid pathology in cognitively normal elderly individuals; identify risk factors for amyloid pathology; identify prognostic markers for cognitive decline in cognitively normal subjects with amyloid pathology (Fig. 1); and determine the contribution of genetic and environmental influences on these markers.

Methods

Project

The European Medical Information Framework for AD

The study is part of the Innovative Medicine Initiative European Medical Information Framework for AD

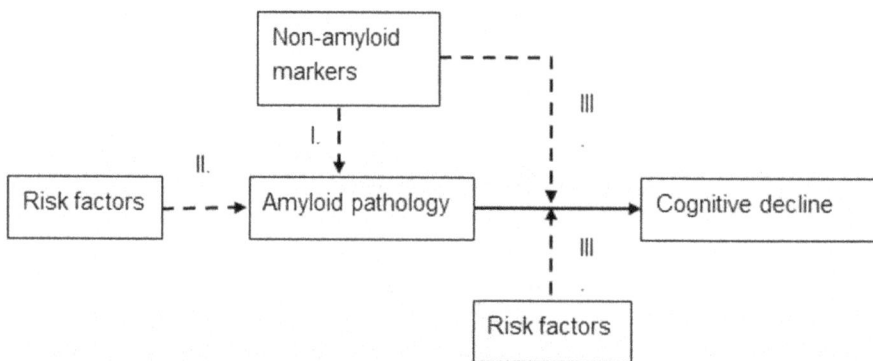

Fig. 1 Hypothetical model of amyloid pathology. Hypothetical model for evaluating risk factors for amyloid pathology, for cognitive decline in subjects with amyloid pathology and other markers that might be involved in early AD pathology. (I) Markers for amyloid pathology in cognitively healthy elderly individuals; (II) risk factors for amyloid pathology; (III) prognostic markers for cognitive decline in cognitively normal subjects with amyloid pathology

(EMIF-AD) project, which aims to facilitate the development of treatment for AD in nondemented subjects (http://www.emif.eu/) by discovering and validating diagnostic markers, prognostic markers, and risk factors for AD in nondemented subjects using existing data resources where possible.

Sample selection

We included 81 cognitively normal participants from the ACPRC. The ACPRC originally comprised over 6000 adults from the North of England, UK, who underwent detailed batteries of cognitive function biannually until 2003 [26]. In 1999 and 2000, active members of this cohort were invited and consented to provide a deoxyribonucleic acid (DNA) sample to the Dyne-Steel DNA Archive for study of Cognitive Genetics in later life. In 2003, a subsample of 500 Manchester volunteers underwent detailed physical examination and provided samples of saliva, serum, and plasma. Over time, the cohort has reduced in size through attrition, largely by mortality, to a number of approximately 660 volunteers. Since 2003, study participants have been assessed biannually with a smaller battery of tests and rating scales in order to diagnose pathological cognitive impairment and emotional problems. The current study coincides with the fourth wave of follow-up investigations. In Amsterdam, monozygotic twins were recruited from the NTR [29]. The NTR started recruiting adolescent and adult twins and their relatives in 1987 and had included over 200,000 participants by 2012 [27]. Twins who gave consent for the NTR also allow researchers to approach them for participation in scientific studies. From 1991 onward, participants completed extensive questionnaires every 2 or 3 years and DNA was collected in the NTR-Biobank project [30]. Smaller subgroups of participants underwent biomarker collection such as laboratory tests, electroencephalogram, or magnetic resonance imaging (MRI) [31–33]. The current study is a new NTR sub study.

Ethical considerations

The National Research Ethics Service Committee North West—Greater Manchester South performed ethical approval of the study in Manchester. The Medical Ethics Review Committee of the VU University Medical Center performed approval of the study in Amsterdam. Research was performed according to the principles of the Declaration of Helsinki and in accordance with the Medical Research Involving Human Subjects Act and codes on 'good use' of clinical data and biological samples as developed by the Dutch Federation of Medical Scientific Societies. All participants gave written informed consent.

Inclusion criteria

Inclusion criteria for the PreclinAD cohort were age 60 years and older, a delayed recall score above – 1.5 SD of demographically adjusted normative data on the Consortium to Establish a Registry for Alzheimer's Disease 10-word list [34, 35], a Telephone Interview for Cognitive Status-modified score of 23 or higher [36], a 15-item Geriatric Depression Scale score < 11 [37], and a Clinical Dementia Rating score of 0 [38] (Additional file 1: Table S1).

Exclusion criteria

To avoid possible interference with normal cognition, subjects with the following medical conditions, at present or in the past, were excluded: diagnosis of mild cognitive impairment (MCI), probable AD or other neurodegenerative disorders such as Huntington disease, cortical basal degeneration, multiple system atrophy, Creutzfeldt-Jakob disease, primary progressive aphasia or Parkinson's disease, stroke resulting in physical impairment, epilepsy with current use of antiepileptic drugs, brain infection (e.g., herpes simplex encephalitis), brain tumor, severe head trauma with loss of consciousness longer than 5 min, cancer with terminal life expectancy, untreated vitamin B12 deficiency, diabetes mellitus, thyroid disease, schizophrenia, bipolar disorders, or recurrent psychotic disorders. Furthermore, a history of recreational drug use, alcohol consumption > 35 units per week (1 unit = 10 ml or 8 g of pure alcohol), use of high-dose benzodiazepine, lithium carbonate, antipsychotics (including atypical agents), high-dose antidepressants, or Parkinson's disease medication were exclusion criteria. Finally, subjects who were not able to attend the hospital due to physical morbidity or illness or who had a contraindication for MRI (e.g., metal implants, pacemaker, etc.) were excluded (Additional file 1: Table S1).

Data collection

Neuropsychological testing battery and questionnaires

During a 4-h screening research facility visit (Manchester) or home visit (Amsterdam), participants underwent extensive neuropsychological testing and questionnaires. A complete overview of the neuropsychological testing battery and questionnaires is presented in Additional file 2: Table S2 and Additional file 3: Table S3, respectively. In short, we assessed memory function with the Rey auditory verbal learning task [39], visual association task [40], face–name associative memory examination [41], Rey complex figure recall [42], CANTAB paired associate learning [43], and digit span [44]. We also tested verbal fluency, naming [45], visuo-constructional skills, and executive functions [42, 46, 47] (see Additional file 2: Table S2). Using questionnaires we assessed social and physical activities [48–50], sleep quality [51, 52], activities of daily living [53, 54], memory complaints [55], and psychiatric symptoms [56] (see Additional file 3: Table S3).

Physical examination

Data on waist circumference, hip circumference, body mass index, resting blood pressure, heart rate, and grip strength of the dominant hand were collected for all participants (Table 1). In Manchester, an ankle/brachial pressure index and a 4-min walking test were also performed. In Amsterdam, a trained physician performed exploratory neurological examination. In addition, bioelectrical impedance analysis, repeated resting blood pressure measurement, and lead 1 of an electrocardiogram (measured by holding a Diagnostick [57] for 1 min) were performed and a color photograph of the face of each participant was taken. See Table 1 and Additional file 4: Table S4 for all biomarker data availability.

Blood collection

For all participants, 50 ml of blood was collected in the morning, after 2 h of fasting, including EDTA blood for DNA isolation, plasma, and buffy coat, clotted blood for serum, and Paxgene tubes for RNA isolation. Immediate plasma analysis was performed for complete blood count, hemoglobin A1C, 2-h fasting glucose, liver enzymes, lipid spectrum, C-reactive protein, erythrocyte sedimentation rate, thyroid stimulating hormone, and vitamin B12. EDTA tubes with anticoagulated whole blood were centrifuged at $1300–2000 \times g$ for 10 min, and plasma and remaining buffy coat were, like whole blood for collecting serum, aliquoted according to the standardized operating procedures of the BIOMAR-KAPD project [58] in aliquots of 0.25–0.5 ml and stored locally until analysis. All samples were stored at – 80 °C within 2 h. Two 2.5-ml Paxgene tubes were stored at room temperature for a minimum of 2 h and a maximum of 72 h, before they were frozen at – 20 °C until RNA isolation. The EDTA whole blood tube for DNA analysis was stored at – 20 °C until isolation.

DNA and RNA collection

Extraction of DNA and RNA from peripheral blood samples was performed at both sites. In addition, at the Amsterdam site, buccal cells were collected for zygosity, genome-wide association studies, and epigenetics [59]. Amsterdam participants were genotyped on the Affymetrix Axiom array and the Affymetrix 6 array [60]; these were first cross-chip imputed following the protocols described by Fedko et al. [61] and then imputed into HRC with the Michigan Imputation server [62]. The APOE genotypes were assessed using isoforms in Manchester as described by Ghebranious et al. [63]. In Amsterdam, the APOE genotype was assessed using imputed dosages of

the SNPs rs429358 (APOE ε4, imputation quality = 0.956) and rs7412 (APOE ε2, imputation quality = 0.729) [64].

Ultrasound carotid artery

In Manchester, a duplex ultrasound scan of the left and right carotid arteries was performed to collect data on velocity, vessel thickness, stenosis, and plaques rated according to the North American Symptomatic Carotid Endarterectomy Trial guidelines [65]. In Amsterdam, a duplex ultrasound scan of the right carotid artery was performed to assess intima media thickness and distension using ArtLab software [66–68].

Magnetic resonance imaging

Acquisition protocol In Manchester, brain scans were performed at the Wellcome Trust Manchester Clinical Research Facility (Central Manchester University Hospital NHS Foundation Trust). All MRI investigations were performed on a 3 T Philips Achieva scanner using a 32-channel head coil. Participants underwent an MRI protocol that included 3D-T1, 3D fluid-attenuated inversion recovery (FLAIR), pseudocontinuous arterial spin labeling (ASL), and quantitative magnetization transfer scans. In Amsterdam, brain scans were also obtained using a 3 T Philips Achieva scanner equipped with an eight-channel head coil. The MRI protocol included structural 3D-T1, FLAIR, pseudocontinuous ASL, susceptibility weighted imaging (SWI), diffusion tensor imaging (DTI), and 6 min of resting state functional MRI (rs-fMRI). The MRI settings are presented in Additional file 5: Table S5.

Visual assessment All MRI scans were reviewed for incidental findings by an experienced neuroradiologist, and visually rated by a single experienced rater (MtK) who was blinded to demographic information and twin pairing at the moment of rating. White matter hyperintensities were visually assessed on the FLAIR images using the 4-point Fazekas scale (none, punctuate, early confluent, confluent) [69]. Lacunes were defined as deep lesions from 3 to 15 mm with CSF-like signal on T1-weighted and FLAIR images. Microbleeds were assessed on SWI scans and defined as rounded hypointense homogeneous foci of up to 10 mm in the brain parenchyma. Medial temporal lobe atrophy was assessed on coronal reconstructions of the T1-weighted images using a 5-point visual rating scale [70]. Global cortical atrophy was rated on transversal FLAIR images using a 4-point scale [71]. Posterior cortical atrophy was assessed using a 4-point visual rating scale [72].

Amyloid positron emission tomography

[18F]flutemetamol In both centers, [18F]flutemetamol was used as a fibrillar amyloid radiotracer.

Table 1 Sample characteristics

Demographic	n	Combined sample (n = 285)	n	Amsterdam site (n = 204)	n	Manchester site (n = 81)
Age (years)	285	75.0 (9.7) (range 60–95)	204	70.8 (7.8) (range 60–94)	81	85.7 (4.3)*** (range 79–95)
Gender (% female)	285	182 (64%)	204	119 (58%)	81	63 (78%)**
Education (years)	278	14.8 (4.2)	204	14.9 (4.5)	74	14.2 (3.0)
NART	285	41.9 (6.0)	204	41.2 (6.4)	81	43.7 (4.3)***
MMSE	281	28.9 (1.2)	204	28.9 (1.2)	77	28.7 (1.3)
TICS-m	282	28.3 (3.2)	204	28.3 (3.0)	78	28.5 (3.7)
CERAD 10-word recall	285	22.8 (3.3)	204	22.0 (3.0)	81	24.8 (3.3)***
GDS	282	1.0 (1.5)	204	0.7 (1.2)	78	1.9 (1.7)***
CDR total	284	0 (0.1)	204	0	80	0.03 (0.1)*
CDR sum of boxes	284	0.03 (0.1)	204	0	80	0.1 (0.3)**
APOE e4 carrier	282	85 (30%)	202	66 (33%)	80	19 (24%)
APOE4 genotype	282		202		80	
e2e2		2 (1%)		2 (1%)		–
e2e3		24 (9%)		12 (6%)		12 (15%)
e2e4		9 (3%)		6 (3%)		3 (4%)
e3e3		171 (61%)		122 (60%)		49 (61%)
e3e4		69 (25%)		54 (27%)		15 (19%)
e4e4		7 (3)		6 (3%)		1 (1%)
Family history dementia	273	106 (39%)	203	92 (45%)	70	14 (20%)***
Diabetes type II	–	–	204	13 (6%)	–	–
Current smoker	281	23 (8%)	203	21 (10%)	78	2 (3%)
Alcohol use present	282	224 (79%)	204	158 (77%)	78	66 (85%)
Blood pressure (mmHg)	281	152 (21)/80 (12)	202	155 (21)/83 (11)	79	143 (19)/70 (10)***
Pulse rate (beats/min)	279	66 (11)	202	65 (11)	77	69 (10)**
Height (m)	283	1.66 (0.10)	204	1.69 (0.09)	79	1.60 (0.08)***
Weight (kg)	283	73.1 (14.0)	204	75.7 (13.6)	79	66.6 (13.0)***
Body mass index	283	26.3 (4.0)	204	26.4 (3.8)	79	26.1 (4.3)
Waist circumference (cm)	282	93.4 (13.6)	203	94.7 (12.0)	79	89.9 (16.6)**
Hip circumference (cm)	234	101.9 (11.4)	155	102.6 (9.8)	79	100.5 (14.0)
Grip strength (kg)	283	28.5 (11.3)	204	30.9 (10.9)	79	22.2 (9.8)***
CSF Aβ1–42 (pg/ml)	–	–	126	889 (314)	–	–
CSF Aβ1–40 (pg/ml)	–	–	126	9592 (2844)	–	–
Ratio CSF Aβ1–42/1–40	–	–	126	0.10 (0.03)	–	–
CSF total-tau (pg/ml)	–	–	126	412 (143)	–	–
CSF p-tau 181 (pg/ml)	–	–	126	76 (44)	–	–
Visual read PET abnormal	272	58 (22%)	196	32 (16%)	76	26 (34%)**
Fazekas score	279	1.3 (0.9)	199	1.2 (0.8)	80	1.7 (0.8)***
Medial temporal lobe atrophy score (average left and right)	277	0.7 (0.7)	197	0.6 (0.7)	80	0.9 (0.6)*
Parietal atrophy (average left and right)	279	1.1 (0.7)	199	1.1. (0.7)	80	1.2 (0.6)*

Data presented as mean (standard deviation) or n (%)

NART National Adult Reading Test, MMSE Mini-Mental State Examination, TICS-m Modified Telephone Interview for Cognitive Status, CERAD Consortium to Establish A Registry for Alzheimer's Disease, GDS Geriatric Depression Scale, CDR Clinical Dementia Rating, APOE Apolipoprotein E, CSF cerebrospinal fluid, Aβ amyloid beta, p-tau phosphorylated tau, PET positron emission tomography

***$p < 0.001$, **$p < 0.01$, *$p < 0.05$, group difference assessed with t test or chi-square test

[^{18}F]flutemetamol is an ^{11}C-Pittsburgh compound B (PiB) derivative radiolabeled with ^{18}F and has structural similarity to PiB, which is a frequently used compound for in-vivo detection of amyloid plaques [73]. In Manchester, the tracer [^{18}F]flutemetamol was produced at the Wolfson Molecular Imaging Centre (WMIC) Good Manufacturing Practice radiochemistry facility using General Electric Healthcare's (GEHC) FASTlab and cassettes. For Amsterdam, the same tracer was produced at the Cyclotron Research Center of the University of Liège (Liège, Belgium). GEHC was responsible for production and transportation of [^{18}F]flutemetamol. Prior [^{18}F]flutemetamol studies showed good brain uptake and radiation dosimetry similar to other radiopharmaceuticals in clinical use, test–retest variability for image quantitation differentiation between healthy participants and patients with AD, and the ability to detect brain Aβ [73].

Acquisition protocol At both sites, all participants were scanned dynamically from 0 to 30 min and then again from 90 to 110 min after intravenous injection of 185 MBq ($\pm$ 10%) [^{18}F]flutemetamol. The initial scan (0–30 min) was shortened or omitted if it was not accepted or tolerated by the participant. The second time window (90–110 min) is the recommended interval for assessment of amyloid biomarker abnormality. In Manchester, all PET scans were performed on a high-resolution research tomograph brain scanner (HRRT; Siemens/CTI, Knoxville, TN, USA) at the WMIC of the University of Manchester. Two 7-min transmission scans using a ^{137}Cs point source were acquired for subsequent attenuation and scatter correction; one prior to the first emission scan, and another following the second emission scan [74, 75]. In Amsterdam, all PET scans were performed using a Philips Ingenuity Time-of-Flight PET–MRI scanner at the Department of Radiology & Nuclear Medicine of the VU University Medical Center. Immediately prior to each part of the PET scan, a dedicated MR sequence (atMR) was performed for attenuation correction of the PET image [76]. For both sites, the first dynamic emission scan was reconstructed into 18 frames with progressive increase in frame length (6 × 5 s, 3 × 10 s, 4 × 60 s, 2 × 150 s, 2 × 300 s, 1 × 600 s). The second part of the scan consisted of 4 × 5-min frames. During scanning, the head was immobilized to reduce movement artifacts using laser beams.

Visual assessment All [^{18}F]flutemetamol amyloid PET scans were checked for movement and the frames were summed to obtain a static image (90–110 min). PET images were visually read as abnormal or normal by an experienced reader (SFC in Manchester and BNMvB in Amsterdam), blinded to clinical and demographic data,

according to GEHC guidelines described in the summary of product characteristics [77].

CSF collection (Amsterdam site only)

Up to 20 ml of CSF was obtained by lumbar puncture in Sarstedt polypropylene syringes using a Spinocan 25-gauge needle in one of the intervertebral spaces between L3 and S1. One milliliter was immediately processed for leukocyte count, erythrocyte count, glucose, and total protein. The remaining CSF was mixed and centrifuged at 1300–2000 × g for 10 min at 4 °C. Supernatants were stored in aliquots of 0.25–0.5 ml and frozen within 2 h at – 80 °C and stored for future biomarker discovery studies [78]. Levels of amyloid β1–40 and β1–42 were analyzed using kits from ADx Neurosciences/Euroimmun according to the manufacturer's instructions. All samples were measured in kits from the same lot.

Magnetoencephalography (Amsterdam site only)

Magnetoencephalography (MEG) measurements were recorded using a 306-channel, whole-head MEG system (ElektaNeuromag Oy, Helsinki, Finland) in a magnetically shielded room (Vacuumschmelze GmbH, Hanau, Germany). Participants were instructed to lie on a bed with their eyes closed but to stay awake and reduce eye movements in order to minimize artifacts. Participants were scanned for 5 min with eyes closed, 2 min with eyes open, and another 5 min with eyes closed. On MEG we used source-reconstructed time series (https://doi.org/10.1016/j.neuroimage.2011.11.005) to extract both frequency spectrum properties (relative band power and peak frequency) and functional connectivity between regions, as well as network topology using modern network theory (synchronization likelihood, modularity, path length, phase lag index) [79, 80]. These analysis techniques were applied using BrainWave software (http://home.kpn.nl/stam7883/brainwave.html) [81] and inhouse MATLAB scripts (MATLAB Release 2012a; The MathWorks, Inc., Natick, MA, USA).

Ophthalmological markers (Amsterdam site only)

Exploratory eye examination An exploratory eye examination including measurement of best corrected visual acuity, refractive error, and intra-ocular pressure (noncontact tonometry) was performed. In a subsample (n = 50), slit lamp examination by a trained physician was performed as well.

Ocular coherence tomography Ocular coherence tomography (OCT) was performed using the Heidelberg Spectralis. With OCT we measured retinal nerve fiber layer tissue, total macular thickness, and the thickness of macular individual retinal layers using the built-in segmentation software from the Spectralis [82], which might correlate with cerebral amyloid pathology [83]. With the same device, fundus autofluorescence was performed to try to detect degenerative retinal abnormalities possibly related to amyloid pathology [83, 84].

Retinal imaging Using a nonmydriatic camera (Topcon), two digital images (mostly 50°, and some 30°) per eye were taken of the retina—one centered to the macula, and the other to the optic nerve head—after pupil dilation with tropicamide. On the digitalized fundoscopy image we measured retinal vascular parameters using the Singapore I vessel Assessment software [85].

Data management
Data were stored in the online database CASTOR (https://castoredc.com/) with restricted access. Each site provided clinical information and sample information to the database according to a predefined case report form. Blood and CSF samples, PET and MRI scans, and MEG data are stored locally until centralized analysis.

Follow-up visit
A follow-up visit including neuropsychological testing, questionnaires at both sites, and physical examination, blood sampling, buccal cell collection, and lumbar puncture in a subset will be performed after 21 months ± 3 months.

Follow-up started in February 2017 and is still ongoing. So far 241 individuals have been invited, and of those 221 (92%) participated in the follow-up.

For the twin pairs, an additional follow-up visit after 4 years is planned, starting in January 2019. This follow-up includes amyloid-PET, tau-PET, MRI, lumbar puncture, neuropsychological testing, questionnaires, physical examination, blood sampling, and buccal cell collection.

Statistical approaches
Group analysis
The main outcome measure will be the presence of amyloid pathology as a dichotomous and continuous outcome measure. We aim to identify for each diagnostic modality the best set of predictors for amyloid pathology using step forward selection. The best predictors for each modality will be combined in a single risk score, based on the β value of these predictors in the regression model. Analysis will be performed using multivariate multilevel generalized estimating equation analysis with correction for age, gender, education, and twin status (Amsterdam only) [86]. In addition, as there are differences between the cohorts, we will correct for cohort in the analysis and test interactions of predictor variables with cohort to check whether pooling the data may introduce a bias.

Results
Inclusion
Manchester
From the ACPRC, 321 subjects in total were invited by letter to participate in the PreclinAD study. From this selection, 81 subjects were included for participation (see Fig. 2a).

Amsterdam
In total 517 twins from the NTR were invited by letter. Of these, 100 complete pairs (99 MZ, one dizygotic, as confirmed with DNA analysis) and four singletons, of which the co-twin did not meet the inclusion criteria due to cognitive impairment of other neurological conditions, were included (see Fig. 2b). This also included one twin who appeared to be demented at baseline hospital visit, even though this subject passed the inclusion criteria at first, and one subject from a monozygotic triplet, which we included due to the unique opportunity to analyze a genetically identical triplet, but this subject did not meet the inclusion criteria due to MCI. All participants, except for one twin pair, have European descent. When analyzing genetic data this twin pair will be excluded from the analysis.

Demographics and biomarkers
Participants were on average 74.8 years old, 64% female, and 30% APOE ε4 carriers; for further baseline characteristics see Table 1. Participants tested in Manchester were older compared to Amsterdam participants (85.7 vs 70.8 years, $p < 0.001$) and more often female (78 vs 58%, $p < 0.01$). Manchester participants also had a higher intelligence score according to the Adult Reading Task (43.7 vs 41.2, $p < 0.001$), less often a family member with dementia (20 vs 45%, $p < 0.001$), lower blood pressure, (143/70 vs 155/83 mmHg, $p < 0.001$), and higher white matter lesion load according to the Fazekas score (1.7 vs 1.2, $p < 0.001$) (Table 1).

Amyloid data were available for 275 participants (Manchester $n = 76$, Amsterdam $n = 199$). In Amsterdam, 123 participants had both CSF and PET available, 73 PET only, and three CSF only. For 10 participants we were unable to assess their amyloid status: six participants were not able to attend the hospital after inclusion, one participant did not undergo PET due to meningiomas on MRI, two participants suffered from claustrophobia during the hospital visit, and one participant had a panic attack before injection of the PET tracer. Dynamic PET scans were present in 261 participants: four participants failed their dynamic scan due to logistic problems, and in seven participants quality control of the images failed.

Amyloid pathology
Of the 272 participants with a static PET amyloid measure available, 58 (21%) had an abnormal PET scan as

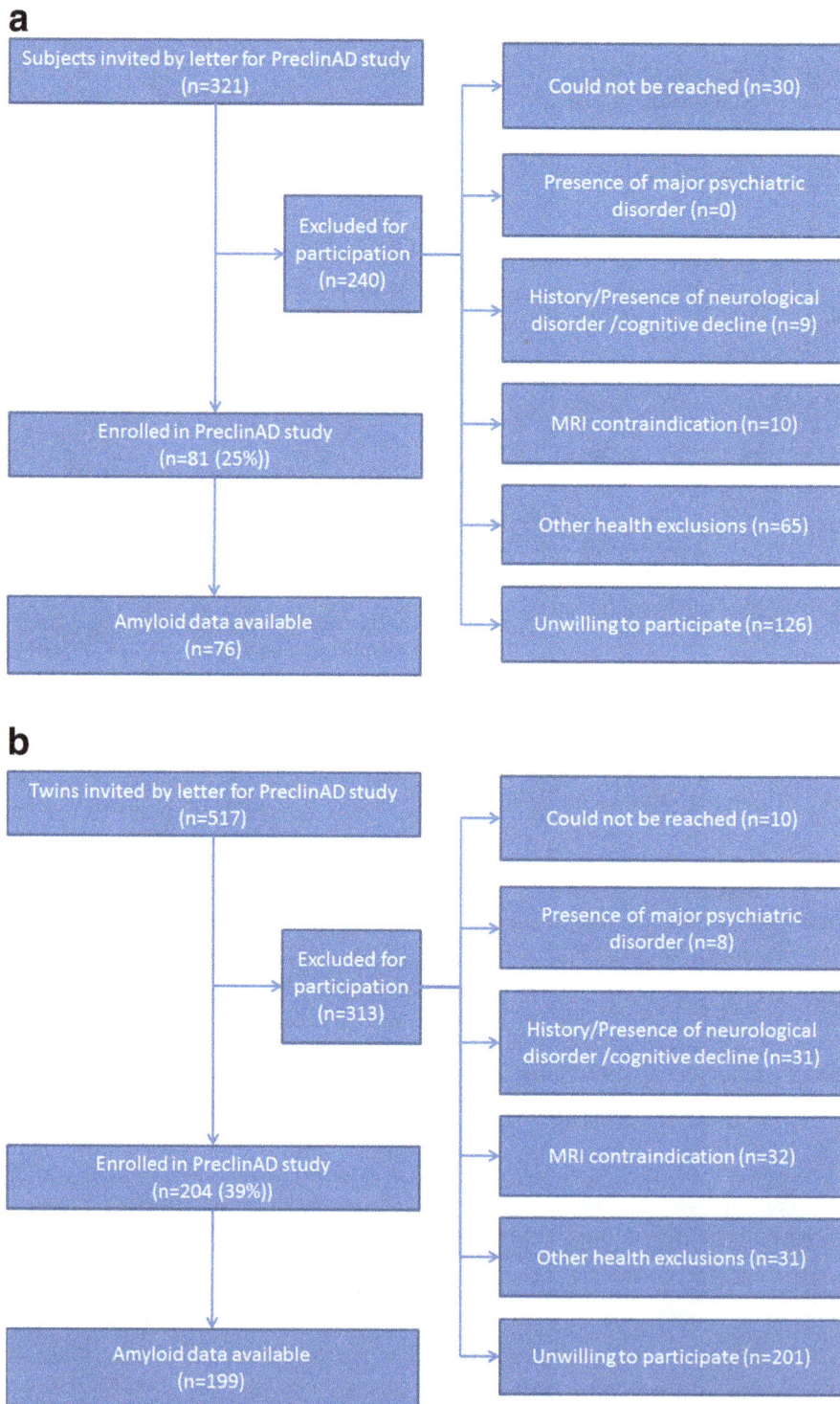

Fig. 2 Inclusion flow chart for participants from **a** Manchester invited subjects selected from a sample of 660 subjects who were part of Manchester and Newcastle Age and Cognitive Performance Research Cohort (ACPRC, Manchester) at time of recruitment and **b** from Amsterdam invited twins selected from a sample of 678 monozygotic twins who were actively registered in Netherlands Twin Register (Amsterdam) at time of recruitment

visually read on a summed static PET image. An abnormal PET was less common in Amsterdam (16%) than in Manchester (34%) ($p < 0.001$). The prevalence of abnormal amyloid PET scans was higher in older age groups (Fig. 3).

Discussion

The PreclinAD study is a prospective cohort study of 285 cognitively normal elderly individuals with extensive phenotyping for amyloid pathology, neurodegeneration markers, cognition, and lifestyle factors.

We noted some differences in baseline characteristics between the Manchester and Amsterdam sites. This could mainly be explained by the higher age in the Manchester substudy. The prevalence of amyloid pathology increased with age, although the prevalence was somewhat lower than would be expected based on a large subject-level meta-analysis, in particular in the age range below 80 years [4]. This might be explained by the relatively healthy sample of participants, due to the strict inclusion and exclusion criteria.

The Amsterdam sub study is the first to assess a wide range of AD markers in a large sample of cognitively normal monozygotic twin pairs above age 60 years. The uniqueness of studying a cohort of twin pairs sharing 100% of their genetic material enables us to further explore the nature of the relation between AD markers. If MZ twin pairs are highly similar for AD markers, this suggests involvement of shared genetic and/or shared environmental factors, whereas within-pair differences indicate the involvement of unique environmental factors [87]. The strength of the MZ twin within-pair difference model further enables us to identify environmental risk factors (e.g., smoking, alcohol use, diet, sleep, physical activity, cognitive activity, and education) that, either directly or indirectly through epigenetic mechanisms, explain observed differences in AD markers within pairs. This may provide clues for novel preventive and therapeutic strategies. However, this model also has the disadvantage that, because MZ twins are genetically identical, we have to correct for twin dependency in all analysis, which may reduce statistical power [86]. Further, we did not include dizygotic twins in the current study, because this optimizes power for twin difference analysis, thereby strengthening the search for environmental risk factors influencing AD development. However, this has the disadvantage that the relative contribution of shared genetic and shared environmental factors to within-pair correlations cannot be estimated. Still, previous studies in elderly twins suggested that the contribution of shared environment at older age is highly limited, possibly because subjects have already been living apart for a longer period of time [88, 89].

A strength of our study, compared to other studies on preclinical AD, is that participants have been recruited from cohorts that have been ongoing for up to 20 years, which provides the possibility to test biomarkers, cognition, and lifestyle collected in the past as predictors for AD biomarkers. Our study design also has several limitations. First, although acquisition protocols were harmonized across sites, they were not always identical (e.g., use of HRRT vs PET-MR). For this reason, site will be used as a covariate in all analyses. Some of the biomarkers were only acquired at the Amsterdam site, which will reduce the statistical power for the analysis of these markers.

Conclusions

We collected a large European cognitively normal sample with an extensive panel of AD biomarkers available

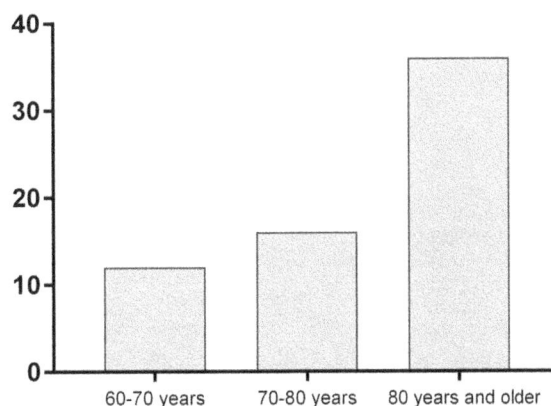

Percentage of subjects with abnormal PET by agegroup

Fig. 3 Amyloid abnormality on PET scan per age group ($n = 58$, 22%). Abnormal PET scan visually read on summed static PET images: 12% of subjects aged 60–70 years, 16% of subjects between 70 and 80 years, and 36% of subjects 80 years and older had abnormal PET scan

at baseline, with clinical follow-up planned after 2 years, to identify healthy elderly individuals at risk for amyloid pathology and future cognitive decline. Results from this study will improve understanding of the pathophysiology of AD and thereby help to adapt the design of secondary prevention trials.

Abbreviations

ACPRC: Manchester and Newcastle Age and Cognitive Performance Research Cohort; AD: Alzheimer's disease; APOE: Apolipoprotein E; ASL: Arterial spin labeling; CSF: Cerebrospinal fluid; DTI: Diffusion tensor imaging; EDTA: Ethylene diamine tetra-acetic acid; EMIF-AD: European Medical Information Framework for AD; FLAIR: 3D fluid-attenuated inversion recovery; GEHC: General Electric Healthcare; HRRT: High-resolution research tomograph; MCI: Mild cognitive impairment; MEG: Magnetoencephalography; MRI: Magnetic resonance imaging; MZ: Monozygotic; NTR: Netherlands Twins Register; OCT: Ocular coherence tomography; PET: Positron emission tomography; rs-fMRI: Resting state functional MRI; SWI: Susceptibility weighted imaging; WMIC: Wolfson Molecular Imaging Centre

Acknowledgements

The authors want to thank all PreclinAD participants for their efforts to join and complete this demanding study. Thanks to Heleen Labuschagne, Leoni Goossens, Lisanne Labuschagne, Naomi Prent, Diederick de Leeuw, Jasper van Dam, Eva Postma, Esmee Runhardt, and Djoeke Rondagh for help with EMIF-AD data collection.

Funding

This work has received support from the EU/EFPIA Innovative Medicines Initiative Joint Undertaking EMIF grant agreement n°115372. This work also received in-kind sponsoring of the Diagnostick device from Applied Biomedical Systems BV, the CANTAB device from Cambridge Cognition, the CSF assay from ADx NeuroSciences, and the PET tracer from GE Health Care.

Authors' contributions

PJV and KH conceived the study and designed the protocol. EK, SFC, MtK, AdB, JT, CA, H-TN, JAvdK, and LW collected data. EK, SFC, MtK, MY, and RH performed image analysis. EK and AdB performed statistical analysis. EK, SFC, MtK, and AdB drafted the manuscript. JT, CA, LW, H-TN, JAvdK, MY, MD, SDM, AH, FHB, CET, EHS, ACM, FDV, RH, NP, AAL, FB, BNMvB, DIB, PS, KH, and PJV edited the manuscript for critical content. PJV and KH provided overall study supervision. All authors read and approved the final version of the manuscript

Consent for publication

Not applicable.

Competing interests

CET has functioned on advisory boards of Fujirebio and Roche, received nonfinancial support in the form of research consumables from ADxNeurosciences and Euroimmun, and performed contract research or received grants from Janssen Prevention Center, Boehringer, Brainsonline, AxonNeurosciences, EIP farma, and Roche. FB is supported by the NIHR UCLH Biomedical Research Center and has received consulting fees or honoraria from Novartis, Roche, Bayer-Schering, Biogen-IDEC, Genzyme-Sanofi, TEVA, Merck-Serono, Jansen Research, IXICO Ltd, GeNeuro, and Apitope Ltd. AH reports reimbursements for conference from Elekta Oy. BNMvB is a trainer for the visual interpretation of [18F]flutemetamol PET scans, and does not receive personal compensation for this. The remaining authors declare that they have no competing interests

Author details

[1]Alzheimer Center, Department of Neurology, VU University Medical Center, Neuroscience Amsterdam, PO Box 7057, 1007 MB Amsterdam, The Netherlands. [2]Wolfson Molecular Imaging Centre, Division of Neuroscience and Experimental Psychology, University of Manchester, Manchester, UK. [3]Department of Biological Psychology, VU University, Neuroscience Amsterdam, Amsterdam, The Netherlands. [4]Department of Ophthalmology, VU University Medical Center, Neuroscience Amsterdam, Amsterdam, The Netherlands. [5]Department of Radiology & Nuclear Medicine, VU University Medical Center, Neuroscience Amsterdam, Amsterdam, The Netherlands. [6]Neurochemistry Laboratory, Department of Clinical Chemistry, VU University Medical Center, Neuroscience Amsterdam, Amsterdam, The Netherlands. [7]Department of Clinical Neurophysiology, VU University Medical Center, Neuroscience Amsterdam, Amsterdam, The Netherlands. [8]Department of Internal Medicine, VU University Medical Center, Neuroscience Amsterdam, Amsterdam, The Netherlands. [9]Wolfson Molecular Imaging Centre, Division of Informatics, Imaging and Data Sciences, Faculty of Medicine, Biology and Health, University of Manchester, Manchester, UK. [10]Institutes of Neurology & Healthcare Engineering, UCL, London, UK. [11]Department of Psychiatry and Neuropsychology, School for Mental Health and Neuroscience, Alzheimer Center Limburg, Maastricht University, Maastricht, The Netherlands.

References

1. Braak H, Braak E. Diagnostic criteria for neuropathologic assessment of Alzheimer's disease. Neurobiol Aging. 1997;18(4 Suppl):S85–8.
2. Bateman RJ, Xiong C, Benzinger TL, Fagan AM, Goate A, Fox NC, Marcus DS, Cairns NJ, Xie X, Blazey TM, et al. Clinical and biomarker changes in dominantly inherited Alzheimer's disease. N Engl J Med. 2012;367(9):795–804.
3. Villemagne VL, Burnham S, Bourgeat P, Brown B, Ellis KA, Salvado O, Szoeke C, Macaulay SL, Martins R, Maruff P, et al. Amyloid beta deposition, neurodegeneration, and cognitive decline in sporadic Alzheimer's disease: a prospective cohort study. Lancet Neurol. 2013;12:357–67.
4. Jansen WJ, Ossenkoppele R, Knol DL, Tijms BM, Scheltens P, Verhey FR, Visser PJ, Amyloid Biomarker Study G, Aalten P, Aarsland D, et al. Prevalence of cerebral amyloid pathology in persons without dementia: a meta-analysis. JAMA. 2015;313:1924–38.
5. Price JL, Morris JC. Tangles and plaques in nondemented aging and "preclinical" Alzheimer's disease. Ann Neurol. 1999;45:358–68.
6. Mintun MA, Larossa GN, Sheline YI, Dence CS, Lee SY, Mach RH, Klunk WE, Mathis CA, DeKosky ST, Morris JC. [11C]PIB in a nondemented population: potential antecedent marker of Alzheimer disease. Neurol. 2006;67:446–52.
7. Aizenstein HJ, Nebes RD, Saxton JA, Price JC, Mathis CA, Tsopelas ND, Ziolko SK, James JA, Snitz BE, Houck PR, et al. Frequent amyloid deposition without significant cognitive impairment among the elderly. Arch Neurol. 2008;65:1509–17.
8. Rowe CC, Ellis KA, Rimajova M, Bourgeat P, Pike KE, Jones G, Fripp J, Tochon-Danguy H, Morandeau L, O'Keefe G, et al. Amyloid imaging results from the Australian Imaging, Biomarkers and Lifestyle (AIBL) study of aging. Neurobiol Aging. 2010;31:1275–83.
9. Chételat G, La Joie R, Villain N, Perrotin A, de La Sayette V, Eustache F, Vandenberghe R. Amyloid imaging in cognitively normal individuals, at-risk populations and preclinical Alzheimer's disease. NeuroImage. 2013;2:356–65.
10. Dubois B, Feldman HH, Jacova C, Hampel H, Molinuevo JL, Blennow K, DeKosky ST, Gauthier S, Selkoe D, Bateman R, et al. Advancing research diagnostic criteria for Alzheimer's disease: the IWG-2 criteria. Lancet Neurol. 2014;13:614–29.
11. McKhann GM, Knopman DS, Chertkow H, Hyman BT, Jack CRJ, Kawas CH, Klunk WE, Koroshetz WJ, Manly JJ, Mayeux R, et al. The diagnosis of dementia due to Alzheimer's disease: recommendations from the National Institute on Aging-Alzheimer's Association workgroups on diagnostic guidelines for Alzheimer's disease. Alzheimers Dement. 2011;7:263–9.

12. Dickerson BC, Wolk DA. MRI cortical thickness biomarker predicts AD-like CSF and cognitive decline in normal adults. Neurology. 2011;78:84–90.

13. Lunnon K, Sattlecker M, Furney SJ, Coppola G, Simmons A, Proitsi P, Lupton MK, Lourdusamy A, Johnston C, Soininen H, et al. A blood gene expression marker of early Alzheimer's disease. J Alzheimers Dis. 2013;33:737–53.

14. Hye A, Riddoch-Contreras J, Baird AL, Ashton NJ, Bazenet C, Leung R, Westman E, Simmons A, Dobson R, Sattlecker M, et al. Plasma proteins predict conversion to dementia from prodromal disease. Alzheimers Dement. 2014;10(6):799–807. e792

15. Fjell AM, Walhovd KB, Fennema-Notestine C, McEvoy LK, Hagler DJ, Holland D, Blennow K, Brewer JB, Dale AM. Brain atrophy in healthy aging is related to CSF levels of Abeta1–42. Cereb Cortex. 2010;20:2069–79.

16. Corder EH, Saunders AM, Strittmatter WJ, Schmechel DE, Gaskell PC, Small GW, Roses AD, Haines JL, Pericak-Vance MA. Gene dose of apolipoprotein E type 4 allele and the risk of Alzheimer's disease in late onset families. Science. 1993;261(5123):921–3.

17. Jack CRJ, Wiste HJ, Weigand SD, Knopman DS, Vemuri P, Mielke MM, Lowe V, Senjem ML, Gunter JL, Machulda MM, et al. Age, sex, and APOE epsilon4 effects on memory, brain structure, and beta-amyloid across the adult life span. JAMA Neurol. 2015;72:511–9.

18. Wirth M, Villeneuve S, La Joie R, Marks SM, Jagust WJ. Gene-environment interactions: lifetime cognitive activity, APOE genotype, and beta-amyloid burden. J Neurosci. 2014;34(25):8612–7.

19. Vos SJ, Xiong C, Visser PJ, Jasielec MS, Hassenstab J, Grant EA, Cairns NJ, Morris JC, Holtzman DM, Fagan AM. Preclinical Alzheimer's disease and its outcome: a longitudinal cohort study. Lancet Neurol. 2013;12:957–65.

20. Buckley RF, Hanseeuw B, Schultz AP, Vannini P, Aghjayan SL, Properzi MJ, Jackson JD, Mormino EC, Rentz DM, Sperling RA, et al. Region-specific association of subjective cognitive decline with tauopathy independent of global β-amyloid burden. JAMA Neurol. 2017;74(12):1455–63.

21. Lim YY, Maruff P, Pietrzak RH, Ellis KA, Darby D, Ames D, Harrington K, Martins RN, Masters CL, Szoeke C, et al. Aβ and cognitive change: examining the preclinical and prodromal stages of Alzheimer's disease. Alzheimers Dement. 2014;10(6):743–51. e741

22. Landau SM, Lu M, Joshi AD, Pontecorvo M, Mintun MA, Trojanowski JQ, Shaw LM, Jagust WJ. Alzheimer's Disease Neuroimaging Initiative. Comparing PET imaging and CSF measurements of Aβ. Ann Neurol. 2013; 74(6):826–36.

23. Zwan M, van Harten A, Ossenkoppele R, Bouwman F, Teunissen C, Adriaanse S, Lammertsma A, Scheltens P, van Berckel B, van der Flier W. Concordance between cerebrospinal fluid biomarkers and [11C]PIB PET in a memory clinic cohort. J Alzheimers Dis. 2014;41:801–7.

24. Mattsson N, Insel PS, Donohue M, Landau S, Jagust WJ, Shaw LM, Trojanowski JQ, Zetterberg H, Blennow K, Weiner MW, et al. Independent information from cerebrospinal fluid amyloid-beta and florbetapir imaging in Alzheimer's disease. Brain. 2015;138(Pt 3):772–83.

25. Palmqvist S, Mattsson N, Hansson O, Alzheimer's Disease Neuroimaging Initiative. Cerebrospinal fluid analysis detects cerebral amyloid-beta accumulation earlier than positron emission tomography. Brain. 2016;139(Pt 4):1226–36.

26. PMA R, et al. The University of Manchester longitudinal study of cognition in normal healthy old age, 1983 through 2003. Aging Neuropsychol C. 2004; 11:245–79.

27. Willemsen G, Vink JM, Abdellaoui A, den Braber A, van Beek JH, Draisma HH, van Dongen J, van 't Ent D, Geels LM, van Lien R, et al. The adult Netherlands twin register: twenty-five years of survey and biological data collection. Twin Res Hum Genet. 2013;16(1):271–81.

28. Gatz M, Reynolds CA, Fratiglioni L, Johansson B, Mortimer JA, Berg S, Fiske A, Pedersen NL. Role of genes and environments for explaining Alzheimer disease. Arch Gen Psychiatry. 2006;63(2):168–74.

29. Boomsma DI, de Geus EJ, Vink JM, Stubbe JH, Distel MA, Hottenga JJ, Posthuma D, van Beijsterveldt TC, Hudziak JJ, Bartels M, et al. Netherlands Twin Register: from twins to twin families. Twin Res Hum Genet. 2006;9(6): 849–57.

30. Willemsen G, de Geus EJ, Bartels M, van Beijsterveldt CE, Brooks AI, Estourgie-van Burk GF, Fugman DA, Hoekstra C, Hottenga JJ, Kluft K, et al. The Netherlands Twin Register biobank: a resource for genetic epidemiological studies. Twin Res Hum Genet. 2010;13(3):231–45.

31. van Beijsterveldt CE, van Baal GC, Molenaar PC, Boomsma DI, de Geus EJ. Stability of genetic and environmental influences on P300 amplitude: a longitudinal study in adolescent twins. Behav Genet. 2001;31(6):533–43.

32. Posthuma D, Meulenbelt I, de Craen AJ, de Geus EJ, Slagboom PE, Boomsma DI, Westendorp RG. Human cytokine response to ex vivo amyloid-beta stimulation is mediated by genetic factors. Twin Res Hum Genet. 2005;8(2):132–7.

33. den Braber A, van 't Ent D, Cath DC, Veltman DJ, Boomsma DI, de Geus EJ. Brain activation during response interference in twins discordant or concordant for obsessive compulsive symptoms. Twin Res Hum Genet. 2012;15(3):372–83.

34. Morris JC, Heyman A, Mohs RC, Hughes JP, van Belle G, Fillenbaum G, Mellits ED, Clark C. The Consortium to Establish a Registry for Alzheimer's Disease (CERAD). Part I Clinical and neuropsychological assessment of Alzheimer's disease. Neurol. 1989;39:1159–65.

35. Aebi C. Validierung der neuropsychologischen Testbatterie CERAD-NP: eine Multi-Center Studie [Validation of the CERAD neuropsychological assessment battery: a multi-centre study]. Basel: University of Basel; 2002.

36. de Jager CA, Budge MM, Clarke R. Utility of TICS-M for the assessment of cognitive function in older adults. Int J Geriatr Psychiatry. 2003;18:318–24.

37. Yesavage JA, Brink TL, Rose TL, Lum O, Huang V, Adey M, Leirer VO. Development and validation of a geriatric depression screening scale: a preliminary report. J Psychiatr Res. 1982;17:37–49.

38. Morris JC. The Clinical Dementia Rating (CDR): current version and scoring rules. Neurol. 1993;43:2412–4.

39. Rey A. L'examen clinique en psychologie. Paris: Presses Universitaires de France; 1964.

40. Lindeboom J, Schmand B, Tulner L, Walstra G, Jonker C. Visual association test to detect early dementia of the Alzheimer type. J Neurol Neurosurg Psychiatry. 2002;73:126–33.

41. Rentz DM, Amariglio RE, Becker JA, Frey M, Olson LE, Frishe K, Carmasin J, Maye JE, Johnson KA, Sperling RA. Face-name associative memory performance is related to amyloid burden in normal elderly. Neuropsychologia. 2011;49:2776–83.

42. Meyers JE, Bayless JD, Meyers KR. Rey complex figure: memory error patterns and functional abilities. Appl Neuropsychol. 1996;3:89–92.

43. Robbins TW, James M, Owen AM, Sahakian BJ, McInnes L, Rabbitt P. Cambridge Neuropsychological Test Automated Battery (CANTAB): a factor analytic study of a large sample of normal elderly volunteers. Dementia. 1994;5:266–81.

44. Wechsler D. Manual for the Wechsler adult intelligence scale. San Antonio: The Psychological Corporation; 1997.

45. McKenna P, Warrington EK. Testing for nominal dysphasia. J Neurol Neurosurg Psychiatry. 1980;43:781–8.

46. Tombaugh TN. Trail Making Test A and B: normative data stratified by age and education. Arch Clin Neuropsychol. 2004;19:203–14.

47. Wechsler D. Wechsler adult intelligence scale—revised manual. New York: Psychological Corporation; 1981.

48. Jakobsson U. Using the 12-item short form health survey (SF-12) to measure quality of life among older people. Aging Clin Ex Res. 2007;19:457–64.

49. Landau SM, Marks SM, Mormino EC, Rabinovici GD, Oh H, O'Neil JP, Wilson RS, Jagust WJ. Association of lifetime cognitive engagement and low beta-amyloid deposition. Arch Neurol. 2012;69:623–9.

50. Washburn RA, Smith KW, Jette AM, Janney CA. The Physical Activity Scale for the Elderly (PASE): development and evaluation. J Clin Epidemiol. 1993; 46:153–62.

51. Boeve BF, Molano JR, Ferman TJ, Smith GE, Lin SC, Bieniek K, Haidar W, Tippmann-Peikert M, Knopman DS, Graff-Radford NR, et al. Validation of the Mayo Sleep Questionnaire to screen for REM sleep behavior disorder in an aging and dementia cohort. Sleep Med. 2011;12:445–53.

52. Netzer NC, Stoohs RA, Netzer CM, Clark K, Strohl KP. Using the Berlin Questionnaire to identify patients at risk for the sleep apnea syndrome. Ann Intern Med. 1999;131:485–91.

53. Sikkes SA, Knol DL, Pijnenburg YA, de Lange-de Klerk ES, Uitdehaag BM, Scheltens P. Validation of the Amsterdam IADL Questionnaire©, a new tool to measure instrumental activities of daily living in dementia. Neuroepidemiol. 2013;41:35–41.

54. Pfeffer RI, Kurosaki TT, Harrah CHJ, Chance JM, Filos S. Measurement of functional activities in older adults in the community. J Gerontol. 1982;37:323–9.

55. Saykin AJ, Wishart HA, Rabin LA, Santulli RB, Flashman LA, West JD, McHugh TL, Mamourian AC. Older adults with cognitive complaints show brain atrophy similar to that of amnestic MCI. Neurology. 2006;67:834–42.

56. Kaufer DI, Cummings JL, Ketchel P, Smith V, MacMillan A, Shelley T, Lopez OL, DeKosky ST. Validation of the NPI-Q, a brief clinical form of the neuropsychiatric inventory. J Neuropsychiatry Clin Neurosci. 2000;12:233–9.

57. Kaasenbrood F, Hollander M, Rutten FH, Gerhards LJ, Hoes AW, Tieleman RG. Yield of screening for atrial fibrillation in primary care with a hand-held, single-lead electrocardiogram device during influenza vaccination. Europace. 2016;18(10):1514–20.

58. Teunissen CE, Tumani H, Engelborghs S, Mollenhauer B. Biobanking of CSF: international standardization to optimize biomarker development. Clin Biochem. 2014;47(4–5):288–92.

59. Meulenbelt I, Droog S, Trommelen GJ, Boomsma DI, Slagboom PE. High-yield noninvasive human genomic DNA isolation method for genetic studies in geographically dispersed families and populations. Am J Hum Genet. 1995;57(5):1252–4.

60. Ehli EA, Abdellaoui A, Fedko IO, Grieser C, Nohzadeh-Malakshah S, Willemsen G, de Geus EJ, Boomsma DI, Davies GE, Hottenga JJ. A method to customize population-specific arrays for genome-wide association testing. Eur J Hum Genet. 2017;25(2):267–70.

61. Fedko IO, Hottenga JJ, Medina-Gomez C, Pappa I, van Beijsterveldt CE, Ehli EA, Davies GE, Rivadeneira F, Tiemeier H, Swertz MA, et al. Estimation of genetic relationships between individuals across cohorts and platforms: application to childhood height. Behav Genet. 2015;45(5):514–28.

62. Das S, Forer L, Schonherr S, Sidore C, Locke AE, Kwong A, Vrieze SI, Chew EY, Levy S, McGue M, et al. Next-generation genotype imputation service and methods. Nat Genet. 2016;48(10):1284–7.

63. Ghebranious N, Ivacic L, Mallum J, Dokken C. Detection of ApoE E2, E3 and E4 alleles using MALDI-TOF mass spectrometry and the homogeneous mass-extend technology. Nucleic Acids Res. 2005;33(17):e149.

64. van der Lee SJ, Wolters FJ, Ikram MK, Hofman A, Ikram MA, Amin N, van Duijn CM. The effect of APOE and other common genetic variants on the onset of Alzheimer's disease and dementia: a community-based cohort study. Lancet Neurol. 2018;17(5):434–44.

65. Moneta GL, Edwards JM, Chitwood RW, Taylor LMJ, Lee RW, Cummings CA, Porter JM. Correlation of North American Symptomatic Carotid Endarterectomy Trial (NASCET) angiographic definition of 70% to 99% internal carotid artery stenosis with duplex scanning. J Vasc Surg. 1993;17: 152–7. discussion 157–159

66. Cardenas VA, Reed B, Chao LL, Chui H, Sanossian N, Decarli CC, Mack W, Kramer J, Hodis HN, Yan M, et al. Associations among vascular risk factors, carotid atherosclerosis, and cortical volume and thickness in older adults. Stroke. 2012;43:2865–70.

67. Wendell CR, Waldstein SR, Ferrucci L, O'Brien RJ, Strait JB, Zonderman AB. Carotid atherosclerosis and prospective risk of dementia. Stroke. 2012;43: 3319–24.

68. van Sloten TT, Schram MT, van den Hurk K, Dekker JM, Nijpels G, Henry RM, Stehouwer CD. Local stiffness of the carotid and femoral artery is associated with incident cardiovascular events and all-cause mortality. J Am College Cardiol. 2014;63:1739–47.

69. Fazekas F, Chawluk JB, Alavi A, Hurtig HI, Zimmerman RA. MR signal abnormalities at 1.5 T in Alzheimer's dementia and normal aging. AJR. 1987; 149:351–6.

70. Scheltens P, Launer LJ, Barkhof F, Weinstein HC, van Gool WA. Visual assessment of medial temporal lobe atrophy on magnetic resonance imaging: interobserver reliability. J Neurol. 1995;242:557–60.

71. Pasquier F, Leys D, Weerts JG, Mounier-Vehier F, Barkhof F, Scheltens P. Inter- and intraobserver reproducibility of cerebral atrophy assessment on MRI scans with hemispheric infarcts. Eur Neurol. 1996;36:268–72.

72. Koedam ELGE, Lehmann M, van der Flier WM, Scheltens P, Pijnenburg YAL, Fox N, Barkhof F, Wattjes MP. Visual assessment of posterior atrophy development of a MRI rating scale. Eur Radiol. 2011;21:2618–25.

73. Curtis C, Gamez JE, Singh U, Sadowsky CH, Villena T, Sabbagh MN, Beach TG, Duara R, Fleisher AS, Frey KA, et al. Phase 3 trial of flutemetamol labeled with radioactive fluorine 18 imaging and neuritic plaque density. JAMA Neurol. 2015;72(3):287–94.

74. Sibomana M, et al. Simultaneous measurement of transmission and emission contamination using a collimated 137Cs point source for the HRRT. In: IEEE Symposium Conference Record Nuclear Science 2004. Rome: IEEE; 2004. https://doi.org/10.1109/NSSMIC.2004.1462795.

75. Sibomana M, et al. New attenuation correction for the HRRT using transmission scatter and total variation regularization. Orlando: IEEE Nuclear Science Symposium Conference Record (NSS/MIC); 2009. https://doi.org/10.1109/NSSMIC.2009.5401730.

76. Hu ZON, Renisch S, et al. MR-based attenuation correction for a whole-body sequential PET/MR system. In: IEEE Nucl Sci Symp Conference; 2009. p. 3508–12.

77. Healthcare G. EPAR product information—summary of product characteristics. 2014.

78. del Campo M, Mollenhauer B, Bertolotto A, Engelborghs S, Hampel H, Simonsen AH, Kapaki E, Kruse N, Le Bastard N, Lehmann S, et al. Recommendations to standardize preanalytical confounding factors in Alzheimer's and Parkinson's disease cerebrospinal fluid biomarkers: an update. Biomark Med. 2012;6(4):419–30.

79. Stam CJ. Use of magnetoencephalography (MEG) to study functional brain networks in neurodegenerative disorders. J Neurol Sci. 2010;289:128–34.

80. de Haan W, van der Flier WM, Koene T, Smits LL, Scheltens P, Stam CJ. Disrupted modular brain dynamics reflect cognitive dysfunction in Alzheimer's disease. NeuroImage. 2012;59:3085–93.

81. Demuru M, Gouw AA, Hillebrand A, Stam CJ, van Dijk BW, Scheltens P, Tijms BM, Konijnenberg E, Ten Kate M, den Braber A, et al. Functional and effective whole brain connectivity using magnetoencephalography to identify monozygotic twin pairs. Sci Rep. 2017;7(1):9685.

82. Mayer MA, Hornegger J, Mardin CY, Tornow RP. Retinal nerve fiber layer segmentation on FD-OCT scans of normal subjects and glaucoma patients. Biomed Opt Express. 2010;1:1358–83.

83. Koronyo Y, Salumbides BC, Black KL, Koronyo-Hamaoui M. Alzheimer's disease in the retina: imaging retinal abeta plaques for early diagnosis and therapy assessment. Neurodegener Dis. 2012;10:285–93.

84. Nandakumar N, Buzney S, Weiter JJ. Lipofuscin and the principles of fundus autofluorescence: a review. Semin Ophthalmol. 2012;27:197–201.

85. Frost S, Kanagasingam Y, Sohrabi H, Vignarajan J, Bourgeat P, Salvado O, Villemagne V, Rowe CC, Macaulay SL, Szoeke C, et al. Retinal vascular biomarkers for early detection and monitoring of Alzheimer's disease. Transl Psychiatry. 2013;3:e233.

86. Minica CC, Dolan CV, Kampert MM, Boomsma DI, Vink JM. Sandwich corrected standard errors in family-based genome-wide association studies. Eur J Hum Genet. 2015;23(3):388–94.

87. Vitaro FBM, Arseneault L. The discordant MZ-twin method: one step closer to the holy grail of causality. Int J Behav Dev. 2009;33(4):376–82.

88. Blokland GA, de Zubicaray GI, McMahon KL, Wright MJ. Genetic and environmental influences on neuroimaging phenotypes: a meta-analytical perspective on twin imaging studies. Twin Res Hum Genet. 2012;15(3):351–71.

89. Fennema-Notestine C, McEvoy LK, Notestine R, Panizzon MS, Yau WW, Franz CE, Lyons MJ, Eyler LT, Neale MC, Xian H, et al. White matter disease in midlife is heritable, related to hypertension, and shares some genetic influence with systolic blood pressure. Neuroimage Clin. 2016;12:737–45.

Vascular Endothelial Growth Factor remains unchanged in cerebrospinal fluid of patients with Alzheimer's disease and vascular dementia

Ananya Chakraborty[1]([iD]), Madhurima Chatterjee[2], Harry Twaalfhoven[2], Marta Del Campo Milan[2], Charlotte E. Teunissen[2], Philip Scheltens[3], Ruud D. Fontijn[1], Wiesje M. van Der Flier[3,4] and Helga E. de Vries[1*]

Abstract

Background: Increasing evidence suggests that cerebral vascular dysfunction is associated with the early stages of Alzheimer's disease (AD). Vascular endothelial growth factor (VEGF) is one of the key players involved in the development and maintenance of the vasculature. Here, we hypothesized that VEGF levels in cerebrospinal fluid (CSF) may be altered in AD patients with vascular involvement, characterized by the presence of microbleeds (MB), and in vascular dementia (VaD) patients compared to controls.

Methods: VEGF levels were determined by electrochemilumiscence Meso Scale Discovery (MULTI-SPOT Assay System) in CSF from age-matched groups of controls with subjective cognitive decline ($n = 21$), AD without MB ($n = 25$), AD with MB ($n = 25$), and VaD ($n = 21$) patients.

Results: The average level of VEGF in the different groups was 2.8 ± 1 pg/ml CSF. Adjusted for age and gender, no significant differences were detected between groups ($p > 0.5$). However, we detected a significant correlation between the concentration of VEGF in the CSF and age ($r = 0.22$, $p = 0.03$). In addition, males ($n = 54$) revealed higher VEGF levels in their CSF compared to females ($n = 38$) (males $= 3.08 \pm 0.769$ pg/ml (mean $\pm$ SD), females $= 2.6 \pm 0.59$; $p = 0.006$), indicating a gender-related regulation.

Conclusion: Our study suggests that VEGF levels in the CSF do not reflect the cerebral vascular alterations in either AD or VaD patients. The observed associations of VEGF with age and gender may indicate that VEGF reflects normal aging and that males and females may differ in their aging process.

Keywords: Vascular endothelial growth factor, Alzheimer's disease, Vascular dementia, Biomarker, Cerebrospinal fluid, Cerebral vascular dysfunction

Background

Cerebrovascular disease is a major contributor to cognitive decline and dementia in old age [1], and vascular dysfunction may contribute to early onset of dementia and progression thereof [2]. Vascular damage, including that of the blood–brain barrier (BBB), is believed to be the result of impaired cerebral blood flow (CBF), which in turn induces hypoperfusion of the brain, resulting in hypoxia [2–5]. In addition, alterations in cerebral hemodynamics may impair glucose transport to the brain and reduce cerebral perfusion, propagating the process of neurodegeneration [6–8]. Postmortem reports further suggest the loss of structural integrity of the cerebrovasculature in Alzheimer's disease (AD) patients compared to their age-matched peers [9, 10]. Additionally, an increased risk of morbidity is reported in AD patients with vascular diseases, such as atherosclerosis and stroke [11]. However to date, diagnostic tools to assess altered vascular function of the CNS in AD are limited.

* Correspondence: he.devries@vumc.nl
[1]Department of Molecular Cell Biology and Immunology, Amsterdam Neuroscience, VU University Medical Center, De Boelelaan 1108, 1007 MB Amsterdam, The Netherlands
Full list of author information is available at the end of the article

Neuropathologically, AD is characterized by the presence of neurofibrillary tangles (NFT) and senile plaques, formed by deposits of beta-amyloid (Aβ) in the brain parenchyma [12]. Many patients with VaD also have AD-related pathology, often referred to as mixed pathology. This vascular pathology includes ischemic changes, which if severe enough may also cause vascular dementia (VaD) on their own. In addition, Aβ may accumulate in the walls of cerebral vessels, a process that reflects a direct link between Alzheimer pathology and vessel pathology and is referred to as cerebral amyloid angiopathy (CAA) [13]. CAA may lead to intracerebral hemorrhage, and on MRI microbleeds are often regarded as an indication of underlying CAA [14].

Current body fluid diagnostic biomarkers for AD used in the clinic include the determination of levels of CSF Aβ42, which reflects the presence of parenchymal senile plaque aggregates, in combination with increased levels of total tau (tTau) and phosphorylated tau (pTau) that reflect NFT [15–17]. So far, there is no established fluid biomarker that reflects changes in vasculature. Thus, there is an urgent need to identify and validate new biomarkers that allow monitoring of pathological vascular alterations.

A potential candidate to detect vascular alterations in AD is vascular endothelial growth factor (VEGF). In general, VEGF is essential for the maintenance of the optimal function of the vasculature, but under pathological conditions high levels of VEGF may induce the formation of pathological vessels through angiogenesis [18]. In the CNS, VEGF can be locally produced and secreted by astrocytes and subsequently bind to endothelial VEGF receptors 1 and 2, which in turn activate downstream pathways that regulate cell survival, angiogenesis, and vascular cell permeability [19, 20]. After, for instance, an ischemic stroke or upon CNS injury, VEGF production is induced and may cause cerebral angiogenesis, increased BBB permeability, and dysfunction [21]. Additionally, reduction of the expression of VEGF was reported in cerebral capillaries in postmortem brain tissue derived from patients with AD, indicative of pathological vessel formation [22, 23]. Interestingly, oncological studies have shown that VEGF may serve as a serum biomarker for angiogenic processes that are associated with the progression of different forms of cancer, such as colorectal tumors [24]. In AD, one study showed increased serum VEGF levels in AD patients of microbleeds whereas another study demonstrates [25] lower levels of serum VEGF in patients compared to age-matched controls [26], illustrating its suitability as a potential biomarker for AD.

We hypothesized that VEGF levels in CSF may be altered in AD patients with vascular involvement as evidenced by microbleeds and in VaD patients where vascular pathology is essential to the disease, compared to AD patients without microbleeds and controls.

Methods
Patients
We selected patients from the Amsterdam Dementia Cohort [27]. Fifty patients with AD (25 patients with microbleeds and 25 without microbleeds matched for age and gender) and 21 patients with VaD were included and 21 patients with subjective cognitive decline without microbleeds, matched for age and gender, served as the control group. All patients underwent extensive dementia screening at baseline, including physical and neurological examination. Global cognitive functioning was assessed using the Mini-Mental State Examination (MMSE). In addition, our diagnostic workup includes a standardized neuropsychological test battery [27]. Tests included the visual association test (VAT) and the Dutch version of Rey auditory verbal learning task (memory), animal fluency (language), and the trail making test and digit span (attention and executive functions). Diagnoses were made in consensus by a multidisciplinary team. Diagnosis of AD cases was performed following the NIA-AA guidelines [28]. NINDS-AIREN [29] criteria were used to diagnose VaD patients. Individuals who presented with cognitive complaints at our memory clinic but performed normal on clinical investigations (i.e., criteria for MCI, dementia, or any psychiatric disorder not met) served as controls. All subjects gave written consent and the ethical review board of VU Medical Center approved of this study.

MRI assessment
MRI rating was performed blinded to the patients' clinical data. MBs were defined as rounded hypointense homogeneous foci up to 10 mm in size in the brain parenchyma on T2*-weighted images. MBs were counted in four lobar regions (frontal, parietal, temporal, and occipital) and in two nonlobar regions: basal ganglia (including thalamus) and infratentorial. To assess the vascular alteration, MRI analysis of cerebral vessels was performed. White matter hyperintensities (WMH) were assessed using the age-related white matter change scale [30]. In addition, the presence of large-vessel and lacunar infarcts was assessed. Large-vessel infarcts were rated as present or absent based on hyperintensity of the lesion on both fluid-attenuated inversion recovery (FLAIR) and T2-weighted sequences. Lacunar infarcts were defined as deep lesions from 3 to 15 mm with low signal on fluid-attenuated inversion recovery and T1 sequences and high signal on T2-weighted images. Lacunar infarcts were scored as present or absent. Furthermore, two widely used visual rating scales for the assessment of atrophy were used. Medial temporal lobe atrophy (MTA) was rated using a 5-point rating scale (0–4) [31]. In the analysis, the average MTA score for the left and right sides was used. Global cortical atrophy was assessed on the fluid-attenuated inversion

recovery sequence. The global cortical atrophy scale ranges from 0 to 3. On both scales, maximal atrophy is represented by the highest score.

Meso Scale Discovery MULTI-SPOT assay system

CSF was collected and stored according to JPND-BIOMARKAPD guidelines [32]. AD CSF biomarkers (Aβ42, total Tau and phospho Tau$_{181}$) were analyzed as a part of the routine diagnosis (Innotest; Fujirebio, Ghent, Belgium) [33].

The VEGF levels in CSF were determined using a Meso Scale Discovery (MSD) cytokine-V-PLEX single cytokine assay (cytokine panel1 human), following the manufacturer's protocol. The kit was validated for the analysis of VEGF in CSF in earlier studies [34, 35]. Briefly, MSD plates were precoated with capture antibodies on a defined spot. CSF samples were diluted twice using sample dilution buffer and 50 μl of CSF samples were added to each well. The samples were incubated for 2 h while shaking. Plates were washed with 150 μl of washing buffer three times, after which 25 μl of detection antibodies conjugated with electrochemiluminescent labels (MSD SULFO-TAG) were added and were subsequently kept for incubation for 2 h with shaking. Plates were washed again three times using 150 μl of washing buffer and 150 μl reading buffer was added to each well. The MSD buffer added created a chemical environment for electrochemiluminescence. The plates were subsequently analyzed using a MSD imager (Sector Imager 2400) where a high voltage was applied, enabling the captured labels to emit light.

Statistics

Statistical analysis was performed using SPSS version 20 (IBM,Chicago, IL, USA). The data were checked for normality using the Kolmogorov–Smirnov test. VEGF levels in males versus females and APOEε4 carrier versus noncarriers were analyzed using Student's t test after correcting for age. The four groups were compared using ANCOVA with correction for age and sex. Correlations were performed using Spearman's correlation test. Statistical significance was defined at (two-tailed) $p < 0.05$.

Results

Patient demographics

The demographic and clinical variables are presented in Table 1. The groups differed on Mini Mental State Examination (MMSE) scores and CSF levels of Aβ42, tTau, and pTau (Additional file 1: Figure S1). As per the study design, there was no difference in age and sex between the groups. VEGF levels in the CSF were correlated with age ($r = 0.22$, $p = 0.03$) (Fig. 1a). Additionally, VEGF concentrations were higher in males ($n = 54$) than in females ($n = 38$; $p = 0.006$, adjusted for age) (Fig. 1b).

VEGF levels in the CSF are comparable in controls, AD, and vAD patients and do not correlate with classical AD biomarkers

CSF VEGF levels in controls and AD–MB, AD+MB, and VaD patients were 2.7 ± 1.1, 2.8 ± 1.2, 2.7 ± 0.7, and 3.1 ± 1.3 pg/ml. ANOVA revealed that there were no significant differences in the CSF VEGF levels between diagnostic groups (Fig. 2 and Table 2 and Additional file 2: Table S1). Adjustment for age and sex did not change this result ($F(3,83) = 0.807$, $p = 0.493$). Furthermore, VEGF levels in the CSF did not correlate with MMSE scores ($r = -0.02$, $p = 0.79$; Fig. 3a), CSF Aβ42 ($r = -0.07$, $p = 0.46$; Fig. 3b), CSF tTau ($r = 0.07$, $p = 0.53$; Fig. 3c), or CSF pTau ($r = 0.04$, $p = 0.70$; Fig. 3d) levels. Additionally, we found that VEGF levels were similar in APOEε4 carriers and noncarriers ($p = 0.71$).

Discussion

The main finding of our study is that VEGF in CSF has similar concentrations across all diagnostic groups, indicating that VEGF in CSF does not help to recognize vascular involvement in patients presenting at a memory clinic. VEGF levels in the CSF were associated with increasing age

Table 1 Demographic details of patients

	Control	AD–MB	AD+MB	VaD
N	21	25	25	21
Sex, female:male	10:11	10:15	11:14	7:15
MMSE[a]	28.5 ± 1.4	21.7 ± 4.3	18.44 ± 5.5	23.50 ± 3.9
Age	65.9 ± 6.1	67.8 ± 6.3	67 ± 7.7	68.6 ± 6.6
Aβ42 (pg/ml)	803 (1057–675)	500 (612–423)	408 (491–304)	606 (868–424)
tTau (pg/ml)	313 (442–240)	615 (743–430)	567 (784–396)	361 (498–196)
pTau (pg/ml)	53 (73–46.50)	85 (109–66.5)	89 (105–68.5)	50 (65–31)
VEGF (pg/ml)	2.7 (3.4–2.3)	2.8 (3.6–2.4)	2.7 (3.2–2.5)	3.1 (3.9–2.6)

MMSE scores and age presented as mean ± standard deviation. Cerebrospinal fluid biomarkers presented as median (interquartile range)
Aβ42 beta-amyloid, *AD–MD* Alzheimer's disease without microbleeds, *AD+MB* Alzheimer's disease with microbleeds, *MMSE* Mini-Mental State Examination, *pTau* phosphorylated tau, *tTau* total tau, *VaD* vascular dementia, *VEGF* vascular endothelial growth factor
[a]A 30-point questionnaire to assess cognitive health

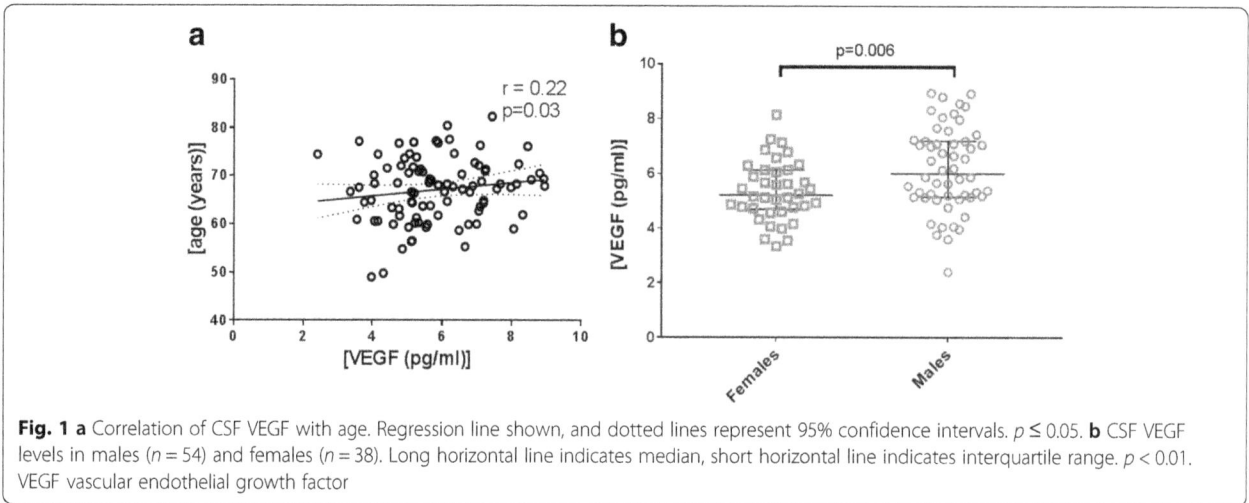

Fig. 1 a Correlation of CSF VEGF with age. Regression line shown, and dotted lines represent 95% confidence intervals. $p \leq 0.05$. **b** CSF VEGF levels in males ($n = 54$) and females ($n = 38$). Long horizontal line indicates median, short horizontal line indicates interquartile range. $p < 0.01$. VEGF vascular endothelial growth factor

and with gender, as males had higher levels of VEGF compared to age-matched females.

Our results showed a modest correlation between increasing age and concentrations of VEGF in CSF. Similar to many ageing disorders like atherosclerosis and cardiovascular diseases [36], cerebral vascular distress is also associated with age [37]. The observed association of age and increased levels of VEGF in the CSF may result from an age-related increase of cerebral vascular distress, although a longitudinal study is needed to further understand the relation between VEGF levels in the CSF and increasing age.

We detected that VEGF levels in CSF in males are higher compared to females. A previous study has shown that males have higher concentrations of vascular biomarkers

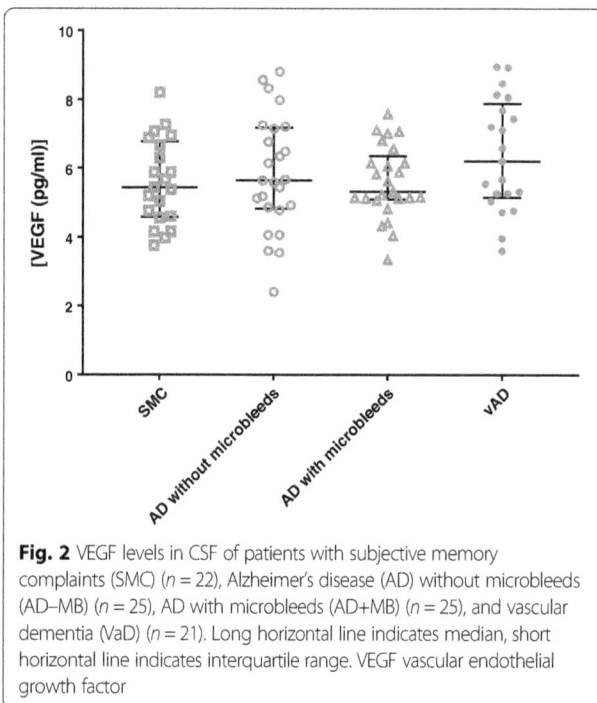

Fig. 2 VEGF levels in CSF of patients with subjective memory complaints (SMC) ($n = 22$), Alzheimer's disease (AD) without microbleeds (AD–MB) ($n = 25$), AD with microbleeds (AD+MB) ($n = 25$), and vascular dementia (VaD) ($n = 21$). Long horizontal line indicates median, short horizontal line indicates interquartile range. VEGF vascular endothelial growth factor

such as E-selectin and vascular cell adhesion molecule-1(VCAM-1) in their CSF [38], which is in accordance with our study. A recent imaging study indicated that cerebrovascular diseases lead to enhanced hippocampal atrophy, independent of Aβ deposition, especially in males [39], suggesting a gender-dependent regulation of vascular function under pathological conditions. Our results may also result from a higher incidence of subclinical cerebrovascular diseases in males than females. This is concordant with an earlier epidemiological study showing that males are at a higher risk of cerebrovascular diseases than females, specifically in those who are middle aged or early old aged [40]. Our finding that CSF VEGF levels are similar across all diagnostic groups is consistent with a previous study in which comparable VEGF levels in the CSF were observed in AD patients ($n = 23$) and controls ($n = 27$) [41]. In general, we did not observe any correlations of VEGF levels with MMSE scores or with the CSF levels of Aβ42, pTau, and tTau, which is in line with previous studies [42]. Our results are also in accordance with data from the ADNI [43], where no differential levels of VEGF were found among control ($n = 90$), mild cognitive impairment ($n = 130$), and AD ($n = 59$) groups at baseline, indicating that VEGF in the CSF may not reflect cerebral vascular distress. Further longitudinal studies are needed to establish whether the correlation between VEGF levels with CSF biomarker Aβ42, pTau, and tTau possibly changes over time during the development of disease. Increased intrathecal VEGF levels in AD ($n = 17$)

Table 2 Multiple group comparisons of cerebrospinal fluid vascular endothelial growth factor levels[a]

	Sum of squares	df	Mean square	F	p
Contrast	1.227	3	0.409	0.881	0.455
Error	39.946	86	0.464		

[a]Controls, Alzheimer's disease without microbleeds, Alzheimer's disease with microbleeds, and vascular dementia compared using analysis of covariance adjusted for age and sex

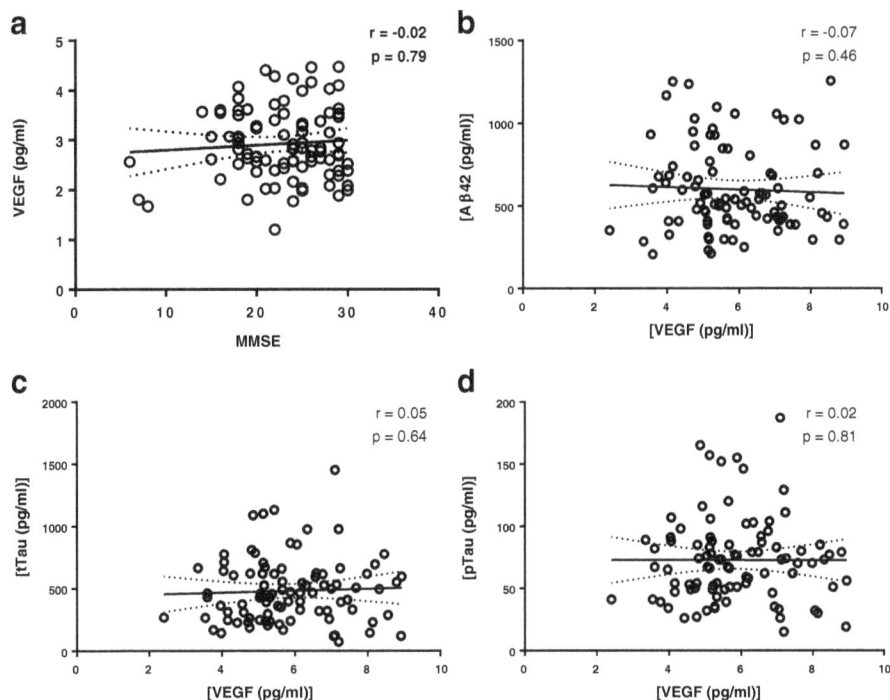

Fig. 3 Correlation of CSF VEGF with (**a**) Mini-Mental State Examination (MMSE), (**b**) beta-amyloid (Aβ42), (**c**) total tau (tTau), and (**d**) phosphorylated tau (pTau). Regression line shown, and dotted lines represent 95% confidence intervals. $p \leq 0.05$. VEGF vascular endothelial growth factor

and VaD ($n = 19$) patients were detected compared to controls ($n = 18$), although this study was limited by the relatively small sample size [44]. Other potential explanations for the differential outcome on the use of VEGF as a biomarker for vascular pathology may be the differences in technologies used and the included sample sizes. Finally, it should be noted that levels of soluble VEGFR1 and VEGFR2, the former of which was shown to be altered in the brain of AD patients [45], modulate angiogenic response of VEGF and, possibly, VEGF levels in CSF.

In this study, for the first time, VEGF levels in CSF were analyzed in four different diagnostic groups including AD patients with and without microbleeds. We used a well-defined cohort where the patients were selected carefully in a specialized memory clinic. Although we had a well-characterized case–control study, the present study was limited by a small sample size. It should be explored further whether VEGF changes longitudinally in AD+MB patients and in VaD patients.

Conclusion

The present study illustrates that VEGF levels are not altered in the CSF of patients with AD with microbleeds or with VaD. We found higher concentrations, however, in males and with increasing age, suggesting that VEGF may play an important role in cerebral vascular changes related to aging.

Abbreviations

AD: Alzheimer's disease; ADNI: Alzheimer's Disease Neuroimaging Initiative; CSF: Cerebrospinal fluid; MB: Microbleeds; MMSE: Mini-Mental State Examination; VaD: Vascular dementia; VEGF: Vascular endothelial growth factor

Funding

This work was supported by a Erasmus Mundus Foundation and European Neuroscience Campus (ENC) joint doctoral fellowship.

Authors' contributions

AC, WMvDF, CET, MDCM and HEdV conceived of and designed the study. All authors acquired and/or interpreted data. AC and HT performed the experiment. AC and MC performed statistical analysis. PS, WMvDF helped with patient selection. AC, MC, WMvDF, RDF and HEdV drafted the manuscript. All authors read and approved the final manuscript.

Competing interests

The authors declare that they have no competing interests.

Author details

[1]Department of Molecular Cell Biology and Immunology, Amsterdam Neuroscience, VU University Medical Center, De Boelelaan 1108, 1007 MB Amsterdam, The Netherlands. [2]Department of Clinical Chemistry, VU University Medical Center, Amsterdam, The Netherlands. [3]Alzheimer Centre and Department of Neurology, Amsterdam Neuroscience, VU University Medical Center, Amsterdam, The Netherlands. [4]Department of Epidemiology and Biostatistics, Amsterdam Neuroscience, VU University Medical Centrer, Amsterdam, The Netherlands.

References

1. Knopman DS: Cerebrovascular disease and dementia. Br J Radiol 2007, 80 Spec No 2:S121–S127.
2. de la Torre JC. The vascular hypothesis of Alzheimer's disease: bench to bedside and beyond. Neurodegener Dis. 2010;7:116–21.
3. de la Torre JC. Vascular basis of Alzheimer's pathogenesis. Ann N Y Acad Sci. 2002;977:196–215.
4. de la Torre JC. Alzheimer disease as a vascular disorder: nosological evidence. Stroke. 2002;33:1152–62.
5. Vagnucci AH Jr, Li WW. Alzheimer's disease and angiogenesis. Lancet. 2003; 361:605–8.
6. Roher AE, Debbins JP, Malek-Ahmadi M, Chen K, Pipe JG, Maze S, Belden C, Maarouf CL, Thiyyagura P, Mo H, et al. Cerebral blood flow in Alzheimer's disease. Vasc Health Risk Manag. 2012;8:599–611.
7. Kisler K, Nelson AR, Montagne A, Zlokovic BV. Cerebral blood flow regulation and neurovascular dysfunction in Alzheimer disease. Nat Rev Neurosci. 2017;18:419–34.
8. Sierra-Marcos A. Regional cerebral blood flow in mild cognitive impairment and Alzheimer's disease measured with arterial spin labeling magnetic resonance imaging. Int J Alzheimers Dis. 2017;2017:5479597.
9. Montagne A, Nation DA, Pa J, Sweeney MD, Toga AW, Zlokovic BV. Brain imaging of neurovascular dysfunction in Alzheimer's disease. Acta Neuropathol. 2016;131:687–707.
10. Carrano A, Hoozemans JJ, van der Vies SM, van Horssen J, de Vries HE, Rozemuller AJ. Neuroinflammation and blood-brain barrier changes in capillary amyloid angiopathy. Neurodegener Dis. 2012;10:329–31.
11. Viswanathan A, Rocca WA, Tzourio C. Vascular risk factors and dementia: how to move forward? Neurology. 2009;72:368–74.
12. Bloom GS. Amyloid-beta and tau: the trigger and bullet in Alzheimer disease pathogenesis. JAMA Neurol. 2014;71:505–8.
13. Thal DR, Ghebremedhin E, Rub U, Yamaguchi H, Del Tredici K, Braak H. Two types of sporadic cerebral amyloid angiopathy. J Neuropathol Exp Neurol. 2002;61:282–93.
14. Charidimou A, Shoamanesh A, Al-Shahi Salman R, Cordonnier C, Perry LA, Sheth KN, Biffi A, Rosand J, Viswanathan A. Cerebral amyloid angiopathy, cerebral microbleeds and implications for anticoagulation decisions: the need for a balanced approach. Int J Stroke. 2018;13(2):117–120.
15. Buerger K, Ewers M, Pirttila T, Zinkowski R, Alafuzoff I, Teipel SJ, DeBernardis J, Kerkman D, McCulloch C, Soininen H, Hampel H. CSF phosphorylated tau protein correlates with neocortical neurofibrillary pathology in Alzheimer's disease. Brain. 2006;129:3035–41.
16. Strozyk D, Blennow K, White LR, Launer LJ: CSF Aβ 42 levels correlate with amyloid-neuropathology in a population-based autopsy study. Neurology 2003, 60:652–656.
17. Scheltens P, Blennow K, Breteler MM, de Strooper B, Frisoni GB, Salloway S, Van der Flier WM. Alzheimer's disease. Lancet. 2016;388:505–17.
18. Neufeld G, Cohen T, Gengrinovitch S, Poltorak Z. Vascular endothelial growth factor (VEGF) and its receptors. FASEB J. 1999;13:9–22.
19. Koch S, Claesson-Welsh L. Signal transduction by vascular endothelial growth factor receptors. Cold Spring Harb Perspect Med. 2012;2:a006502.
20. Rosenstein JM, Krum JM, Ruhrberg C. VEGF in the nervous system. Organogenesis. 2010;6:107–14.
21. Zhang ZG, Zhang L, Jiang Q, Zhang R, Davies K, Powers C, Bruggen N, Chopp M. VEGF enhances angiogenesis and promotes blood-brain barrier leakage in the ischemic brain. J Clin Invest. 2000;106:829–38.
22. Provias J, Jeynes B. Reduction in vascular endothelial growth factor expression in the superior temporal, hippocampal, and brainstem regions in Alzheimer's disease. Curr Neurovasc Res. 2014;11:202–9.
23. Inai T, Mancuso M, Hashizume H, Baffert F, Haskell A, Baluk P, Hu-Lowe DD, Shalinsky DR, Thurston G, Yancopoulos GD, McDonald DM. Inhibition of vascular endothelial growth factor (VEGF) signaling in cancer causes loss of endothelial fenestrations, regression of tumor vessels, and appearance of basement membrane ghosts. Am J Pathol. 2004;165:35–52.
24. Murukesh N, Dive C, Jayson GC. Biomarkers of angiogenesis and their role in the development of VEGF inhibitors. Br J Cancer. 2010;102:8–18.
25. Zhang JB, Li MF, Zhang HX, Li ZG, Sun HR, Zhang JS, Wang PF. Association of serum vascular endothelial growth factor levels and cerebral microbleeds in patients with Alzheimer's disease. Eur J Neurol. 2016;23:1337–42.

26. Mateo I, Llorca J, Infante J, Rodriguez-Rodriguez E, Fernandez-Viadero C, Pena N, Berciano J, Combarros O. Low serum VEGF levels are associated with Alzheimer's disease. Acta Neurol Scand. 2007;116:56–8.
27. van der Flier WM, Pijnenburg YA, Prins N, Lemstra AW, Bouwman FH, Teunissen CE, van Berckel BN, Stam CJ, Barkhof F, Visser PJ, et al. Optimizing patient care and research: the Amsterdam Dementia Cohort. J Alzheimers Dis. 2014;41:313–27.
28. McKhann G, Drachman D, Folstein M, Katzman R, Price D, Stadlan EM. Clinical diagnosis of Alzheimer's disease: report of the NINCDS-ADRDA Work Group under the auspices of Department of Health and Human Services Task Force on Alzheimer's Disease. Neurology. 1984;34:939–44.
29. Roman GC, Tatemichi TK, Erkinjuntti T, Cummings JL, Masdeu JC, Garcia JH, Amaducci L, Orgogozo JM, Brun A, Hofman A, et al. Vascular dementia: diagnostic criteria for research studies. Report of the NINDS-AIREN International Workshop. Neurology. 1993;43:250–260.
30. Wahlund LO, Barkhof F, Fazekas F, Bronge L, Augustin M, Sjogren M, Wallin A, Ader H, Leys D, Pantoni L, et al. A new rating scale for age-related white matter changes applicable to MRI and CT. Stroke. 2001;32:1318–22.
31. Scheltens P, Launer LJ, Barkhof F, Weinstein HC, van Gool WA. Visual assessment of medial temporal lobe atrophy on magnetic resonance imaging: interobserver reliability. J Neurol. 1995;242:557–60.
32. Reijs BL, Teunissen CE, Goncharenko N, Betsou F, Blennow K, Baldeiras I, Brosseron F, Cavedo E, Fladby T, Froelich L, et al. The Central Biobank and Virtual Biobank of BIOMARKAPD: a resource for studies on neurodegenerative diseases. Front Neurol. 2015;6:216.
33. Mulder C, Verwey NA, van der Flier WM, Bouwman FH, Kok A, van Elk EJ, Scheltens P, Blankenstein MA. Amyloid-beta(1-42), total tau, and phosphorylated tau as cerebrospinal fluid biomarkers for the diagnosis of Alzheimer disease. Clin Chem. 2010;56:248–53.
34. Lee JW, Devanarayan V, Barrett YC, Weiner R, Allinson J, Fountain S, Keller S, Weinryb I, Green M, Duan L, et al. Fit-for-purpose method development and validation for successful biomarker measurement. Pharm Res. 2006;23:312–28.
35. Andreasson U, Perret-Liaudet A, van Waalwijk van Doorn LJ, Blennow K, Chiasserini D, Engelborghs S, Fladby T, Genc S, Kruse N, Kuiperij HB, et al. A practical guide to immunoassay method validation. Front Neurol. 2015;6:179.
36. Niccoli T, Partridge L. Ageing as a risk factor for disease. Curr Biol. 2012;22: R741–52.
37. Peters R. Ageing and the brain. Postgrad Med J. 2006;82:84–8.
38. Li G, Shofer JB, Petrie EC, Yu CE, Wilkinson CW, Figlewicz DP, Shutes-David A, Zhang J, Montine TJ, Raskind MA, et al. Cerebrospinal fluid biomarkers for Alzheimer's and vascular disease vary by age, gender, and APOE genotype in cognitively normal adults. Alzheimers Res Ther. 2017;9:48.
39. Jack CR Jr, Wiste HJ, Weigand SD, Knopman DS, Vemuri P, Mielke MM, Lowe V, Senjem ML, Gunter JL, Machulda MM, et al. Age, sex, and APOE epsilon4 effects on memory, brain structure, and beta-amyloid across the adult life span. JAMA Neurol. 2015;72:511–9.
40. Chene G, Beiser A, Au R, Preis SR, Wolf PA, Dufouil C, Seshadri S. Gender and incidence of dementia in the Framingham Heart Study from mid-adult life. Alzheimers Dement. 2015;11:310–20.
41. Blasko I, Lederer W, Oberbauer H, Walch T, Kemmler G, Hinterhuber H, Marksteiner J, Humpel C. Measurement of thirteen biological markers in CSF of patients with Alzheimer's disease and other dementias. Dement Geriatr Cogn Disord. 2006;21:9–15.
42. Hoglund K, Kern S, Zettergren A, Borjesson-Hansson A, Zetterberg H, Skoog I, Blennow K. Preclinical amyloid pathology biomarker positivity: effects on tau pathology and neurodegeneration. Transl Psychiatry. 2017;7:e995.
43. Hohman TJ, Bell SP, Jefferson AL, Alzheimer's Disease Neuroimaging Inititative. The role of vascular endothelial growth factor in neurodegeneration and cognitive decline: exploring interactions with biomarkers of Alzheimer disease. JAMA Neurol. 2015;72:520–9.
44. Tarkowski E, Issa R, Sjogren M, Wallin A, Blennow K, Tarkowski A, Kumar P. Increased intrathecal levels of the angiogenic factors VEGF and TGF-beta in Alzheimer's disease and vascular dementia. Neurobiol Aging. 2002;23:237–243.
45. Harris R, Miners JS, Allen S, Love S. VEGFR1 and VEGFR2 in Alzheimer's Disease. J Alzheimers Dis. 2018;61:741–752.

Exome sequencing in an Italian family with Alzheimer's disease points to a role for seizure-related gene 6 (*SEZ6*) rare variant R615H

Lara Paracchini[1], Luca Beltrame[1], Lucia Boeri[2], Federica Fusco[3], Paolo Caffarra[4], Sergio Marchini[1], Diego Albani[3]*[iD] and Gianluigi Forloni[3]

Abstract

Background: The typical familial form of Alzheimer's disease (FAD) accounts for about 5% of total Alzheimer's disease (AD) cases. Presenilins (*PSEN1* and *PSEN2*) and amyloid-β (A4) precursor protein (*APP*) genes carry all reported FAD-linked mutations. However, other genetic loci may be involved in AD. For instance, seizure-related gene 6 (*SEZ6*) has been reported in brain development and psychiatric disorders and is differentially expressed in the cerebrospinal fluid of AD cases.

Methods: We describe a targeted exome sequencing analysis of a large Italian kindred with AD, negative for *PSEN* and *APP* variants, that indicated the *SEZ6* heterozygous mutation R615H is associated with the pathology.

Results: We overexpressed R615H mutation in H4-SW cells, finding a reduction of amyloid peptide Aβ(1–42). *Sez6* expression decreased with age in a mouse model of AD (3xTG-AD), but independently from transgene expression.

Conclusions: These results support a role of exome sequencing for disease-associated variant discovery and reinforce available data on *SEZ6* in AD models.

Keywords: Alzheimer's disease, *SEZ6*, Exome sequencing, Rare variants

Background

Alzheimer's disease (AD) is a multifactorial neurodegenerative disorder whose onset is mostly sporadic [1]. The genetic background has a major role in AD, and DNA variants may contribute, ranging from predisposing risk factors (having from medium to large effect size, such as the ε4 allele of the *APOE* gene) [2] to full penetrant causal mutations in a few genes, namely presenilins (*PSEN1* and *PSEN2*) and the amyloid-β (A4) precursor protein (*APP*) [3, 4]. *PSEN1/2* and *APP* gene mutations have been linked to early-onset, autosomal dominant familial forms of Alzheimer's disease (FAD) [5, 6]. Recently, large-scale whole-exome sequencing has found rare variants reported to contribute to AD risk, such as

in the *PLCG2*, *ABI3*, and *TREM2* genes [7]. These findings indicate the involvement in familiar forms of AD of variants belonging to genes other than *PSEN1/2* and *APP*, which may have a causal or predisposing role, as recently reported for *SORL1* gene [8].

We report an Italian family with several cases of AD (having an onset between 60 and 70 years) negative for *PSEN1/2* or *APP* mutations and whose available affected members were found to bear *SEZ6* gene rare missense variant R615H. We describe the genetic, *in vitro*, and *in vivo* findings further supporting a role for *SEZ6* in AD molecular mechanisms.

Methods
Family and patient description
The family's pedigree is reported in Fig. 1. We extracted DNA for exome sequencing analysis from the members indicated by the code PR (seven subjects). We had

* Correspondence: diego.albani@marionegri.it
[3]Department of Neuroscience, Istituto di Ricerche Farmacologiche Mario Negri IRCCS, Via La Masa 19, 20156 Milan, Italy
Full list of author information is available at the end of the article

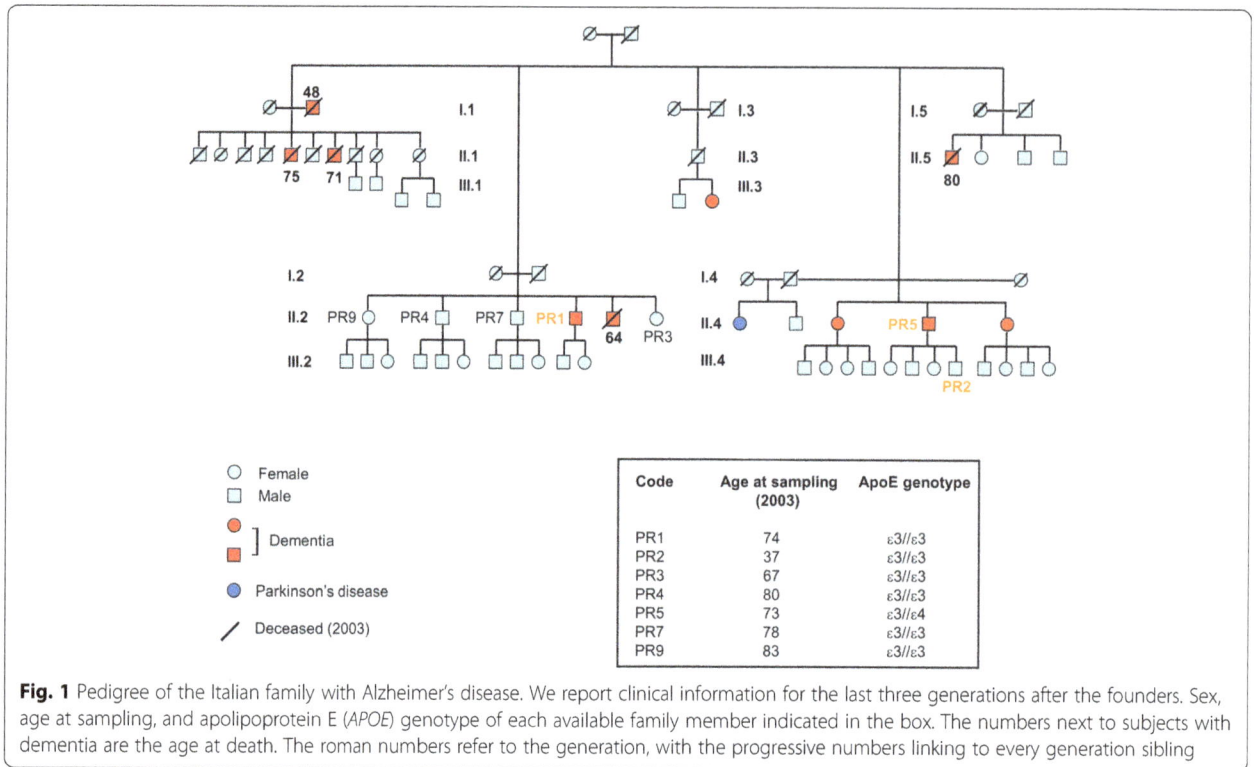

Fig. 1 Pedigree of the Italian family with Alzheimer's disease. We report clinical information for the last three generations after the founders. Sex, age at sampling, and apolipoprotein E (*APOE*) genotype of each available family member indicated in the box. The numbers next to subjects with dementia are the age at death. The roman numbers refer to the generation, with the progressive numbers linking to every generation sibling

clinical details about three generations after the founder. Ten dementia cases were reported in the whole pedigree, with an additional member having Parkinson's disease. The age of onset of neurodegenerative disorders ranged from 60 to 70 years. In the first generation, one early-onset dementia case was reported (age at death, 48 years). In the second generation, 8 of 25 siblings (32%) were diagnosed with AD, with an additional case in the third generation (age at onset 64 years). The remaining siblings of this generation were cognitively normal, aged between 35 and 45 years. Apolipoprotein E genotype (*APOE*) of available patients was in all cases ε3//ε3 apart from PR5 (ε3//ε4). Two siblings of PR5, diagnosed with AD, had dementia too, but they were unavailable for sampling.

Sporadic AD cases (*n* = 9) and cognitively normal elderly control subjects (*n* = 191) were included for independent evaluation of the *SEZ6*(R615H) variant frequency by digital droplet PCR (ddPCR).

Patients and healthy control subjects were recruited by the same clinical center, and AD was diagnosed according to international criteria. Healthy control subjects were spouses of patients coming to clinical attention, and they had no sign of neurodegenerative disorders and Mini Mental State Examination (MMSE) scores in the normal range [9].

Exome sequencing and *APOE* genotyping

The full-exome sequencing of 4811 disease-associated genes (clinical exome) was done starting from 50 ng of DNA diluted in Tris-HCl 10 mM, pH 8.5 (TruSight One Sequencing Panel; Illumina, San Diego, CA, USA), following the manufacturer's instructions. Briefly, capture-based libraries were prepared by pooling three samples per time. The libraries' concentrations were calculated using a Qubit® dsDNA High-Sensitivity Assay Kit (Invitrogen, Carlsbad, CA, USA), and the distribution of DNA fragments for each library was evaluated using a high-sensitivity DNA kit and a 2100 Bioanalyzer (Agilent Technologies, Santa Clara, CA, USA). Each library was run on a MiSeq platform (Illumina) using a 2 × 150-bp (300 cycles) configuration on a V3 sequencing flow cell.

Data analysis was performed according to best practice from the bioinformatics community. Raw sequence fragments (reads) were aligned to the reference genome (human, build hg19) with the Burrows-Wheeler alignment tool [10], followed by post-processing to recalibrate base call quality scores. Variants were called with the Genome Analysis Toolkit [11–13], using the HaplotypeCaller method, then annotated with the Variant Effect Predictor [14] and loaded into a specialized database [15] for further analysis. *In silico* mutation impact predictions were extracted from the dbNSFP database [16]. For computation, we used the "bcbio" pipeline (https://github.com/chapmanb/bcbio-nextgen) running on a high-performance computing platform as part of the Cloud4CaRE project. Data files were uploaded to the European Nucleotide Archive with accession number pending.

Selection of candidate variants used the following criteria: (a) depth at least 30×; (b) low frequency in the general population (< 1% in the 1000 Genomes Project); (c) at least a damaging predicted effect as reported from the dbNSFP; and (d) present in all family members affected by AD or their offspring. The *APOE* genotype was assessed by restriction fragment length polymorphism using the CfoI (Roche, Basel, Switzerland) restriction enzyme, as previously described [17].

Exome sequencing validation by digital droplet PCR
ddPCR experiments were done with the Bio-Rad QX200TM ddPCR system (Bio-Rad Laboratories, Hercules, CA, USA). The mutational assay for *SEZ6* R615H was carried out according to the manufacturer's instructions. Briefly, the TaqMan™ reaction mix, composed of 2× ddPCR Supermix for probes (no deoxyuridine triphosphate), 20× custom target probes for mut SEZ6 (probe sequence: CTACGG**TCA**TGGGCAG-FAM), and 20× reference probes for wild-type SEZ6 (probe sequence: CTACGG**TCG**TGGGCA-HEX), was assembled at a final concentration of 450 nM and 20 ng of DNA in a volume of 20 µl. This reaction mix was added to a DG8 cartridge together with 60 µl of droplet generation oil for probe and used for droplet generation (QX200 droplet generator; Bio-Rad Laboratories). Droplets were then manually transferred to 96-well PCR plates and placed on a thermal cycler (T100 Thermal Cycler; Bio-Rad Laboratories) for the PCR amplification (thermal cycling conditions: 95 °C for 5 min, 95 °C for 30 s, and 55 °C for 1 min, 40 cycles; 98 °C for 10 min and 4 °C infinite; ramping rate 2 °C/s). The PCR plate was then transferred into the QX100 Droplet Reader for the fluorescence measurement of FAM and HEX probes. The numbers of positive and negative droplets were used to calculate the concentrations (copies/µl) of the target and the reference *SEZ6* DNA sequence and their Poisson-based 95% CIs, excluding reactions with fewer than 10,000 total events (positive and negative) (QuantaSoft Analysis pro software 1.0.596; Bio-Rad Laboratories).

For family members and patients with sporadic AD, experiments were run in duplicate; the assay on the healthy population was run once.

Cloning and overexpression of *SEZ6*(R615H) in H4-SW cells
pSEZ6(R615H) cloning
Synthetic *SEZ6*(R615H) complementary DNA was provided by GenScript® in pCDNA3.1(+) vector and expanded in competent *Escherichia coli* cells (strain JM109; Promega, Madison, WI, USA). After purification, p*SEZ6*(R615H) was verified through the unique enzymatic restriction site PmeI (New England Biolabs, Hitchin, UK) and agarose gel electrophoresis.

Cell culture
H4-SW neuroglioma cells overexpressing human *APP* gene harboring the Swedish (SW) mutation [18] were grown in DMEM supplemented with 10% FBS, 2 mM L-glutamine, and antibiotics (100 U/ml penicillin, 100 µg/ml streptomycin, 300 µg/ml hygromycin B, 10 µg/ml blasticidin-S).

Transient transfection was done using FuGENE® HD Transfection Reagent (Promega), and cells were selected with G418 (1200 µg/ml) after 48 h. For clonal selection of *SEZ6*(R615H) mutants, we picked colonies and analyzed DNA and protein extracts by PCR and Western blotting. Finally, a single-point mutation (G→A) leading to R615H substitution was checked by Sanger sequencing.

PCR for *SEZ6*(R615H) expression in H4-SW cells
PCR was run in a 20-µl mixture containing 50 ng of DNA, 0.5 mM each of forward primer 5′-CTACGGTCATGGGCAGGATTG-3′, which contains the single-point mutation (G→A), and the reverse oligonucleotide primer 5′- ATCATGGCAGGTGAGGATGGACT-3′ (metabion, Planegg, Germany); 1× PCR buffer 200 mM Tris-HCl, 500 mM KCl (Thermo Fisher Scientific, Waltham, MA, USA); 2.5 mM deoxynucleotide triphosphate (Thermo Fisher Scientific); 25 mM MgCl$_2$ (Thermo Fisher Scientific); and 1 unit of Taq polymerase (Thermo Fisher Scientific). Amplification was done with an initial denaturation at 95 °C for 2 min, followed by 30 cycles of denaturation at 95 °C for 30 s, annealing at 61.7 °C for 30 s, extension at 72 °C for 70 s, and a final 5-min extension at 72 °C. The resulting PCR fragments were resolved by 1% agarose gel electrophoresis (Sigma-Aldrich, St. Louis, MO, USA).

Western blotting for SEZ6 overexpression in H4-SW cells
To assess protein overexpression of *SEZ6* in H4-SW, protein extracts (18 µg) were separated on 8% SDS-PAGE gel and transferred to a nitrocellulose membrane. Blots were developed using horseradish peroxidase-conjugated secondary antibodies and the ECL chemiluminescence system (MerckMillipore, Burlington, MA, USA). All blots were normalized to α-tubulin and quantified using ImageJ software (National Institutes of Health, Bethesda, MD, USA). The following antibodies were used: anti-α-tubulin (1:7500; Abcam, Cambridge, UK) and anti-SEZ6 (1:1000; Aviva Systems Biology, San Diego, CA, USA).

DNA sequencing
To verify the presence of the single point mutation, we amplified the region containing the mutated base by PCR with forward primer 5′- GAGATCACAGACTCGGCTG-3′ and the reverse primer 5′- ATCATGGCAGGTGAGGATGGACT-3′ (metabion). The total amount of the generated PCR product was purified using the Wizard SV Gel PCR Clean-Up System (Promega) and

sent to a Sanger sequencing service (Eurofins Genomics, Ebersberg, Germany). Output data were analyzed using Chromas Lite 2.01 software.

Aβ(1–42) and Aβ(1–40) in H4-SW cells expressing SEZ6(R615H)

A specific sandwich enzyme-linked immunosorbent assay (ELISA) (Immuno-Biological Laboratories Co., Gunma, Japan) was used to measure Aβ(1–42) and Aβ(1–40) concentrations in conditioned media from cultured H4-SW cells. A total of 150×10^3 cells were seeded in a six-well plate and grown overnight. The next day, the medium was changed, and after 48 h it was collected and immediately frozen after the addition of a broad-spectrum protease inhibitor (Sigma-Aldrich). An aliquot of 100 μl was used for ELISA to assess each value in triplicate.

Western blot analysis for Sez6 brain expression in 3xTG-AD mice

For Sez6 brain expression analysis, we used 3xTG-AD mice at 3, 9, and 19 months of age. This triple-transgenic model harbors human PS1(M146 V), APP(SW), and MAPT(P301L) transgenes, and starting from around 9 months of age, mice develop at brain level amyloid plaques and protein tau tangles. They also show early signs of synaptic dysfunction (starting from around 3 months of age), including long-term potentiation alteration [19]. Strain, age, and sex-matched nontransgenic animals were used as controls. Mice were housed at 23 °C room temperature with food and water *ad libitum* and a 12-h/12-h light/dark cycle. To obtain brain protein extract, the cortex was dissected from a single brain hemisphere and homogenized with ice-cold lysis buffer (pH 7.4) containing 1% Triton X-100 and a broad-range protease inhibitor cocktail. Cortex protein extract (20 μg) was analyzed as described above.

Statistics

Data analysis was done using Prism® version 6.0 software (GraphPad Software, La Jolla, CA, USA). In vitro and in vivo data were compared using one-way analysis of variance followed by Tukey's post hoc test. Two-tailed levels of significance were used, and $p < 0.05$ was considered significant.

Results

Exome sequencing and APOE genotyping

To identify variants linked to dementia phenotype, we sequenced DNA samples from family members (healthy and AD cases) and unrelated patients with sporadic AD for a set of over 4000 genes reported as implicated in rare and genetic diseases. Our initial analysis identified 15,745 variants passing our quality control filters (variant depth 30× or more). Many of these were common

polymorphisms present in the general population, so we selected only those rare in the European population (< 1% frequency), lowering the count to 612 (Additional file 1: Table S1).

To further narrow the search for variants of interest, we used *in silico* analysis to restrict our findings to those predicted as damaging for protein, finding 138 variants (Additional file 1: Table S1). The majority (96.4%) of possible damaging variants were common between both familial and sporadic AD samples. On the contrary, five variants (3.6%) were exclusive to the family samples (Table 1). In particular, a missense variant in the SEZ6 neuronal gene (c.1844G>A, R615H) was present only in the two available AD cases (PR1 and PR5) and in a first-degree relative (PR2, son of PR5). This variant was localized on one of the extracellular CUB domains of the protein [20, 21] and was predicted to have a high damaging potential (Combined Annotation Dependent Domain [CADD] score = 23). This prompted us to further focus on this variant.

Validation of exome sequencing SEZ6(R615H) data and variant screening in sporadic AD cases and healthy control subjects

Because the clinical exome results indicated a mutation in SEZ6 gene (c.1844G>A) as unique to the available family members with AD, we performed an independent validation to confirm the result. Using ddPCR, we tested for the SEZ6 variant in exome sequencing-positive family members (n = 3) and in sporadic AD cases (n = 9). To exclude the possibility that the polymorphic variant of SEZ6 identified could be detected at low frequency in the healthy population, too, the mutational assay was also done in a control group of 191 cognitively healthy people.

Figure 2 shows SEZ6 mutational analysis of three family members (PR1, PR2, and PR5) and a representative case of sporadic AD (PR11). Wild-type SEZ6 (green droplets) was detected in all samples, whereas mutated SEZ6 (blue) was detected only in the PR1, PR2 and PR5 samples. A single event with both wild-type and mutated SEZ6 was detected in PR11, probably a polymerase artifact.

Regarding a quantitative measure of the SEZ6 variant, Table 2 reports the concentration as the number of target molecules/μl of wild-type and mutant SEZ6 in all sporadic cases (n = 9), in family members (n = 3), and in healthy individuals (n = 191). Wild-type SEZ6 copies were detected in all groups. The means of wild-type SEZ6 copies/μl were 564, 258, and 130 in the healthy control group, sporadic AD cases, and family members, respectively. A high concentration of mutant SEZ6 was detected in family member samples. The simultaneous presence of the wild-type and the mutated form of

Table 1 Variants exclusive of family members and satisfying the filtering criteria

Chr	Position	Gene	Variant	Amino acid change	(%)	dbSNP ID	Found in (family code)
chr8	144,589,984	ZC3H3	c.1646 C > T	p.Ser549 Leu	0.5%	rs 149,025,999	*PR 1*, PR 2, PR 3, PR 4, *PR 5*, PR 7, PR 9
chr9	738,341	KANK1	c.3391 G > C	p.Ala1131Pro	0.1%	rs 180,816,986	*PR1*, PR3, *PR5*
chr17	27,286,417	**SEZ6**	c.1844 G > A	p.Arg615 His	0.01%	rs 371,753,097	*PR1*, PR2, *PR5*
chr20	57,598,807	TUBB1	c.326 G > A	p.Gly109 Glu	0.2%	rs 41,303,899	*PR1*, PR2, PR3, *PR5*
chr22	24,717,509	SPECC1L	c.562 C > T	p.Leu188 Phe	0.9%	rs 56,168,869	*PR1*, PR2, PR3, *PR5*, PR9

Chr Chromosome number

Percentage population frequency refers to data of the European population frequency derived from the 1000 Genomes Project at the time the manuscript was written. *See* the "Methods" section of text for further details. Chromosome positions refer to the hg19 assembly. The gene of interest (SEZ6) is highlighted in bold, and members affected with AD are Italic

SEZ6, with ratios (mutated *SEZ6* to wild-type *SEZ6*) ranging from 0.95 to 1.1, confirmed the heterozygous nature of the *SEZ6* C>T 27,286,417–27,186,418 substitution.

Aβ peptide generation in H4-SW cells

Three different H4-SW stable clonal lines (C3, C4, and C13) transfected with a pCDNA3.1 plasmid coding for *SEZ6*(R615H) mutant were selected, and the presence of the variant at DNA level was confirmed by allele-specific PCR and sequencing (data not shown). The effect of the R615H substitution on Aβ(1–42) and Aβ(1–40) production by H4-SW cells was assessed in conditioned media from cultured H4-SW(R615H) in comparison to H4-SW cells (untransfected or mock-transfected with an empty pCDNA3.1 vector) (Fig. 3a). The mean concentration of released Aβ(1–42), normalized to cell total protein content, was significantly lower in C4 and C13 than in controls, whereas for the C3 line, there was a trend in the

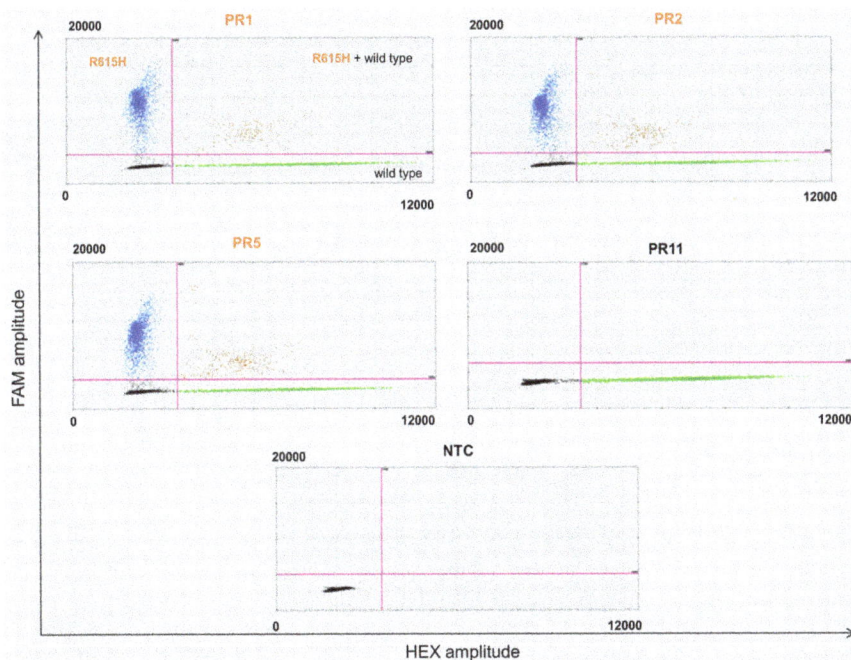

Fig. 2 Digital droplet PCR validation of the exome sequencing data. For each patient, a 2D dot plot is shown, reporting the distribution of fluorescence (on the *y*-axis FAM amplitude, and on the *x*-axis HEX amplitude). FAM and HEX are the fluorescent dyes for the *SEZ6* mutant and *SEZ6* wild type, respectively. On the basis of the fluorescence measurements and the droplet distributions, thresholds (*pink lines*) were set to 5000 for the FAM channel (*y*-axis) and 3000 for the HEX channel (*x*-axis). Negative droplets (*gray*), FAM-positive (*blue*), HEX-positive (*green*), and FAM/HEX double-positive (*orange*) droplets are reported for the four cases and no-template control (NTC) analyzed. Each case represents the sum of independent reactions

Table 2 Mutant *SEZ6* assay by digital droplet PCR in healthy control subjects, patients with sporadic Alzheimer's disease, and family members

Healthy population (n = 191)					Sporadic AD cases (n = 9)					Family members (n = 3)					
Sample	Target	Concentration (copies/μl)	Target	Concentration (copies/μl)	Sample	Target	Concentration (copies/μl)	Target	Concentration (copies/μl)	Sample	Target	Concentration (copies/μl)	Target	Concentration (copies/μl)	RATIO (mut/wt)
6	MUT SEZ6	N.D.	WT SEZ6	17	PR3	MUT SEZ6	N.D.	WT SEZ6	239	PR1	MUT SEZ6	116	WT SEZ6	103	1.13
7	MUT SEZ6	N.D.	WT SEZ6	14		MUT SEZ6	N.D.	WT SEZ6	226		MUT SEZ6	114	WT SEZ6	120	0.95
8	MUT SEZ6	N.D.	WT SEZ6	11	PR4	MUT SEZ6	N.D.	WT SEZ6	220	PR2	MUT SEZ6	130	WT SEZ6	130	1.00
9	MUT SEZ6	N.D.	WT SEZ6	59		MUT SEZ6	N.D.	WT SEZ6	224		MUT SEZ6	131	WT SEZ6	127	1.03
11	MUT SEZ6	N.D.	WT SEZ6	41	PR6	MUT SEZ6	N.D.	WT SEZ6	267	PR5	MUT SEZ6	149	WT SEZ6	153	0.97
12	MUT SEZ6	N.D.	WT SEZ6	49		MUT SEZ6	N.D.	WT SEZ6	261		MUT SEZ6	154	WT SEZ6	152	1.01
13	MUT SEZ6	N.D.	WT SEZ6	36	PR7	MUT SEZ6	N.D.	WT SEZ6	331						
14	MUT SEZ6	N.D.	WT SEZ6	29		MUT SEZ6	N.D.	WT SEZ6	371						
16	MUT SEZ6	N.D.	WT SEZ6	29	PR8	MUT SEZ6	N.D.	WT SEZ6	307						
17	MUT SEZ6	N.D.	WT SEZ6	27		MUT SEZ6	N.D.	WT SEZ6	303						
18	MUT SEZ6	N.D.	WT SEZ6	43	PR9	MUT SEZ6	N.D.	WT SEZ6	254						
19	MUT SEZ6	N.D.	WT SEZ6	30		MUT SEZ6	N.D.	WT SEZ6	266						
21	MUT SEZ6	N.D.	WT SEZ6	35	PR10	MUT SEZ6	N.D.	WT SEZ6	239						
22	MUT SEZ6	N.D.	WT SEZ6	53		MUT SEZ6	N.D.	WT SEZ6	273						
23	MUT SEZ6	N.D.	WT SEZ6	37	PR11	MUT SEZ6	N.D.	WT SEZ6	233						
24	MUT SEZ6	N.D.	WT SEZ6	45		MUT SEZ6	N.D.	WT SEZ6	228						
25	MUT SEZ6	N.D.	WT SEZ6	32	PR12	MUT SEZ6	N.D.	WT SEZ6	212						
27	MUT SEZ6	N.D.	WT SEZ6	26		MUT SEZ6	N.D.	WT SEZ6	190						
28	MUT SEZ6	N.D.	WT SEZ6	47											

Table 2 Mutant *SEZ6* assay by digital droplet PCR in healthy control subjects, patients with sporadic Alzheimer's disease, and family members *(Continued)*

Healthy population (n = 191)					Sporadic AD cases (n = 9)					Family members (n = 3)					RATIO (mut/wt)
Sample	Target	Concentration (copies/µl)	Target	Concentration (copies/µl)	Sample	Target	Concentration (copies/µl)	Target	Concentration (copies/µl)	Sample	Target	Concentration (copies/µl)	Target	Concentration (copies/µl)	
29	MUT SEZ6	N.D.	WT SEZ6	48											
30	MUT SEZ6	N.D.	WT SEZ6	30											
34	MUT SEZ6	N.D.	WT SEZ6	30											
36	MUT SEZ6	N.D.	WT SEZ6	49											
38	MUT SEZ6	N.D.	WT SEZ6	32											
39	MUT SEZ6	N.D.	WT SEZ6	34											
41	MUT SEZ6	N.D.	WT SEZ6	74											
42	MUT SEZ6	N.D.	WT SEZ6	43											
44	MUT SEZ6	N.D.	WT SEZ6	53											
46	MUT SEZ6	N.D.	WT SEZ6	64											
51	MUT SEZ6	N.D.	WT SEZ6	55											
52	MUT SEZ6	N.D.	WT SEZ6	19											
53	MUT SEZ6	N.D.	WT SEZ6	32											
60	MUT SEZ6	N.D.	WT SEZ6	46											
61	MUT SEZ6	N.D.	WT SEZ6	44											
62	MUT SEZ6	N.D.	WT SEZ6	64											
64	MUT SEZ6	N.D.	WT SEZ6	55											
66	MUT SEZ6	N.D.	WT SEZ6	45											
67	MUT SEZ6	N.D.	WT SEZ6	46											

Table 2 Mutant *SEZ6* assay by digital droplet PCR in healthy control subjects, patients with sporadic Alzheimer's disease, and family members *(Continued)*

| Healthy population (n = 191) | | | | | Sporadic AD cases (n = 9) | | | | | Family members (n = 3) | | | | | |
Sample	Target	Concentration (copies/µl)	Target	Concentration (copies/µl)	Sample	Target	Concentration (copies/µl)	Target	Concentration (copies/µl)	Sample	Target	Concentration (copies/µl)	Target	Concentration (copies/µl)	RATIO (mut/wrt)
69	MUT SEZ6	N.D.	WT SEZ6	48											
70	MUT SEZ6	N.D.	WT SEZ6	45											
71	MUT SEZ6	N.D.	WT SEZ6	67											
72	MUT SEZ6	N.D.	WT SEZ6	57											
74	MUT SEZ6	N.D.	WT SEZ6	54											
89	MUT SEZ6	N.D.	WT SEZ6	47											
90	MUT SEZ6	N.D.	WT SEZ6	78											
91	MUT SEZ6	N.D.	WT SEZ6	64.3											
101	MUT SEZ6	N.D.	WT SEZ6	283											
112	MUT SEZ6	N.D.	WT SEZ6	524											
113	MUT SEZ6	N.D.	WT SEZ6	1451											
114	MUT SEZ6	N.D.	WT SEZ6	962											
115	MUT SEZ6	N.D.	WT SEZ6	534											
118	MUT SEZ6	N.D.	WT SEZ6	527											
119	MUT SEZ6	N.D.	WT SEZ6	1691											
120	MUT SEZ6	N.D.	WT SEZ6	359											
129	MUT SEZ6	N.D.	WT SEZ6	186											
130	MUT SEZ6	N.D.	WT SEZ6	258											
133	MUT SEZ6	N.D.	WT SEZ6	232											

Table 2 Mutant *SEZ6* assay by digital droplet PCR in healthy control subjects, patients with sporadic Alzheimer's disease, and family members (*Continued*)

Healthy population (n = 191)					Sporadic AD cases (n = 9)					Family members (n = 3)					RATIO (mut/wt)
Sample	Target	Concentration (copies/μl)	Target	Concentration (copies/μl)	Sample	Target	Concentration (copies/μl)	Target	Concentration (copies/μl)	Sample	Target	Concentration (copies/μl)	Target	Concentration (copies/μl)	
135	MUT SEZ6	N.D.	WT SEZ6	373											
137	MUT SEZ6	N.D.	WT SEZ6	319											
144	MUT SEZ6	N.D.	WT SEZ6	310											
151	MUT SEZ6	N.D.	WT SEZ6	396											
152	MUT SEZ6	N.D.	WT SEZ6	180											
160	MUT SEZ6	N.D.	WT SEZ6	574											
162	MUT SEZ6	N.D.	WT SEZ6	400											
163	MUT SEZ6	N.D.	WT SEZ6	142											
164	MUT SEZ6	N.D.	WT SEZ6	39											
170	MUT SEZ6	N.D.	WT SEZ6	96											
179	MUT SEZ6	N.D.	WT SEZ6	94											
180	MUT SEZ6	N.D.	WT SEZ6	27											
182	MUT SEZ6	N.D.	WT SEZ6	1406											
184	MUT SEZ6	N.D.	WT SEZ6	1994											
185	MUT SEZ6	N.D.	WT SEZ6	161											
192	MUT SEZ6	N.D.	WT SEZ6	14.5											
193	MUT SEZ6	N.D.	WT SEZ6	1740											
197	MUT SEZ6	N.D.	WT SEZ6	185											
198	MUT SEZ6	N.D.	WT SEZ6	250											

Table 2 Mutant *SEZ6* assay by digital droplet PCR in healthy control subjects, patients with sporadic Alzheimer's disease, and family members *(Continued)*

	Healthy population (n = 191)					Sporadic AD cases (n = 9)					Family members (n = 3)					
Sample	Target	Concentration (copies/µl)	Target	Concentration (copies/µl)		Sample	Target	Concentration (copies/µl)	Target	Concentration (copies/µl)	Sample	Target	Concentration (copies/µl)	Target	Concentration (copies/µl)	RATIO (mut/wt)
199	MUT SEZ6	N.D.	WT SEZ6	145												
200	MUT SEZ6	N.D.	WT SEZ6	132												
202	MUT SEZ6	N.D.	WT SEZ6	663												
205	MUT SEZ6	N.D.	WT SEZ6	658												
206	MUT SEZ6	N.D.	WT SEZ6	118												
210	MUT SEZ6	N.D.	WT SEZ6	103												
212	MUT SEZ6	N.D.	WT SEZ6	23												
214	MUT SEZ6	N.D.	WT SEZ6	385												
215	MUT SEZ6	N.D.	WT SEZ6	125												
219	MUT SEZ6	N.D.	WT SEZ6	223												
223	MUT SEZ6	N.D.	WT SEZ6	316												
228	MUT SEZ6	N.D.	WT SEZ6	109												
233	MUT SEZ6	N.D.	WT SEZ6	385												
237	MUT SEZ6	N.D.	WT SEZ6	767												
240	MUT SEZ6	N.D.	WT SEZ6	318												
241	MUT SEZ6	N.D.	WT SEZ6	15												
243	MUT SEZ6	N.D.	WT SEZ6	30												
245	MUT SEZ6	N.D.	WT SEZ6	166												
247	MUT SEZ6	N.D.	WT SEZ6	161												

Table 2 Mutant *SEZ6* assay by digital droplet PCR in healthy control subjects, patients with sporadic Alzheimer's disease, and family members (*Continued*)

Healthy population (n = 191)					Sporadic AD cases (n = 9)					Family members (n = 3)					
Sample	Target	Concentration (copies/µl)	Target	Concentration (copies/µl)	Sample	Target	Concentration (copies/µl)	Target	Concentration (copies/µl)	Sample	Target	Concentration (copies/µl)	Target	Concentration (copies/µl)	RATIO (mut/wrt)
251	MUT SEZ6	N.D.	WT SEZ6	164											
253	MUT SEZ6	N.D.	WT SEZ6	491											
254	MUT SEZ6	N.D.	WT SEZ6	772											
255	MUT SEZ6	N.D.	WT SEZ6	771											
257	MUT SEZ6	N.D.	WT SEZ6	148											
261	MUT SEZ6	N.D.	WT SEZ6	875											
263	MUT SEZ6	N.D.	WT SEZ6	381											
267	MUT SEZ6	N.D.	WT SEZ6	442											
270	MUT SEZ6	N.D.	WT SEZ6	368											
275	MUT SEZ6	N.D.	WT SEZ6	317											
276	MUT SEZ6	N.D.	WT SEZ6	368											
277	MUT SEZ6	N.D.	WT SEZ6	186											
278	MUT SEZ6	N.D.	WT SEZ6	63											
279	MUT SEZ6	N.D.	WT SEZ6	234											
287	MUT SEZ6	N.D.	WT SEZ6	99											
293	MUT SEZ6	N.D.	WT SEZ6	125											
324	MUT SEZ6	N.D.	WT SEZ6	605											
325	MUT SEZ6	N.D.	WT SEZ6	153											
326	MUT SEZ6	N.D.	WT SEZ6	692											

Table 2 Mutant *SEZ6* assay by digital droplet PCR in healthy control subjects, patients with sporadic Alzheimer's disease, and family members *(Continued)*

Healthy population (n = 191)					Sporadic AD cases (n = 9)					Family members (n = 3)					RATIO (mut/wt)
Sample	Target	Concentration (copies/µl)	Target	Concentration (copies/µl)	Sample	Target	Concentration (copies/µl)	Target	Concentration (copies/µl)	Sample	Target	Concentration (copies/µl)	Target	Concentration (copies/µl)	
327	MUT SEZ6	N.D.	WT SEZ6	713											
328	MUT SEZ6	N.D.	WT SEZ6	391											
332	MUT SEZ6	N.D.	WT SEZ6	759											
333	MUT SEZ6	N.D.	WT SEZ6	661											
337	MUT SEZ6	N.D.	WT SEZ6	798											
338	MUT SEZ6	N.D.	WT SEZ6	903											
340	MUT SEZ6	N.D.	WT SEZ6	40											
341	MUT SEZ6	N.D.	WT SEZ6	274											
342	MUT SEZ6	N.D.	WT SEZ6	240											
344	MUT SEZ6	N.D.	WT SEZ6	209											
345	MUT SEZ6	N.D.	WT SEZ6	873											
348	MUT SEZ6	N.D.	WT SEZ6	2330											
350	MUT SEZ6	N.D.	WT SEZ6	387											
351	MUT SEZ6	N.D.	WT SEZ6	430											
353	MUT SEZ6	N.D.	WT SEZ6	360											
360	MUT SEZ6	N.D.	WT SEZ6	473											
361	MUT SEZ6	N.D.	WT SEZ6	553											
362	MUT SEZ6	N.D.	WT SEZ6	2470											
363	MUT SEZ6	N.D.	WT SEZ6	889											

Table 2 Mutant *SEZ6* assay by digital droplet PCR in healthy control subjects, patients with sporadic Alzheimer's disease, and family members *(Continued)*

Healthy population (n = 191)					Sporadic AD cases (n = 9)					Family members (n = 3)					
Sample	Target	Concentration (copies/μl)	Target	Concentration (copies/μl)	Sample	Target	Concentration (copies/μl)	Target	Concentration (copies/μl)	Sample	Target	Concentration (copies/μl)	Target	Concentration (copies/μl)	RATIO (mut/wt)
366	MUT SEZ6	N.D.	WT SEZ6	1990											
367	MUT SEZ6	N.D.	WT SEZ6	452											
368	MUT SEZ6	N.D.	WT SEZ6	1736											
369	MUT SEZ6	N.D.	WT SEZ6	1436											
375	MUT SEZ6	N.D.	WT SEZ6	588											
376	MUT SEZ6	N.D.	WT SEZ6	544											
377	MUT SEZ6	N.D.	WT SEZ6	623											
401	MUT SEZ6	N.D.	WT SEZ6	803											
404	MUT SEZ6	N.D.	WT SEZ6	494											
406	MUT SEZ6	N.D.	WT SEZ6	200											
407	MUT SEZ6	N.D.	WT SEZ6	482											
408	MUT SEZ6	N.D.	WT SEZ6	105											
409	MUT SEZ6	N.D.	WT SEZ6	3260											
418	MUT SEZ6	N.D.	WT SEZ6	190											
422	MUT SEZ6	N.D.	WT SEZ6	1325											
430	MUT SEZ6	N.D.	WT SEZ6	772											
434	MUT SEZ6	N.D.	WT SEZ6	1233											
435	MUT SEZ6	N.D.	WT SEZ6	1844											
440	MUT SEZ6	N.D.	WT SEZ6	90											

Table 2 Mutant *SEZ6* assay by digital droplet PCR in healthy control subjects, patients with sporadic Alzheimer's disease, and family members (*Continued*)

Healthy population (n = 191)					Sporadic AD cases (n = 9)					Family members (n = 3)					
Sample	Target	Concentration (copies/µl)	Target	Concentration (copies/µl)	Sample	Target	Concentration (copies/µl)	Target	Concentration (copies/µl)	Sample	Target	Concentration (copies/µl)	Target	Concentration (copies/µl)	RATIO (mut/wt)
446	MUT SEZ6	N.D.	WT SEZ6	745											
451	MUT SEZ6	N.D.	WT SEZ6	1366											
453	MUT SEZ6	N.D.	WT SEZ6	1185											
454	MUT SEZ6	N.D.	WT SEZ6	2950											
466	MUT SEZ6	N.D.	WT SEZ6	329											
468	MUT SEZ6	N.D.	WT SEZ6	681											
493	MUT SEZ6	N.D.	WT SEZ6	80											
497	MUT SEZ6	N.D.	WT SEZ6	154											
499	MUT SEZ6	N.D.	WT SEZ6	128											
501	MUT SEZ6	N.D.	WT SEZ6	1814											
511	MUT SEZ6	N.D.	WT SEZ6	547											
512	MUT SEZ6	N.D.	WT SEZ6	48.2											
513	MUT SEZ6	N.D.	WT SEZ6	40.8											
514	MUT SEZ6	N.D.	WT SEZ6	1019											
519	MUT SEZ6	N.D.	WT SEZ6	1382											
520	MUT SEZ6	N.D.	WT SEZ6	791											
521	MUT SEZ6	N.D.	WT SEZ6	1858											
522	MUT SEZ6	N.D.	WT SEZ6	2180											
523	MUT SEZ6	N.D.	WT SEZ6	1849											

Table 2 Mutant *SEZ6* assay by digital droplet PCR in healthy control subjects, patients with sporadic Alzheimer's disease, and family members (*Continued*)

Healthy population (n = 191)					Sporadic AD cases (n = 9)					Family members (n = 3)					RATIO (mut/wt)
Sample	Target	Concentration (copies/µl)	Target	Concentration (copies/µl)	Sample	Target	Concentration (copies/µl)	Target	Concentration (copies/µl)	Sample	Target	Concentration (copies/µl)	Target	Concentration (copies/µl)	
531	MUT SEZ6	N.D.	WT SEZ6	2110											
532	MUT SEZ6	N.D.	WT SEZ6	3030											
535	MUT SEZ6	N.D.	WT SEZ6	1096											
537	MUT SEZ6	N.D.	WT SEZ6	1941											
538	MUT SEZ6	N.D.	WT SEZ6	78											
539	MUT SEZ6	N.D.	WT SEZ6	917											
542	MUT SEZ6	N.D.	WT SEZ6	1650											
543	MUT SEZ6	N.D.	WT SEZ6	937											
545	MUT SEZ6	N.D.	WT SEZ6	1423											
546	MUT SEZ6	N.D.	WT SEZ6	818											
549	MUT SEZ6	N.D.	WT SEZ6	1196											
550	MUT SEZ6	N.D.	WT SEZ6	716											
558	MUT SEZ6	N.D.	WT SEZ6	845											
567	MUT SEZ6	N.D.	WT SEZ6	724											
570	MUT SEZ6	N.D.	WT SEZ6	765											
571	MUT SEZ6	N.D.	WT SEZ6	2290											
574	MUT SEZ6	N.D.	WT SEZ6	790											
575	MUT SEZ6	N.D.	WT SEZ6	1399											
578	MUT SEZ6	N.D.	WT SEZ6	1293											

Table 2 Mutant *SEZ6* assay by digital droplet PCR in healthy control subjects, patients with sporadic Alzheimer's disease, and family members *(Continued)*

Healthy population (n = 191)					Sporadic AD cases (n = 9)					Family members (n = 3)					
Sample	Target	Concentration (copies/µl)	Target	Concentration (copies/µl)	Sample	Target	Concentration (copies/µl)	Target	Concentration (copies/µl)	Sample	Target	Concentration (copies/µl)	Target	Concentration (copies/µl)	RATIO (mut/wt)
580	MUT SEZ6	N.D.	WT SEZ6	947											

ND Not detectable

Alzheimer's disease cases are underlined. For each group, patient code, digital droplet PCR target, and the calculated concentration (copies/µl) are reported. For the last group, the ratio, defined as concentration mutant *SEZ6*/concentration wild-type *SEZ6*, is also reported

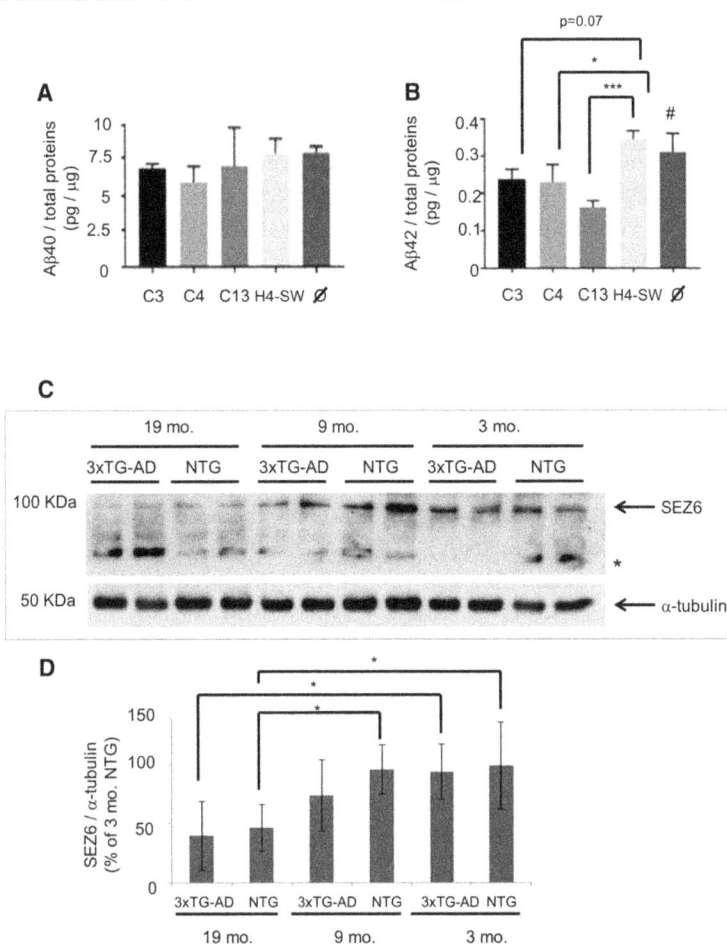

Fig. 3 Evaluation of *SEZ6* relevance for Alzheimer's disease (AD) mechanisms in *in vitro* and *in vivo* models. **a** Quantification by enzyme-linked immunosorbent assay of soluble amyloid-β 1–40 (Aβ$_{1-40}$) in conditioned media from H4-SW clonal lines (C3, C4, and C13) overexpressing *SEZ6*(R615H). The amyloid peptide concentration was normalized to the total protein content of the producing cells of each replicate. Measures are the mean ± SD of three independent wells. *H4-SW* Untransfected control; Ø H4-SW control transfected with pCDNA3.1 empty vector. **b** Same as in (**a**) except for the assessment of Aβ$_{1-42}$ soluble form. * $p < 0.05$; *** $p < 0.001$, one-way analysis of variance (ANOVA) and post hoc test; # $p < 0.05$ vs. C4 and $p < 0.01$ vs. C13, one-way ANOVA and post hoc test. **c** Representative Western blotting for Sez6 protein detection in brain cortical extract from 3xTG-AD mice. Mice were killed at ages 3, 9, or 19 months, and *Sez6* expression was assessed in transgenic and matched nontransgenic (NTG) animals. Each group was composed of three mice, and every animal was loaded in duplicate in the SDS-PAGE experiment. * Unspecific signal. **d** Densitometric quantification of all Western blot analysis data for Sez6 protein cortical expression ($n = 3$ mice/group) using ImageJ software. Each signal was normalized to the corresponding α-tubulin band to control for unequal protein loading. Results are expressed as a percentage of the youngest group (3 months) * $p < 0.05$, one-way ANOVA and post hoc test. *mo.* Months from birth

same direction ($p = 0.07$). The Aβ(1–40) assay showed no differences (Fig. 3b).

Sez6 brain expression in 3xTG-AD mice

Given that few experimental data linked *SEZ6* to AD, we also examined murine *Sez6* expression in a transgenic line model of AD (3xTG-AD), in comparison with age-matched nontransgenic controls (NTG) (Fig. 3c and d). Mice were killed at ages ranging from 3 to 19 months, and Sez6 protein expression was assessed at brain cortical level. Sez6 protein markedly decreased with age, particularly between 3 and 19 months. However, this reduction was common to

both the 3xTG-AD and NTG lines and thus not unique to the AD model.

Discussion

Pathogenic mutations in *APP, PSEN1,* or *PSEN2* genes are linked to FAD [3, 4]. *PSEN1* mutations are responsible for about 60% of the genetic cases of AD, and 286 pathogenic variants have been described in the three above-cited genes [22]. We report an Italian family with AD that we previously screened by denaturing high-performance liquid chromatography (data not shown) for *APP, PSEN1,* or *PSEN2* mutations with no results. Considering that rare variants in other genes have been associated with AD [7], we decided to perform targeted exome-sequencing analysis that yielded a large number of variants; in order to identify those closely related to the disease, we employed a recursive filtering strategy. This strategy was based on the removal of high-frequency (> 1%) variants using a public database (1000 Genomes Project) with *in silico* prediction software (SIFT, PolyPhen2, CADD) to exclude potentially harmless mutations and focus on variants present in FAD but not sporadic AD samples. We gave priority to the *SEZ6*(R615H) variant among those reported in Table 1, considering that *SEZ6* has already been reported as relevant for molecular mechanisms involved in AD pathogenesis, because it is a substrate of the BACE-1 enzyme (β-secretase), affects synapse formation, and is reduced in the cerebrospinal fluid of patients with AD, as revealed by a proteomic study [23–25]. *SEZ6* gene mutations have been also reported in association with febrile seizures, and *SEZ6* was proposed as a candidate gene for epilepsy [26, 27]. Moreover, *SEZ6* mutations were found in cases of childhood-onset schizophrenia [28]. The rare variant R615H (rs371753097, C/T) was reported in the 1000 Genomes Project as absent in Toscani in Italy (TSI) population and had a frequency in the whole project of 0.0002 [29]. Another interesting genetic variant we found by exome sequencing that is deserving of attention is A1131P in the *KANK1* gene [30], which was present in the two AD cases (PR1 and PR5) and in PR3, sibling of PR1. However, PR3 did not have dementia at sampling (age 67 years), and her clinical state is currently unchanged, even though we are not able to exclude a possible later onset. The human *KANK1* gene (alias ANKRD15) was originally described to be a tumor suppressor in renal cell carcinoma, and it encodes an ankyrin repeat domain-containing protein (Kank). It belongs to a family of four homologous members that have a role in actin stress fiber formation and renal pathophysiology [31, 32]. There is no reported interaction of *KANK1* with *SEZ6* or AD-related genes. However, a role of *KANK1* mutation or deletion was reported in cerebral palsy spastic quadriplegic type 2, a central nervous system developmental disorder [33]. Moreover, to the best of our knowledge, no data associate *KANK1* with AD.

In our study's family, we were able to correlate the AD pathology to R615H presence, which was found in the two available AD-affected members and one first-degree relative of an AD case, whose age at sampling in 2003 (PR2, 37 years) was far below the family age of onset (range, 60–70 years) to expect clinical signs. The current clinical diagnosis of PR2 (51 years) is unchanged. We also confirmed that R615H frequency is very low (< 1%) in the Italian population, because we were unable to detect the variant in 200 family-unrelated subjects.

Because it is a common finding that AD pathogenic mutations increase Aβ(1–42) peptide generation [34],

we examined the effect of the R615H variant in a cell model in this respect. In the H4-SW line, we noticed a decrease in Aβ(1–42), whereas Aβ(1–40) was unchanged. However, the increase of Aβ(1–42) in association with FAD-linked mutations is not always replicated. In fact, some presenilin mutants with proved pathologic action did not increase Aβ(1–42) but acted on other Aβ peptide generation or even had no impact on this proteolytic cleavage. In the latter case, the hypothesis is that the mutation affects important functions of presenilin other than the γ-secretase activity [35, 36]. It is worth underlining that we found a peculiar biochemical effect of the *PSEN1* mutation E318G that increased Aβ(1–40) only in cultured skin primary fibroblasts [17]. Our failure to detect an increase of Aβ(1–42) might depend on the reported role of SEZ6 protein as substrate for BACE-1 [23], so its overexpression may be competitive for *APP* in the cell model tested. We need further experiments to clarify the role of the R615H variant in this context.

Finally, we followed *SEZ6* cortical expression in a mouse model of AD (3xTG-AD). Considering that it changed similarly in 3xTG-AD and control mice, we were unable to link this result to AD-specific patterns, but we did notice a decrease of SEZ6 protein with age, in agreement with this gene's reported role in brain development [37, 38]. A damaging mutation (as R615H is predicted to be) may have an impact on the protein activity from birth, with possible neuropathologic outcomes, likely in combination with other triggering factors, also considering the reported role of *SEZ6* in dendritic spine dynamics and cognition [39].

This study has limitations, mainly linked to the unavailability of genomic DNA from all the family's AD-affected members alive at sampling. Moreover, we decided to use a targeted exome-sequencing strategy that, on one hand, gave us clinical data supporting a rational choice of candidate variants to be prioritized, but on the other hand, prevented us from ruling out that additional coding mutations in genes not included in our panel may be linked to AD phenotype, thus acting in synergy with *SEZ6 (R615H)*.

Conclusions

In summary, by using a targeted exome-sequencing approach, we discovered a rare *SEZ6* variant exclusive to AD members of a large Italian family carrying no typical FAD-linked mutations that might have a role in disease onset, in particular taking into account the already described involvement of *SEZ6* in AD pathogenic mechanisms linked to amyloid-β (A4) precursor protein (*APP*) and brain physiology, even though the exact molecular pathway linking *SEZ6* to AD is still unclear.

Acknowledgements
We are grateful to the family that kindly participated in this study. We thank Judith Baggott for English-language editing.

Funding
This work was supported by Fondazione Italo Monzino (Milan, Italy).

Authors' contributions
LP performed the digital droplet PCR assay and exome sequencing. LBe alanyzed genomic data and produced bioinformatics output. FF and LBo prepared the H4-SW clonal lines and measured SEZ6 gene expression in transgenic mice. PC recruited the families with sporadic Alzheimer's disease and control subjects. DA, SM, and GF drafted the manuscript. All authors critically revised the manuscript. All authors read and approved the final manuscript.

Consent for publication
Not applicable, because this article does not contain any individual person's data, images, or videos.

Competing interests
The authors declare that they have no competing interests.

Author details
[1]Department of Oncology, Istituto di Ricerche Farmacologiche Mario Negri IRCCS, Via La Masa 19, 20156 Milan, Italy. [2]Dipartimento di Chimica, Materiali e Ingegneria Chimica "G. Natta", Politecnico di Milano, Piazza Leonardo da Vinci 32, 20133 Milan, Italy. [3]Department of Neuroscience, Istituto di Ricerche Farmacologiche Mario Negri IRCCS, Via La Masa 19, 20156 Milan, Italy. [4]Department of Neuroscience, Istituto di Neurologia, Università di Parma, Via Gramsci 14, 43100 Parma, Italy.

References
1. Chandra V, Schoenberg BS. Inheritance of Alzheimer's disease: epidemiologic evidence. Neuroepidemiology. 1989;8:165–74.
2. Corder EH, Saunders AM, Strittmatter WJ, Schmechel DE, Gaskell PC, Small GW, et al. Gene dose of apolipoprotein E type 4 allele and the risk of Alzheimer's disease in late onset families. Science. 1993;261:921–3.
3. Brunkan AL, Goate AM. Presenilin function and gamma-secretase activity. J Neurochem. 2005;93:769–92.
4. Bertram L, Tanzi RE. The current status of Alzheimer's disease genetics: what do we tell the patients? Pharmacol Res. 2004;50:385–96.
5. Sherrington R, Rogaev EI, Liang Y, Rogaeva EA, Levesque G, Ikeda M, et al. Cloning of a gene bearing missense mutations in early-onset familial Alzheimer's disease. Nature. 1995;375:754–60.
6. Goate A, Chartier-Harlin MC, Mullan M, Brown J, Crawford F, Fidani L, et al. Segregation of a missense mutation in the amyloid precursor protein gene with familial Alzheimer's disease. Nature. 1991;349:704–6.
7. Sims R, van der Lee SJ, Naj AC, Bellenguez C, Badarinarayan N, Jakobsdottir J, et al. Rare coding variants in PLCG2, ABI3, and TREM2 implicate microglial-mediated innate immunity in Alzheimer's disease. Nat Genet. 2017;49:1373–84.
8. Thonberg H, Chiang HH, Lilius L, Forsell C, Lindström AK, Johansson C, et al. Identification and description of three families with familial Alzheimer disease that segregate variants in the SORL1 gene. Acta Neuropathol Commun. 2017;5:43.
9. McKhann G, Drachman D, Folstein M, Katzman R, Price D, Stadlan EM. Clinical diagnosis of Alzheimer's disease: report of the NINCDS-ADRDA Work Group under the auspices of Department of Health and Human Services Task Force on Alzheimer's Disease. Neurology. 1984;34:939–44.
10. Li H, Durbin R. Fast and accurate long-read alignment with Burrows-Wheeler transform. Bioinformatics. 2010;26:589–95.
11. McKenna A, Hanna M, Banks E, Sivachenko A, Cibulskis K, Kernytsky A, et al. The Genome Analysis Toolkit: a MapReduce framework for analyzing next-generation DNA sequencing data. Genome Res. 2010;20:1297–303.
12. DePristo MA, Banks E, Poplin R, Garimella KV, Maguire JR, Hartl C, et al. A framework for variation discovery and genotyping using next-generation DNA sequencing data. Nat Genet. 2011;43:491–8.
13. Van der Auwera GA, Carneiro MO, Hartl C, Poplin R, Del Angel G, Levy-Moonshine A, et al. From FastQ data to high confidence variant calls: the Genome Analysis Toolkit best practices pipeline. Curr Protoc Bioinformatics. 2013;43:11.10.1–33.
14. McLaren W, Gil L, Hunt SE, Riat HS, Ritchie GR, Thormann A, et al. The Ensembl Variant Effect Predictor. Genome Biol. 2016;17:122.
15. Paila U, Chapman BA, Kirchner R, Quinlan AR. GEMINI: integrative exploration of genetic variation and genome annotations. PLoS Comput Biol. 2013;9(7):e1003153.
16. Liu X, Jian X, Boerwinkle E. dbNSFP v2.0: a database of human non-synonymous SNVs and their functional predictions and annotations. Hum Mutat. 2013;34:E2393–402.
17. Albani D, Roiter I, Artuso V, Batelli S, Prato F, Pesaresi M, et al. Presenilin-1 mutation E318G and familial Alzheimer's disease in the Italian population. Neurobiol Aging. 2007;28:1682–8.
18. Haugabook SJ, Yager DM, Eckman EA, Golde TE, Younkin SG, Eckman CB. High throughput screens for the identification of compounds that alter the accumulation of the Alzheimer's amyloid β peptide (Aβ). J Neurosci Methods. 2001;108:171–9.
19. Oddo S, Caccamo A, Shepherd JD, Murphy MP, Golde TE, Kayed R, et al. Triple-transgenic model of Alzheimer's disease with plaques and tangles: intracellular Aβ and synaptic dysfunction. Neuron. 2003;39:409–21.
20. Shimizu-Nishikawa K, Kajiwara K, Sugaya E. Cloning and characterization of seizure-related gene, SEZ-6. Biochem Biophys Res Commun. 1995;216:382–9.
21. Bork P, Beckmann G. The CUB domain: a widespread module in developmentally regulated proteins. J Mol Biol. 1993;231:539–45.
22. Alzheimer Disease & Frontotemporal Dementia Mutation Database (AD&FTDMDB). http://www.molgen.ua.ac.be/ADmutations/. Accessed 21 May 2018.
23. Pigoni M, Wanngren J, Kuhn PH, Munro KM, Gunnersen JM, Takeshima H, et al. Seizure protein 6 and its homolog seizure 6-like protein are physiological substrates of BACE1 in neurons. Mol Neurodegener. 2016;11:67.
24. Zhu K, Xiang X, Filser S, Marinković P, Dorostkar MM, Crux S, et al. B-site amyloid precursor protein cleaving enzyme 1 inhibition impairs synaptic plasticity via seizure protein 6. Biol Psychiatry. 2018;83:428–37.
25. Khoonsari PE, Häggmark A, Lönnberg M, Mikus M, Kilander L, Lannfelt L, et al. Analysis of the cerebrospinal fluid proteome in Alzheimer's disease. PLoS One. 2016;11:e0150672.
26. Yu ZL, Jiang JM, Wu DH, Xie HJ, Jiang JJ, Zhou L, et al. Febrile seizures are associated with mutation of seizure-related (SEZ) 6, a brain-specific gene. J Neurosci Res. 2007;85:166–72.
27. Mulley JC, Iona X, Hodgson B, Heron SE, Berkovic SF, Scheffer IE, et al. The role of seizure-related SEZ6 as a susceptibility gene in febrile seizures. Neurol Res Int. 2011;2011:917565.
28. Ambalavanan A, Girard SL, Ahn K, Zhou S, Dionne-Laporte A, Spiegelman D, et al. De novo variants in sporadic cases of childhood onset schizophrenia. Eur J Hum Genet. 2016;24:944–8.

29. 1000 Genomes Browser. https://www.ncbi.nlm.nih.gov/variation/tools/
     1000genomes/. Accessed 18 July 2017.
30. Sarkar S, Roy BC, Hatano N, Aoyagi T, Gohji K, Kiyama R. A novel ankyrin
     repeat-containing gene (Kank) located at 9p24 is a growth suppressor of
     renal cell carcinoma. J Biol Chem. 2002;277:36585–91.
31. Zhu Y, Kakinuma N, Wang Y, Kiyama R. Kank proteins: a new family of
     ankyrin-repeat domain-containing proteins. Biochim Biophys Acta. 2008;
     1780:128–33.
32. Gee HY, Zhang F, Ashraf S, Kohl S, Sadowski CE, Vega-Warner V, et al. KANK
     deficiency leads to podocyte dysfunction and nephrotic syndrome. J Clin
     Invest. 2015;125:2375–84.
33. Lerer I, Sagi M, Meiner V, Cohen T, Zlotogora J, Abeliovich D. Deletion of
     the ANKRD15 gene at 9p24.3 causes parent-of-origin-dependent inheritance
     of familial cerebral palsy. Hum Mol Genet. 2005;14:3911–20.
34. Suzuki N, Cheung TT, Cai XD, Odaka A, Otvos L Jr, Eckman C, et al. An
     increased percentage of long amyloid β protein secreted by familial
     amyloid β protein precursor (β APP717) mutants. Science. 1994;264:1336–40.
35. Bentahir M, Nyabi O, Verhamme J, Tolia A, Horré K, Wiltfang J, et al.
     Presenilin clinical mutations can affect gamma-secretase activity by different
     mechanisms. J Neurochem. 2006;96:732–42.
36. Szaruga M, Veugelen S, Benurwar M, Lismont S, Sepulveda-Falla D, Lleo A,
     et al. Qualitative changes in human γ-secretase underlie familial Alzheimer's
     disease. J Exp Med. 2015;212:2003–13.
37. Kim MH, Gunnersen JM, Tan SS. Localized expression of the seizure-related
     gene SEZ-6 in developing and adult forebrains. Mech Dev. 2002;118:171–4.
38. Osaki G, Mitsui S, Yuri K. The distribution of the seizure-related gene 6 (Sez-
     6) protein during postnatal development of the mouse forebrain suggests
     multiple functions for this protein: an analysis using a new antibody. Brain
     Res. 2011;1386:58–69.
39. Gunnersen JM, Kim MH, Fuller SJ, De Silva M, Britto JM, Hammond VE, et al.
     Sez-6 proteins affect dendritic arborization patterns and excitability of
     cortical pyramidal neurons. Neuron. 2007;56:621–39.

Synergistic interaction between APOE and family history of Alzheimer's disease on cerebral amyloid deposition and glucose metabolism

Dahyun Yi[1], Younghwa Lee[2], Min Soo Byun[1], Jun Ho Lee[2], Kang Ko[2], Bo Kyung Sohn[3], Young Min Choe[4], Hyo Jung Choi[5], Hyewon Baek[6], Chul-Ho Sohn[7], Yu Kyeong Kim[8], Dong Young Lee[1,2,9*] and for the KBASE research group

Abstract

Background: Recently, the field of gene-gene or gene-environment interaction research appears to have gained growing interest, although it is seldom investigated in Alzheimer's disease (AD). Hence, the current study aims to investigate interaction effects of the key genetic and environmental risks—the apolipoprotein ε4 allele (APOE4) and family history of late-onset AD (FH)—on AD-related brain changes in cognitively normal (CN) middle-aged and older adults.

Methods: [^{11}C] Pittsburg compound-B (PiB) positron emission tomography (PET) imaging as well as [^{18}F] fluoro-2-deoxyglucose (FDG) PET that were simultaneously taken with T1-weighted magnetic resonance imaging (MRI) were obtained from 268 CNs from the Korean Brain Aging Study for Early Diagnosis and Prediction of AD (KBASE). Composite standardized uptake value ratios were obtained from PiB-PET and FDG-PET images in the AD signature regions of interests (ROIs) and analyzed. Voxel-wise analyses were also performed to examine detailed regional changes not captured by the ROI analyses.

Results: A significant synergistic interaction effect was found between the APOE4 and FH on amyloid-beta (Aβ) deposition in the AD signature ROIs as well as other regions. Synergistic interaction effects on cerebral glucose metabolism were observed in the regions not captured by the AD signature ROIs, particularly in the medial temporal regions.

Conclusions: Strong synergistic effects of APOE4 and FH on Aβ deposition and cerebral glucose metabolism in CN adults indicate possible gene-to-gene or gene-to-environment interactions that are crucial for pathogenesis of AD involving Aβ. Other unspecified risk factors—genes and/or environmental—that are captured by the positive FH status might either coexpress or interact with APOE4 to alter AD-related brain changes in CN. Healthy people with both FH and APOE4 need more attention for AD prevention.

Keywords: APOE, Family history of Alzheimer's disease, Cognitively normal adults, Amyloid beta deposition, Cerebral glucose metabolism

* Correspondence: selfpsy@snu.ac.kr
The coinvestigators of the KBASE Research Group are listed in Additional file 1 (Coinvestigators).
[1]Institute of Human Behavioral Medicine, Medical Research Center Seoul National University, Seoul, Republic of Korea
[2]Department of Neuropsychiatry, Seoul National University Hospital, Seoul, Republic of Korea
Full list of author information is available at the end of the article

Background

Decades of research on sporadic late-onset Alzheimer's disease (AD) dementia, the most common form of dementia, have shown that AD dementia is a multifactorial disease with a wide variety of genetic and environmental factors playing a role in the age of onset, risk, and etiology [1]. Numerous heritable and inheritable risk factors have been linked with AD pathogenesis. Nevertheless, to date, only a limited number of studies have investigated the interaction effect between the major risks on in-vivo AD-related brain changes which can reflect the pathogenesis of AD. Information about whether the major risks of AD dementia can synergistically increase AD-specific brain changes before the onset of dementia symptoms will likely help identification of a more urgent target population for the preventive efforts against AD dementia.

The apolipoprotein ε4 allele (APOE4) is a major risk factor for AD dementia and is associated with a decade or more mean age at onset decrease in AD symptoms [2]. Numerous studies have reported a relationship between APOE4 and AD-related brain changes such as increased amyloid-beta (Aβ) deposition and decreased glucose metabolism even in cognitively normal (CN) elderly individuals, although with some inconsistencies in the degree of effects [3–9]. Notably, functional brain abnormalities associated with APOE4 as identified by decreased cerebral glucose metabolism in the AD-related brain regions were found in healthy volunteers even as young as 20–39 years old [10]. Furthermore, a recent meta-analysis has shown strong effects of APOE4 on not only the prevalence of amyloid pathology but also the age of onset of AD dementia [11]. Despite some inconsistencies, the presence of strong effects of APOE4 on Aβ deposition and cerebral glucose metabolism has been repeatedly and undeniably shown.

In recent years, evidence has accumulated for other genetic and environmental factors that influence AD-related brain changes [1]. Having a first-degree family history of AD dementia (FH) is another well-known risk factor for developing AD dementia and is considered to encapsulate both genetic and environmental risk loads [12] as it not only captures heritable genetic susceptibility but also other shared dietary, psychosocial, and somatic factors that are shown to be associated with an individual's risk for developing AD dementia [13–15]. Similar to APOE4, the effects of FH on AD-related brain changes including Aβ deposition and glucose metabolism are present even in CN individuals, although less consistently [16–18].

Previous research shows that FH and APOE4 highly co-occur [19, 20] and, conceivably, their effects on developing AD dementia may overlap. However, given that they reflect different hereditary factors (i.e., genetic only

or both genetic and environmental), it is likely that an interaction of the effects of FH and APOE4 exists for AD-related brain changes such that having both FH and APOE4 will lead to synergistic influences on AD-related brain changes compared to when an individual has only one of the two risk factors. Nonetheless, to the best of our knowledge, no study has examined the synergistic interaction effects of FH and APOE4 on AD-related brain changes, specifically Aβ deposition and glucose metabolism, in cognitively intact adults. In this context, the purpose of the current study was to test the hypothesis that APOE4 and FH have synergistic interaction effects on cerebral Aβ deposition and glucose metabolism in healthy middle-aged and older adults.

Methods

Subjects

This study is a part of the Korean Brain Aging Study for the Early Diagnosis and Prediction of AD (KBASE), an ongoing prospective cohort study that began in 2014 designed to identify novel biomarkers for AD and to explore various lifetime experiences contributing to AD-related brain changes. The current study included 268 community-dwelling CN individuals, between 50 years and 87 years of age, who were recruited as of March 2016. Details on the KBASE study characteristics including recruitment have been described previously [21]. Individuals with medical, psychiatric, and/or neurological conditions or history of conditions that may affect brain structures or functions, such as stroke, head trauma, depression, hydrocephalus, or focal brain lesions on magnetic resonance imaging (MRI) were excluded. All subjects had reliable informants available who provided corroborative information on the family history of medical conditions, including the presence of AD dementia. Subjects had a Clinical Dementia Rating of 0 and performed within the normal range relative to age-, gender-, and education-adjusted normative means on comprehensive neuropsychological assessments [22, 23]. The study was ethically reviewed and all participants provided written informed consent to participate in this study after receiving a complete description of the study, which is approved by Seoul National University Hospital Institutional Review Board.

Assessments

Comprehensive clinical and neuropsychological assessment data were obtained from all participants based on the KBASE assessment protocol that incorporated and expanded upon the Korean version of the Consortium to Establish a Registry for Alzheimer's Disease assessment packet (CERAD-K) [22, 24]. A detailed description of the cognitive assessments has been previously reported [21]. Briefly, the assessments included the Mini-Mental State

Examination in the Korean version of the CERAD assessment packet (MMSE-KC), the CERAD-K verbal memory tests, including Word List Memory, Word List Delayed Recall, Word List Recognition, CERAD-K Constructional Praxis, and CERAD-K nonverbal memory delayed recall, the Trail Making Test A and B, and the Stroop Test (Korean Golden version), Verbal Fluency Tasks (both semantic and phonemic), the CERAD-K confrontational naming test (Modified Korean version of the Boston Naming Test), and the Wechsler Adult Intelligence Scale-revised edition Korean version (WAIS-R-K) Digit Span (forward and backward). Neuropsychological test performances are presented as z scores based on age-, gender-, and education-adjusted normative data [24].

Genomic DNA was extracted from whole blood and APOE genotyping was performed [25]; subjects with at least one ε4 allele were identified as APOE4 carriers. For the majority of participants, cognitive assessments were administered on the same day that the neuroimaging scans were conducted; four individuals underwent cognitive assessment and neuroimaging scans on different dates where the interval was less than 1 month.

Family history of AD

Subjects and reliable informants were administered a semistructured interview by trained psychiatrists or a registered nurse to gather detailed information of any family history of dementia. Participants were asked: 1) if any of their birth parents, natural grandparents, siblings sharing parents, or other relatives had dementia and/or other type of neurological diseases; 2) if so, what was the diagnosis of the affected relative and the age of onset; 3) whether or not the affected family member is deceased; and 4), if deceased, what was the age at death.

Positivity of FH was determined if at least one first-degree relative (parent or sibling) had AD onset at 65 years of age or older and whose diagnosis had been made by a certified clinician. If formal diagnosis for a parent was unavailable due to their old age or age at death that preceded implementation of the established criteria in hospital, participants were asked additional questions to determine if their parent exhibited the symptoms of AD dementia such as cognitive and functional decline consistent with the criteria in the absence of other known causes that could preclude an AD diagnosis; if sufficient information was gathered and findings were deemed consistent with a diagnosis of AD, these subjects were also identified as FH-positive (FH+). If none of the first-degree relatives was identified as having AD dementia, subjects were classified as FH-negative (FH−).

Amyloid-beta imaging

All subjects underwent three-dimensional [11C] Pittsburg compound B (PiB) positron emission tomography (PET)

imaging simultaneously taken with T1-weighted MRI at 3.0 T using a Biograph mMR (PET-MR) scanner (Siemens, Washington DC, USA). Preprocessing steps were performed using Statistical Parametric Mapping 12 (SPM12) (see Additional file 1: Methods for more detail).

Spatial normalization processes were performed on PiB-PET data using Statistical Parametric Mapping 12 (http://www.fil.ion.ucl.ac.uk/spm/software/spm12/) (SPM12) implemented in Matlab 2014a (Mathworks, MA). Static PiB-PET images were coregistered to individual T1 structural images, and transformation parameters for spatial normalization of individual T1 images to a standard MNI (Montreal Neurological Institute) template were calculated, which were then used to spatially normalize the PET images to the MNI template. The spatially normalized PiB-PET images were smoothed with an 8-mm Gaussian filter.

Additional processes were run for PiB-PET data to obtain improved spatial normalization of cerebellar gray matter, which is used as the reference region for intensity normalization (see Additional file 1: Methods section of the online data supplement for more detail).

The PiB retention index as the standardized uptake value ratio (SUVR) for each region of interest (ROI) was calculated by dividing the regional mean value by the individual mean cerebellar uptake values. The automatic anatomic labeling algorithm [26] and a region combining method [27] were applied to set the ROIs to characterize PiB retention level in frontal, lateral parietal, posterior cingulate-precuneus (PC-PRC), and lateral temporal regions. Each participant was classified as Aβ-positive if the SUVR value was > 1.4 in at least one of the four ROIs or as Aβ-negative if the SUVR values of all four ROIs was ≤ 1.4 [27, 28]. For the ROI analyses, a voxel-number weighted average SUVR of a composite global ROI was calculated using the four ROIs (AD$_{PiB}$-ROI).

Cerebral glucose imaging

All subjects also underwent three-dimensional [18F] fluoro-2-deoxyglucose (FDG) PET taken using the same PET-MR scanner as the PiB-PET. The acquisition parameters were similar to the PiB-PET procedures (described in more detail in Additional file 1: Methods).

In terms of spatial normalization processes performed on FDG-PET data, basic preprocessing was the same as for PiB-PET described above. The spatially normalized FDG-PET images were smoothed with a 12-mm Gaussian filter. For FDG-PET images, intensity normalization was performed on spatially normalized images using pons as the reference region, and SUVRs were extracted for ROIs using the standard AAL 116 atlas. For the ROI analyses, a voxel-number weighted average SUVR of a composite ROI (AD$_{FDG}$-ROI) including middle temporal gyrus, posterior cingulate cortex (PCC), and fusiform gyrus was calculated, which are the regions known to be sensitive to metabolic changes associated with AD [17].

Statistical analysis

Analyses were performed with SPSS 23.0 and SPM12. The APOE genotypes were coded as APOE4 carrier (APOE4$^+$) or noncarrier (APOE4$^-$). Differences in clinical and ROI measures between the FH groups as well as the APOE4 groups were examined with independent sample t tests, a general linear model (GLM), and χ^2 tests. Main effects and interaction were examined in the model, adjusting for age and gender effects. Post-hoc tests for an interaction effect were performed using Dunn-Sidak correction for multiple comparisons. In addition, the APOE4 carrier status was added as a covariate for main effects model of FH; likewise, the FH status was added to covariates for the main effects model of APOE4. Results were examined at $p < 0.05$.

To explore the interaction effects with more detailed regional information, the GLM was used to test for regional differences in parametric PiB and FDG SUVR images using SPM12. Results were initially examined at $p < 0.005$,

uncorrected for multiple comparisons. A significant cluster was identified based on a cluster correction procedure available in the Analysis of Functional NeuroImage (3dClustSim, version built 4 November 2016), which performed 10,000 iterations of Monte Carlo simulations on anatomical mask datasets with 1,801,748 voxels. This method, derived from Gaussian Random Field Theory, protects against multiple comparisons [29]. The cluster size threshold to achieve correction for multiple comparisons at $p < 0.05$ was calculated to be $k > 1062$ voxels.

Results

Participant characteristics

Demographic characteristics are shown in Table 1. Of the 268 study participants, 51 (19%) had at least one first-degree family member with a history of late-onset AD. Each participant was identified into one of the four groups: FH$^-$APOE4$^-$, FH$^+$APOE4$^-$, FH$^-$POE4$^+$, or FH$^+$APOE4$^+$. There were no differences between the groups regarding age, gender distribution, education, or cognitive functioning. The total allele frequency of APOE4 in this cohort was 9%, which is consistent with a

Table 1 Subject characteristics by family history and APOE4 groups

	FH$^-$APOE4$^-$	FH$^+$APOE4$^-$	FH$^-$APOE4$^+$	FH$^+$APOE4$^+$	P
n	180	38	37	13	
Age (years), mean (SD)	68.2 (8.2)	65.2 (9.5)	69.6 (9.4)	68.2 (9.5)	0.41
Gender, female/male (% female)	97/83 (53.9)	15/23 (39.5)	20/17 (54.1)	6/7 (46.2)	0.12
Education (years), mean (SD)	11.9 (4.9)	13.4 (4.1)	11.0 (4.1)	12.2 (4.4)	0.15
APOE4 dosage, n of ε4/ε4 (%)	0 (0)	0 (0)	0 (0)	2 (15)	
MMSE (raw score), mean (SD)	27.0 (2.4)	27.5 (2.4)	26.2 (2.9)	27.3 (2.5)	0.11
Neuropsychological test performance (z score, mean (SD))					
Immediate Verbal Memory Free Recall	0.88 (0.96)	0.86 (0.98)	0.60 (1.02)	0.81 (0.73)	0.46
Delayed Verbal Memory Free Recall	0.41 (0.87)	0.54 (0.89)	0.29 (0.90)	0.53 (0.62)	0.60
Delayed Verbal Memory Recognition	0.19 (0.78)	0.28 (0.65)	−0.003 (0.84)	0.27 (0.69)	0.40
Delayed Nonverbal Memory	0.33 (0.92)	0.49 (0.74)	0.05 (0.82)	0.45 (0.58)	0.14
Semantic Fluency	0.30 (1.12)	0.51 (1.18)	−0.09 (0.80)	0.75 (1.58)	0.05
Confrontational Naming	0.52 (0.89)	0.65 (0.63)	0.35 (0.87)	0.87 (0.58)	0.22
Constructional Praxis	−0.04 (0.93)	0.21 (0.66)	−0.08 (1.13)	−0.10 (1.04)	0.46
Stroop Color-Word	0.23 (1.04)	0.45 (0.91)	−0.001 (0.76)	0.27 (0.91)	0.27
Trail Making Test A	0.65 (1.93)	1.03 (0.46)	0.48 (1.91)	0.85 (0.50)	0.54
Trail Making Test B[a]	0.89 (1.04)	1.40 (0.85)	0.94 (1.14)	0.96 (0.73)	0.11
Digit Span Forward	0.36 (1.07)	0.52 (0.90)	−0.04 (0.98)	0.58 (0.92)	0.08
Digit Span Backward	0.12 (1.23)	0.52 (1.34)	−0.24 (0.86)	0.38 (1.81)	0.06
Amyloid-beta positive, n (%)	19 (11)	5 (13)	7 (19)	5 (38)*	0.03

APOE4 apolipoprotein ε4 allele, APOE4$^+$ APOE4 carrier, APOE4$^-$ APOE4 noncarrier, FH parental or sibling (first-degree relative) family history of late-onset AD (age of onset ≥ 65 years), FH$^+$ positive FH, FH$^-$ negative FH, MMSE Mini-Mental State Examination, SD standard deviation

[a]35% of FH$^-$APOE4$^-$, 24% of FH$^+$APOE4$^-$, 59% of FH$^-$APOE4$^+$, and 38% of FH$^+$APOE4$^+$ did not complete the Trail Making Test B due to cognitive reasons, participation refusal, or illiteracy

*Significantly different from the other groups based on post-hoc analyses, multiple comparisons corrected (P = 0.0067). Homozygote APOE4 carriers were not among the five amyloid-beta-positive individuals

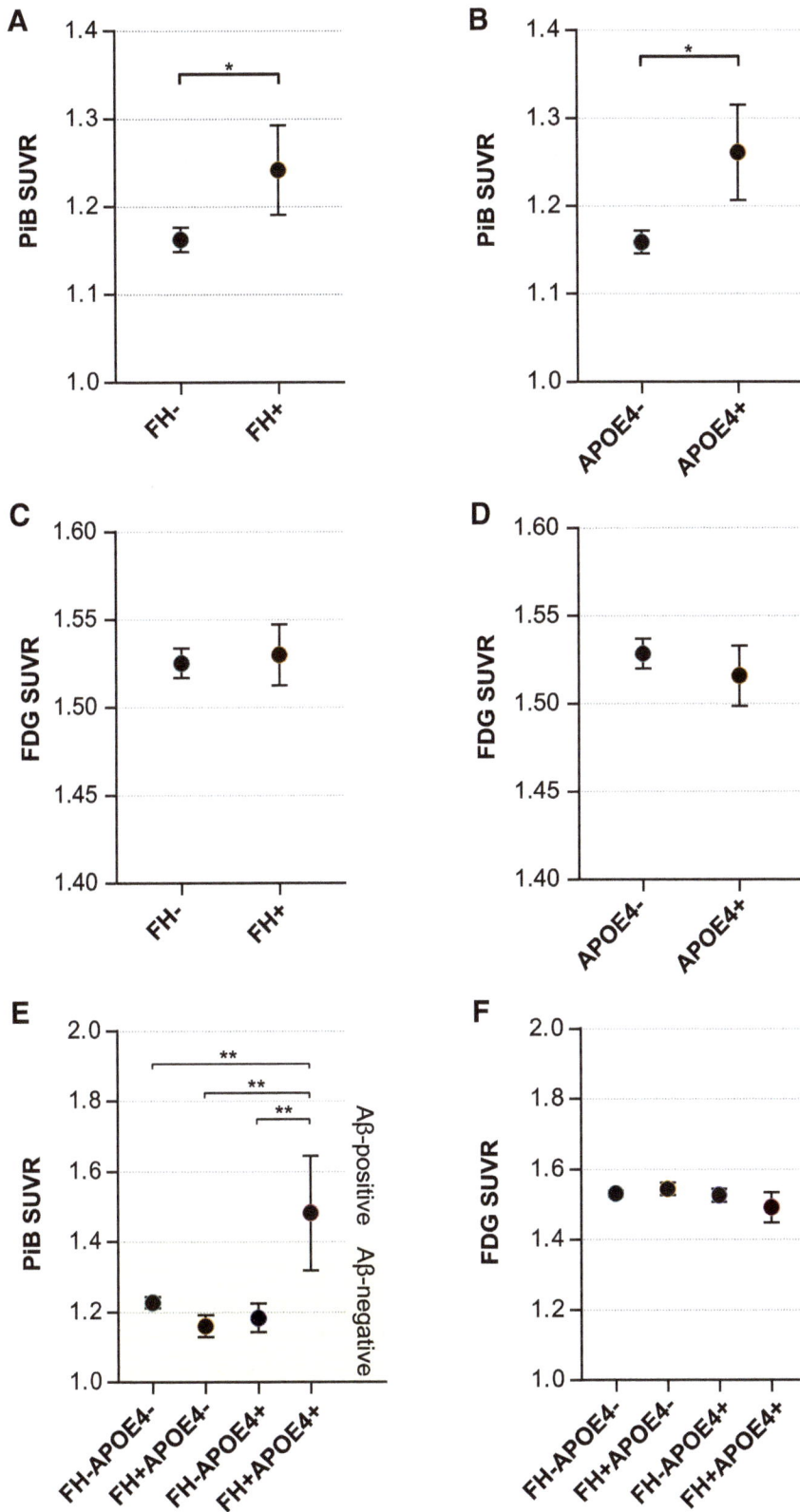

Fig. 1 (See legend on next page.)

(See figure on previous page.)
Fig. 1 Mean PiB retention and FDG uptake SUVRs. **a** AD$_{PiB}$-ROI between FH$^-$ and FH$^+$. **b** AD$_{PiB}$-ROI between APOE4$^-$ and APOE4$^+$. **c** AD$_{FDG}$-ROI between FH$^-$ and FH$^+$. **d** AD$_{FDG}$-ROI between APOE$^-$ and APOE4$^+$. **e** Interaction effect of FH and APOE on PiB retention. **f** Interaction effect of FH and APOE on FDG uptake. The green shaded area in **e** denotes below the PiB SUVR threshold of 1.4. Error bars indicate standard error. *$P < 0.05$; **significant difference in the post-hoc analyses adjusted for multiple comparisons using Dunn-Sidak correction ($P_B < 0.0085$). Aβ amyloid beta, APOE4 apolipoprotein ε4 allele, APOE4$^+$ APOE4 carriers, APOE4$^-$ APOE4 noncarriers, FDG [^{18}F] fluoro-2-deoxyglucose, FH family history of Alzheimer's disease, FH$^+$ individuals with FH, FH$^-$ individuals without FH, L left hemisphere, PiB [^{11}C] Pittsburg compound B, R right hemisphere, SUVR standardized uptake value ratio

previous report on APOE polymorphism among Koreans [30]. There were two APOE4 homozygote carriers in the entire sample, both of whom were FH$^+$. The proportion of Aβ-positive subjects was significantly higher in the FH$^+$APOE4$^+$ group than the other groups.

Independent association of FH and APOE4 on cerebral amyloid deposition

Significant differences between FH$^-$ and FH$^+$ were found for the AD$_{PiB}$-ROI (Additional file 1: Table S3 (Model-A)) and remained the same when the effect was additionally adjusted for APOE4 status (Fig. 1a; Additional file 1: Table S3 (Model-B)).

Significant differences in Aβ deposition levels were found in the AD$_{PiB}$-ROI between the APOE4$^+$ and APOE4$^-$ groups (Additional file 1: Table S3 (Model-C)). Significant differences remained the same when FH status was added as a covariate (Fig. 1b; Additional file 1: Table S3 (Model-D)). Overall, PiB retention was higher in FH$^+$ compared with FH$^-$ and in APOE4$^+$ compared with APOE4$^-$.

Independent association of FH and APOE4 on cerebral glucose metabolism

There were no significant differences found in the AD$_{FDG}$-ROI between the FH groups (Additional file 1: Table S3 (Model-A)) or the APOE4 groups (Additional file 1: Table S3 (Model-C)). Results remained the same when APOE4 status was added as a covariate (Fig. 1c; Additional file 1: Table S3 (Model-B)) or when FH status was added as a covariate (Fig. 1d; Additional file 1: Table S3 (Model-D)).

FH-APOE4 interaction effects: ROI analyses

A significant FH-APOE4 interaction effect was found for the AD$_{PiB}$-ROI ($F = 11.51$, $p < 0.001$, $R^2 = 0.112$) in addition to significant main effects of FH and APOE4 (Additional file 1: Table S1); the FH$^+$APOE4$^+$ group showed significantly higher Aβ deposition compared with the other groups (Fig. 1e). However, there were no main or interaction effects on regional cerebral glucose metabolism (rCMglc) between FH and APOE4 (Fig. 1f; Additional file 1: Table S1). The interaction effects remained significant when two APOE4 homozygote individuals were excluded (Additional file 1: Table S6).

FH-APOE4 interaction effects: voxel-wise analyses

Voxel-wise analyses were conducted between the FH$^+$APOE4$^+$ group and the other groups to further explore detailed brain regions showing the interaction effects on Aβ deposition and rCMglc. Compared with FH$^+$APOE4$^-$, FH$^+$APOE4$^+$ showed increased Aβ deposition in the left postcentral gyrus, left superior frontal gyrus, and left precuneus (Fig. 2a); compared with FH$^-$APOE4$^+$, FH$^+$APOE4$^+$ showed increased Aβ deposition in the left postcentral and supramarginal gyri and left superior frontal gyrus (Fig. 2b); and compared with FH$^-$APOE4$^-$, FH$^+$APOE4$^+$ showed increased Aβ deposition in the left middle frontal and temporal gyri, right inferior parietal lobule, left postcentral gyrus, and left posterior cingulate gyrus (Fig. 2c). There were no regions in any of the comparisons where FH$^+$APOE4$^+$ showed lower Aβ deposition levels (Additional file 1: Table S4).

Although there were no significant interaction effects of FH and APOE4 on rCMglc found from the ROI analyses, voxel-wise analyses were conducted for explorative purposes since subtle changes in CN adults may not have been captured by the AD$_{FDG}$-ROI. Compared with FH$^+$APOE4$^-$, FH$^+$APOE4$^+$ showed decreased rCMglc in the right entorhinal area and left hippocampus (Fig. 3a); compared with FH$^-$APOE4$^+$, FH$^+$APOE4$^+$ showed decreased rCMglc in the right entorhinal area and inferior temporal gyrus (Fig. 3b); and compared with FH$^-$APOE4$^-$, FH$^+$APOE4$^+$ showed decreased rCMglc in the right entorhinal area (Fig. 3c). There were no regions with significant differences in any of the comparisons where FH$^+$APOE4$^+$ showed hypermetabolism compared with the other groups (Additional file 1: Table S4).

Discussion

The present study examined whether APOE4 and FH have synergistic interaction effects on cerebral Aβ deposition and glucose metabolism in healthy middle-aged and older adults. The most notable finding was a significant increase in Aβ deposition if an individual was an APOE4 carrier with a positive family history for AD. While the synergistic interaction effect of FH and APOE4 on cerebral glucose metabolism was not found in the ROI analyses, voxel-wise analyses revealed that the synergistic interaction effect on glucose metabolism was in fact present in the temporal regions, including

A FH+APOE4+ > FH+APOE4-

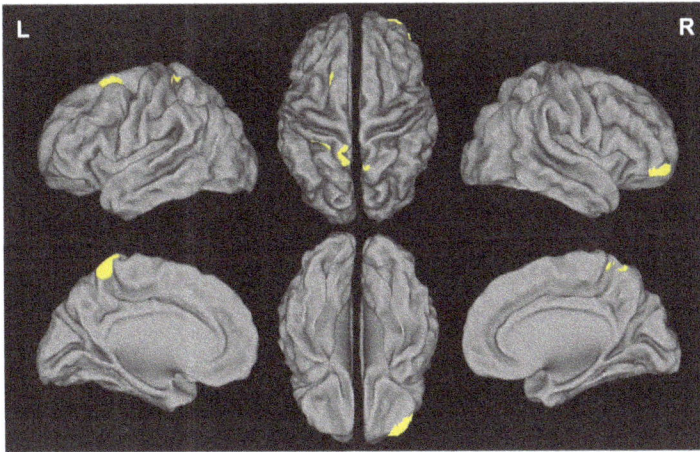

B FH+APOE4+ > FH-APOE4+

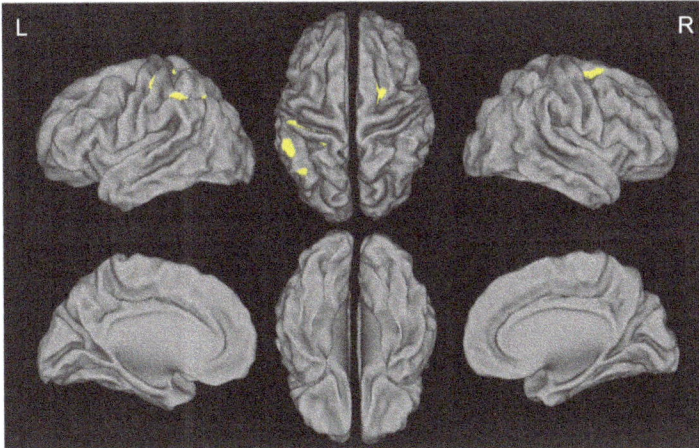

C FH+APOE4+ > FH-APOE4-

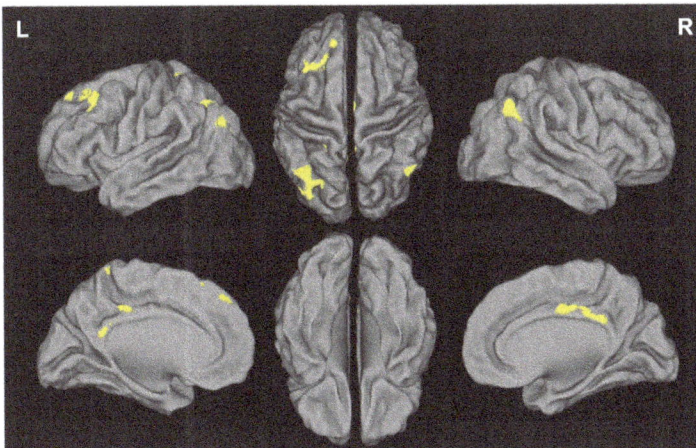

Fig. 2 (See legend on next page.)

the hippocampi. To the best of our knowledge, there is no previous study examining the interaction effects of APOE4 and FH on both Aβ deposition and rCMglc.

A body of literature devoted to investigating the genetic risks of AD has largely focused on either APOE4 or FH. The current findings on the interaction effects of FH and APOE4 on Aβ deposition and rCMglc further delineate the nature of the relationship between the two risk factors on signature AD brain changes. As can be inferred from the interaction effects, differences in the proportions of FH⁺ individuals included in the study samples may account, at least in part, for varied magnitudes of the effects of APOE4 reported in the literature. Conceivably, the commonly reported effects of APOE4 on AD brain biomarkers in the literature may actually be the effects seen in FH⁺APOE4⁺ compared with other groups. A similar argument can be made regarding the investigations of the effects of FH on AD brain biomarkers since the effects of FH were only seen in APOE4 carriers. Given the significant synergistic interaction effect, a simple application of statistical adjustment to achieve independency of the effects of either one of the risk factors may be misrepresenting.

A question arises as to the role played by a family history of AD in APOE4 carriers. The results from the current study strongly suggest that the APOE4 carriers with a family history of AD are more susceptible to alterations of the signature AD brain biomarkers before the onset of any cognitive symptoms. A positive family history status may represent other susceptibility genes that

are either coexpressed or interacting with APOE4. It has been posited that gene-gene interactions account for much of the unexplained variances in AD status [31] and that these interactions are widespread and common [32]. For example, clusterin (CLU; involved in AD pathogenesis directly by influencing Aβ aggregation and clearance [33, 34]) is found to interact with APOE4 [35, 36]. Bridging integrator 1, whose role is implicated in tauopathy [37], is thought to interact with the CLU [38]. In addition to the known genetic risks for AD possibly interacting with each other, there is a possibility that FH⁺ is capturing additional genetics that are considered unrelated to AD but interact with the AD genetic risks. Delineation of the role of genetics in the diagnosis and risk prediction in late-onset AD is complicated since up to 75% of APOE4 carriers do not develop AD and up to 50% of individuals with AD are APOE4 noncarriers [39, 40]. A twin study that examined genetic and environmental influences on AD reported that additive genetic influences explain 79% of the variance in the AD phenotype as opposed to 21% explained by nonshared environmental influences; when shared environmental influences were added to the analysis model, however, the variance in the AD phenotype explained by additive genetic influences changed to 58%, and 42% of the variance was explained by environmental influences (both shared (19%) and nonshared (23%)) [12]. Furthermore, a more recent study using the Alzheimer's Disease Genetics Consortium data and Genome-wide Complex Trait Analysis method reported that 53.24% of phenotypic variance was explained by genetics [41]. Given that

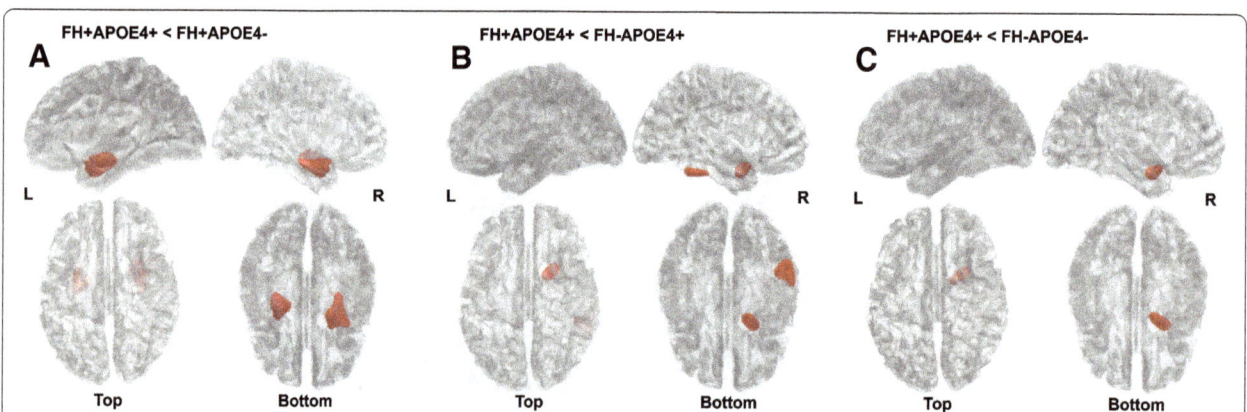

Fig. 3 Regions showing significant difference in cerebral glucose metabolism from voxel-wise analyses. **a** FH⁺APOE4⁺ compared with FH⁺APOE4⁻. **b** FH⁺APOE4⁺ compared with FH⁻APOE4⁺. **c** FH⁺APOE4⁺ compared with FH⁻APOE4⁻. APOE4 apolipoprotein ε4 allele, APOE4⁺ APOE4 carriers, APOE4⁻ APOE4 noncarriers, FH family history of Alzheimer's disease, FH⁺ individuals with FH, FH⁻ individuals without FH, L left hemisphere, R right hemisphere

environmental factors likely can explain the variance unaccounted for by genetic risks, involvement of a family's shared environments (captured by FH+) needs to be considered carefully as they may interact with APOE4 and other genetic risks. Shared environmental factors, which are seldom reported in association with Aβ, include a family's socioeconomic status, place of living (e.g., urban versus rural), lifestyle or dietary habits, parents' educational attainment and intellectual environment, and exposure to pollution [42–46]. Cognitive activity during the early life stage, for example, has been found to be associated with reduced neurodegeneration in AD signature regions in later life [47]. Although the abovementioned environmental factors may not individually show strong effects on AD, a combination of the environmental factors with APOE4 or other genetic risks may exhibit meaningful influences on AD neuropathology.

While independent main effects of APOE4 and FH were observed on Aβ deposition, there were no differences in cerebral glucose metabolism between the FH groups or the APOE4 groups in the brain regions typically affected in clinical AD patients in the current sample of cognitively normal elderly whose degree of degeneration is not yet progressed enough to be detected. In line with the findings by Lowe et al. [5] who showed that most of the APOE4-related differences in hypometabolism are mediated by amyloid accumulation, hypometabolism associated with APOE4 or FH in the AD signature regions in the current sample was only observed in individuals with high Aβ deposition (Additional file 1: Figure S1, Table S5), suggesting that the effects of APOE4 or FH on cerebral glucose metabolism only begin to show when the disease is progressed. Moreover, the hypometabolic pattern observed, particularly in the medial temporal regions, in association with FH+ and APOE4+ status (Fig. 3) is noteworthy given that these regions are where phosphorylated tau (p-tau) pathology is first to develop prior to accumulation of neurofibrillary tangles [8]. Taken together, the current cross-sectional observation in the CN likely reflects early observation of abnormal Aβ biomarkers prior to the onset of changes in glucose metabolism in the AD signature regions, which supports the amyloid pathological cascade model [48].

A strength of the current study is that the study participants were recruited from the community and that the sample includes a large number of APOE4+ and FH+ individuals despite relatively lower proportions (18% and 19%, respectively) compared with previous studies (24–43% and up to 66%, respectively) [5, 6, 8, 9, 16, 18]. The studies based on the Alzheimer's Disease Neuroimaging Initiative (ADNI) data, for instance, frequently recruited from family members of AD patients such that the samples included a large proportion of FH+ individuals, and these samples included a large proportion of Aβ-positive CN individuals

(e.g., 47%) [1, 5, 49], which is considerably higher than the current sample (13%). The current findings on the independent effects of APOE4 and FH on Aβ deposition and glucose metabolism are therefore relatively robust from differences in the proportions of APOE4+ or the number of FH+ individuals included in the total sample.

Similar to previous studies on FH, steps were taken to ensure that AD diagnosis in the subjects' parents was accurate, such as including only the subjects whose parent's AD diagnosis was made by a clinician according to the established criteria. Also, in a few cases where parents were deceased before formal diagnosis was available in clinics (i.e., parents of our old-old participants), a thorough interview was conducted with family members by a psychiatrist with expertise in dementia research to sufficiently address the inclusion/exclusion criteria of the AD diagnosis. Nonetheless, our cohort may have included a few participants whose parents did not have AD but instead had other types of dementia since the information obtained regarding those parents without a formal diagnosis is subject to recall bias. In the future, an investigation into possible protective effects of the APOE ε2 allele will allow further understanding of its role in the interaction effect of APOE and FH.

Conclusions

The current study was the first attempt to elucidate the interaction effects between FH and APOE4 on cerebral Aβ deposition and glucose metabolism in cognitively healthy adults. The strong synergistic effects of APOE4 and FH on brain Aβ deposition and hypometabolism that were found indicate possible gene-to-gene or gene-to-environment interactions that are important for the pathogenesis of AD. Such a synergistic effect also indicates that individuals with both FH and APOE4 are the population that needs more attention with regard to preventive interventions.

Abbreviations
Aβ: Amyloid-beta; AD: Alzheimer's disease; AD$_{FDG}$-ROI: Composite global region of interest of FDG uptake; AD$_{PiB}$-ROI: Composite global region of interest of PiB retention; APOE4: Apolipoprotein ε4 allele; CERAD-K: Consortium to Establish a Registry for Alzheimer's Disease, Korean version; CLU: Clusterin; CN: Cognitively normal; FDG: [^{18}F] fluoro-2-deoxyglucose; FH: Family history of Alzheimer's disease; GLM: General linear model; KBASE: Korean Brain Aging Study for the Early Diagnosis and Prediction of AD; MNI: Montreal Neurological Institute; MRI: Magnetic resonance imaging; PCC: Posterior cingulate cortex; PC-PRC: Posterior cingulate-precuneus; PET: Positron emission tomography; PiB: [^{11}C] Pittsburg compound B; rCMglc: Regional cerebral glucose metabolism; ROI: Region of interest; SUVR: Standardized uptake value ratio

Acknowledgments
We thank all study participants and their families for their contribution.

Funding
This study was supported by a grant from the Ministry of Science and ICT, Republic of Korea (grant no. NRF-2014M3C7A1046042). The funding source had no role in the study design, data collection, data analysis, data interpretation, writing of the manuscript, or decision to submit it for publication.

Authors' contributions
DY was responsible for the acquisition, analysis, and interpretation of data, and drafting and critically revising the manuscript for intellectual content. YL, MSB, JHL, and KK were responsible for the acquisition, analysis, and interpretation of data. BKS, YMC, HJC, HB, CHS, and YKK participated in analysis and interpretation of data. DYL was responsible for the study concept and design, acquisition of data, analysis, and interpretation of data, and drafting and critically revising the manuscript for intellectual content. All authors read and approved the final manuscript.

Consent for publication
Not applicable.

Competing interests
The authors declare that they have no competing interests.

Author details
[1]Institute of Human Behavioral Medicine, Medical Research Center Seoul National University, Seoul, Republic of Korea. [2]Department of Neuropsychiatry, Seoul National University Hospital, Seoul, Republic of Korea. [3]Department of Psychiatry, Sanggye Paik Hospital, Inje University College of Medicine, Seoul, Republic of Korea. [4]Department of Neuropsychiatry, University of Ulsan College of Medicine, Ulsan University Hospital, Ulsan, Republic of Korea. [5]Department of Neuropsychiatry, SMG-SNU Boramae Medical Center, Seoul, Republic of Korea. [6]Department of Neuropsychiatry, Kyunggi Provincial Hospital for the Elderly, Yongin, Republic of Korea. [7]Department of Radiology, Seoul National University College of Medicine & Seoul National University Hospital, Seoul, Republic of Korea. [8]Department of Nuclear Medicine, SMG-SNU Boramae Medical Center, Seoul, Republic of Korea. [9]Department of Psychiatry, Seoul National University College of Medicine, 101 Daehak-ro, Jongno-gu, Seoul 03080, Republic of Korea.

References
1. Chetelat G, La Joie R, Villain N, Perrotin A, de La Sayette V, Eustache F, Vandenberghe R. Amyloid imaging in cognitively normal individuals, at-risk populations and preclinical Alzheimer's disease. Neuroimage Clin. 2013;2:356–65.
2. Corder EH, Saunders AM, Strittmatter WJ, Schmechel DE, Gaskell PC, Small GW, Roses AD, Haines JL, Pericak-Vance MA. Gene dose of apolipoprotein E type 4 allele and the risk of Alzheimer's disease in late onset families. Science. 1993;261(5123):921–3.
3. Jagust WJ, Landau SM, Alzheimer's Disease Neuroimaging Inititative. Apolipoprotein E, not fibrillar beta-amyloid, reduces cerebral glucose metabolism in normal aging. J Neurosci. 2012;32(50):18227–33.
4. Rowe CC, Ellis KA, Rimajova M, Bourgeat P, Pike KE, Jones G, Fripp J, Tochon-Danguy H, Morandeau L, O'Keefe G, et al. Amyloid imaging results from the Australian Imaging, Biomarkers and Lifestyle (AIBL) study of aging. Neurobiol Aging. 2010;31(8):1275–83.
5. Lowe VJ, Weigand SD, Senjem ML, Vemuri P, Jordan L, Kantarci K, Boeve B, Jack CR Jr, Knopman D, Petersen RC. Association of hypometabolism and amyloid levels in aging, normal subjects. Neurology. 2014;82(22):1959–67.
6. Didic M, Felician O, Gour N, Bernard R, Pecheux C, Mundler O, Ceccaldi M, Guedj E. Rhinal hypometabolism on FDG PET in healthy APO-E4 carriers: impact on memory function and metabolic networks. Eur J Nucl Med Mol Imaging. 2015;42(10):1512–21.
7. Knopman DS, Jack CR Jr, Wiste HJ, Lundt ES, Weigand SD, Vemuri P, Lowe VJ, Kantarci K, Gunter JL, Senjem ML, et al. 18F-fluorodeoxyglucose positron emission tomography, aging, and apolipoprotein E genotype in cognitively normal persons. Neurobiol Aging. 2014;35(9):2096–106.
8. Bozoki AC, Zdanukiewicz M, Zhu DC, Alzheimer's Disease Neuroimaging Initiative. The effect of beta-amyloid positivity on cerebral metabolism in cognitively normal seniors. Alzheimers Dement. 2016;12(12):1250–8.
9. Risacher SL, Kim S, Nho K, Foroud T, Shen L, Petersen RC, Jack CR Jr, Beckett LA, Aisen PS, Koeppe RA, et al. APOE effect on Alzheimer's disease biomarkers in older adults with significant memory concern. Alzheimers Dement. 2015;11(12):1417–29.
10. Reiman EM, Chen K, Alexander GE, Caselli RJ, Bandy D, Osborne D, Saunders AM, Hardy J. Functional brain abnormalities in young adults at genetic risk for late-onset Alzheimer's dementia. Proc Natl Acad Sci U S A. 2004;101(1):284–9.
11. Jansen WJ, Ossenkoppele R, Knol DL, Tijms BM, Scheltens P, Verhey FR, Visser PJ, Amyloid Biomarker Study Group, Aalten P, Aarsland D, et al. Prevalence of cerebral amyloid pathology in persons without dementia: a meta-analysis. JAMA. 2015;313(19):1924–38.
12. Gatz M, Reynolds CA, Fratiglioni L, Johansson B, Mortimer JA, Berg S, Fiske A, Pedersen NL. Role of genes and environments for explaining Alzheimer disease. Arch Gen Psychiatry. 2006;63(2):168–74.
13. Ganguli M, Kukull WA. Lost in translation: epidemiology, risk, and Alzheimer disease. Arch Neurol. 2010;67(1):107–11.
14. Migliore L, Coppede F. Genetics, environmental factors and the emerging role of epigenetics in neurodegenerative diseases. Mutat Res. 2009;667(1–2):82–97.
15. Qiu C, De Ronchi D, Fratiglioni L. The epidemiology of the dementias: an update. Curr Opin Psychiatry. 2007;20(4):380–5.
16. Mosconi L, Rinne JO, Tsui WH, Murray J, Li Y, Glodzik L, McHugh P, Williams S, Cummings M, Pirraglia E, et al. Amyloid and metabolic positron emission tomography imaging of cognitively normal adults with Alzheimer's parents. Neurobiol Aging. 2013;34(1):22–34.
17. Mosconi L, Murray J, Tsui WH, Li Y, Spector N, Goldowsky A, Williams S, Osorio R, McHugh P, Glodzik L, et al. Brain imaging of cognitively normal individuals with 2 parents affected by late-onset AD. Neurology. 2014;82(9):752–60.
18. Murray J, Tsui WH, Li Y, McHugh P, Williams S, Cummings M, Pirraglia E, Solnes L, Osorio R, Glodzik L, et al. FDG and amyloid PET in cognitively normal individuals at risk for late-onset Alzheimer's disease. Adv J Mol Imaging. 2014;4(2):15–26.
19. Sager MA, Hermann B, La Rue A. Middle-aged children of persons with Alzheimer's disease: APOE genotypes and cognitive function in the Wisconsin registry for Alzheimer's prevention. J Geriatr Psychiatry Neurol. 2005;18(4):245–9.
20. Scarabino D, Gambina G, Broggio E, Pelliccia F, Corbo RM. Influence of family history of dementia in the development and progression of late-onset Alzheimer's disease. Am J Med Genet B Neuropsychiatr Genet. 2016;171B(2):250–6.
21. Byun MS, Yi D, Lee JH, Choe YM, Sohn BK, Lee JY, Choi HJ, Baek H, Kim YK, Lee YS, et al. Korean brain aging study for the early diagnosis and prediction of Alzheimer's disease: methodology and baseline sample characteristics. Psychiatry Investig. 2017;14(6):851–63.
22. Lee JH, Lee KU, Lee DY, Kim KW, Jhoo JH, Kim JH, Lee KH, Kim SY, Han SH, Woo JI. Development of the Korean version of the consortium to establish a registry for Alzheimer's disease assessment packet (CERAD-K): clinical and neuropsychological assessment batteries. J Gerontol B Psychol Sci Soc Sci. 2002;57(1):47–53.
23. Morris JC. The clinical dementia rating (CDR): current version and scoring rules. Neurology. 1993;43(11):2412–4.
24. Lee DY, Lee KU, Lee JH, Kim KW, Jhoo JH, Kim SY, Yoon JC, Woo SI, Ha J, Woo JI. A normative study of the CERAD neuropsychological assessment battery in the Korean elderly. J Int Neuropsychol Soc. 2004;10(1):72–81.

25. Wenham PR, Price WH, Blandell G. Apolipoprotein E genotyping by one-stage PCR. Lancet. 1991;337(8750):1158–9.

26. Tzourio-Mazoyer N, Landeau B, Papathanassiou D, Crivello F, Etard O, Delcroix N, Mazoyer B, Joliot M. Automated anatomical labeling of activations in SPM using a macroscopic anatomical parcellation of the MNI MRI single-subject brain. Neuroimage. 2002;15(1):273–89.

27. Reiman EM, Chen K, Liu X, Bandy D, Yu M, Lee W, Ayutyanont N, Keppler J, Reeder SA, Langbaum JB, et al. Fibrillar amyloid-beta burden in cognitively normal people at 3 levels of genetic risk for Alzheimer's disease. Proc Natl Acad Sci U S A. 2009;106(16):6820–5.

28. Villeneuve S, Rabinovici GD, Cohn-Sheehy BI, Madison C, Ayakta N, Ghosh PM, La Joie R, Arthur-Bentil SK, Vogel JW, Marks SM, et al. Existing Pittsburgh compound-B positron emission tomography thresholds are too high: statistical and pathological evaluation. Brain. 2015;138(Pt 7):2020–33.

29. Forman SD, Cohen JD, Fitzgerald M, Eddy WF, Mintun MA, Noll DC. Improved assessment of significant activation in functional magnetic resonance imaging (fMRI): use of a cluster-size threshold. Magn Reson Med. 1995;33(5):636–47.

30. Kim KW, Jhoo JH, Lee KU, Lee DY, Lee JH, Youn JY, Lee BJ, Han SH, Woo JI. Association between apolipoprotein E polymorphism and Alzheimer's disease in Koreans. Neurosci Lett. 1999;277(3):145–8.

31. Turton JC, Bullock J, Medway C, Shi H, Brown K, Belbin O, Kalsheker N, Carrasquillo MM, Dickson DW, Graff-Radford NR, et al. Investigating statistical epistasis in complex disorders. J Alzheimers Dis. 2011;25(4):635–44.

32. Shao H, Burrage LC, Sinasac DS, Hill AE, Ernest SR, O'Brien W, Courtland HW, Jepsen KJ, Kirby A, Kulbokas EJ, et al. Genetic architecture of complex traits: large phenotypic effects and pervasive epistasis. Proc Natl Acad Sci U S A. 2008;105(50):19910–4.

33. Harold D, Abraham R, Hollingworth P, Sims R, Gerrish A, Hamshere ML, Pahwa JS, Moskvina V, Dowzell K, Williams A, et al. Genome-wide association study identifies variants at CLU and PICALM associated with Alzheimer's disease. Nat Genet. 2009;41(10):1088–93.

34. Lambert JC, Heath S, Even G, Campion D, Sleegers K, Hiltunen M, Combarros O, Zelenika D, Bullido MJ, Tavernier B, et al. Genome-wide association study identifies variants at CLU and CR1 associated with Alzheimer's disease. Nat Genet. 2009;41(10):1094–9.

35. DeMattos RB, Cirrito JR, Parsadanian M, May PC, O'Dell MA, Taylor JW, Harmony JA, Aronow BJ, Bales KR, Paul SM, et al. ApoE and clusterin cooperatively suppress Abeta levels and deposition: evidence that ApoE regulates extracellular Abeta metabolism in vivo. Neuron. 2004;41(2):193–202.

36. Holtzman DM. In vivo effects of ApoE and clusterin on amyloid-beta metabolism and neuropathology. J Mol Neurosci. 2004;23(3):247–54.

37. Tan MS, Yu JT, Tan L. Bridging integrator 1 (BIN1): form, function, and Alzheimer's disease. Trends Mol Med. 2013;19(10):594–603.

38. Zhou Y, Hayashi I, Wong J, Tugusheva K, Renger JJ, Zerbinatti C. Intracellular clusterin interacts with brain isoforms of the bridging integrator 1 and with the microtubule-associated protein Tau in Alzheimer's disease. PLoS One. 2014;9(7):e103187.

39. Van Cauwenberghe C, Van Broeckhoven C, Sleegers K. The genetic landscape of Alzheimer disease: clinical implications and perspectives. Genet Med. 2016;18(5):421–30.

40. Farrer LA, Cupples LA, Haines JL, Hyman B, Kukull WA, Mayeux R, Myers RH, Pericak-Vance MA, Risch N, van Duijn CM. Effects of age, sex, and ethnicity on the association between apolipoprotein E genotype and Alzheimer disease. A meta-analysis. APOE and Alzheimer disease Meta analysis consortium. JAMA. 1997;278(16):1349–56.

41. Ridge PG, Hoyt KB, Boehme K, Mukherjee S, Crane PK, Haines JL, Mayeux R, Farrer LA, Pericak-Vance MA, Schellenberg GD, et al. Assessment of the genetic variance of late-onset Alzheimer's disease. Neurobiol Aging. 2016;41: 200. e213–200 e220

42. Hendrie HC, Smith-Gamble V, Lane KA, Purnell C, Clark DO, Gao S. The association of early life factors and declining incidence rates of dementia in an elderly population of African Americans. J Gerontol B Psychol Sci Soc Sci. 2018;73(suppl_1):S82–9.

43. Moceri VM, Kukull WA, Emanuel I, van Belle G, Larson EB. Early-life risk factors and the development of Alzheimer's disease. Neurology. 2000;54(2):415–20.

44. Calderon-Garciduenas L, Gonzalez-Maciel A, Reynoso-Robles R, Delgado-Chavez R, Mukherjee PS, Kulesza RJ, Torres-Jardon R, Avila-Ramirez J, Villarreal-Rios R. Hallmarks of Alzheimer disease are evolving relentlessly in metropolitan Mexico City infants, children and young adults. APOE4 carriers have higher suicide risk and higher odds of reaching NFT stage V at </=40 years of age. Environ Res. 2018;164:475–87.

45. Borenstein AR, Copenhaver CI, Mortimer JA. Early-life risk factors for Alzheimer disease. Alzheimer Dis Assoc Disord. 2006;20(1):63–72.

46. Cohen S, Janicki-Deverts D, Chen E, Matthews KA. Childhood socioeconomic status and adult health. Ann N Y Acad Sci. 2010;1186:37–55.

47. Ko K, Byun MS, Yi D, Lee JH, Kim CH, Lee DY. Early-life cognitive activity is related to reduced neurodegeneration in Alzheimer signature regions in late life. Front Aging Neurosci. 2018;10:70.

48. Jack CR Jr, Knopman DS, Jagust WJ, Shaw LM, Aisen PS, Weiner MW, Petersen RC, Trojanowski JQ. Hypothetical model of dynamic biomarkers of the Alzheimer's pathological cascade. Lancet Neurol. 2010;9(1):119–28.

49. Jagust WJ, Bandy D, Chen K, Foster NL, Landau SM, Mathis CA, Price JC, Reiman EM, Skovronsky D, Koeppe RA, et al. The Alzheimer's disease neuroimaging initiative positron emission tomography core. Alzheimers Dement. 2010;6(3):221–9.

Discovery and validation of autosomal dominant Alzheimer's disease mutations

Simon Hsu[1], Brian A. Gordon[2], Russ Hornbeck[2], Joanne B. Norton[1], Denise Levitch[3], Adia Louden[1], Ellen Ziegemeier[3], Robert Laforce Jr.[4], Jasmeer Chhatwal[5], Gregory S. Day[3], Eric McDade[3], John C. Morris[3], Anne M. Fagan[3], Tammie L. S. Benzinger[2,6], Alison M. Goate[7], Carlos Cruchaga[1], Randall J. Bateman[3], Dominantly Inherited Alzheimer Network (DIAN) and Celeste M. Karch[1]* ⓘ

Abstract

Background: Alzheimer's disease (AD) is a neurodegenerative disease that is clinically characterized by progressive cognitive decline. Mutations in amyloid-β precursor protein (*APP*), presenilin 1 (*PSEN1*), and presenilin 2 (PSEN2) are the pathogenic cause of autosomal dominant AD (ADAD). However, polymorphisms also exist within these genes.

Methods: In order to distinguish polymorphisms from pathogenic mutations, the DIAN Expanded Registry has implemented an algorithm for determining ADAD pathogenicity using available information from multiple domains, including genetic, bioinformatic, clinical, imaging, and biofluid measures and in vitro analyses.

Results: We propose that *PSEN1* M84V, *PSEN1* A396T, *PSEN2* R284G, and *APP* T719N are likely pathogenic mutations, whereas *PSEN1* c.379_382delXXXXinsG and *PSEN2* L238F have uncertain pathogenicity.

Conclusions: In defining a subset of these variants as pathogenic, individuals from these families can now be enrolled in observational and clinical trials. This study outlines a critical approach for translating genetic data into meaningful clinical outcomes.

Keywords: APP, PSEN1, PSEN2, Autosomal dominant Alzheimer's disease, Cell-based assays, Pathogenicity algorithm

Background

Alzheimer's disease (AD) is characterized clinically by progressive cognitive decline and neuropathologically by progressive neuronal loss and the accumulation of amyloid plaques and neurofibrillary tangles. Mutations in amyloid-β precursor protein (*APP*), presenilin 1 (*PSEN1*) and presenilin 2 (*PSEN2*) are the pathogenic cause of autosomal dominant AD (ADAD). More than 200 pathogenic mutations have been identified in *APP*, *PSEN1*, and *PSEN2* (reviewed in [1, 2]). PSEN1 and PSEN2 form the catalytic domain of the γ-secretase complex, which is involved in sequential cleavage of APP into amyloid-β (Aβ) peptides.

The Dominantly Inherited Alzheimer Network (DIAN) is an observational study designed to follow families with mutations in *APP*, *PSEN1*, and *PSEN2* that cause ADAD

[3]. The DIAN Expanded Registry (DIAN EXR; www.dianexr.org) is a web-based registry with global outreach to ADAD families and investigators. It functions to identify families with ADAD and to determine the causative mutations through a genetic discovery program. This program includes genetic counseling and testing for known and unknown causes of ADAD. During a period of 6 years (2011 to 2017), the DIAN Clinical/Genetics committee reviewed 150 pedigrees, 76 of which were approved for genetic counseling and testing. Forty-six probands were positive for a coding variant in *APP*, *PSEN1*, or *PSEN2*, including 39 individuals with known pathogenic mutations, 6 with variants of unknown pathogenic significance, and 1 variant that was determined to be an AD risk factor.

In some cases, families are identified with several generations of early-onset AD; however, at the time of enrollment, whether a pathogenic mutation is the cause of disease in these families remains unknown. We performed genetic analyses in research participants from six densely

---
* Correspondence: karchc@wustl.edu
[1]Department of Psychiatry, Washington University School of Medicine, 425 S. Euclid Ave, Campus Box 8134, St. Louis, MO 63110, USA
Full list of author information is available at the end of the article

affected early-onset AD pedigrees and identified variants in *APP*, *PSEN1*, and *PSEN2* with unknown pathogenicity. In all families examined, we lacked sufficient genetic material to perform segregation analyses (e.g., DNA was available from only one or two family members). To assess the pathogenicity of novel variants in *APP*, *PSEN1*, and *PSEN2* when pedigree and clinical data are limited or incomplete, Guerreiro and colleagues [4] proposed a pathogenicity algorithm. In the present study, we modified and expanded this algorithm to evaluate the pathogenicity of these six variants using genetic, biochemical, biomarker, and clinical data.

Methods
Genetic screening
Genomic DNA was extracted from peripheral blood lymphocytes using standard protocols. All coding exons in *APP*, *PSEN1*, and/or *PSEN2* were amplified and sequenced using the BigDye Terminator version 3.1 cycle sequencing kit (Life Technologies, Carlsbad, CA, USA) and analyzed on an ABI 3500 genetic analyzer (Life Technologies). Sequence analysis was performed using Sequencher software (Gene Codes, Ann Arbor, MI, USA).

Bioinformatics
To determine whether *APP*, *PSEN1*, and *PSEN2* variants represented rare or common polymorphisms, we investigated two population-based exome sequencing databases: the Exome Variant Server (EVS) and Exome Aggregation Consortium (ExAC) browser. Polymorphism phenotype v2 (PolyPhen-2; [5]) and Sorting Intolerant From Tolerant (SIFT) were used to predict whether the amino acid change would be disruptive to the encoded protein.

Cerebrospinal fluid
Cerebrospinal fluid (CSF) was collected by lumbar puncture under fasting conditions from the *PSEN1* M84V carrier and noncarrier. CSF $A\beta_{42}$, total tau, and tau phosphorylated at threonine 181 (p-tau$_{181}$) were measured by immunoassay (xMAP; Luminex, Austin, TX, USA) as previously described [6].

PiB imaging
Structural magnetic resonance imaging (MRI) was performed using 3-T scanners and following the Alzheimer's Disease Neuroimaging Initiative (ADNI) protocol [7, 8]. T1-weighted scans were processed through FreeSurfer. Positron emission tomography with Pittsburgh compound B (PiB) was coregistered with MRI images. The standardized uptake value ratio (SUVR) was calculated for each region [9, 10]. Global burden was characterized using a summary measure [9]. These data were collected for a *PSEN1* M84V carrier and noncarrier.

Biochemical analysis
Plasmids and mutagenesis
The full-length *PSEN1* complementary DNA (cDNA) was cloned into pcDNA3.1 Myc/His vector [11]. The M84V, c.379_382delXXXXinsG, or A396T variant was introduced into the *PSEN1* cDNA using the QuikChange II XL Site-Directed Mutagenesis Kit (Agilent Technologies, Santa Clara, CA, USA). Clones were sequenced to confirm the presence of the variant and the absence of additional modifications. *PSEN1* wild type (WT) and the pathogenic *PSEN1* A79V mutation were included as controls.

The full-length *PSEN2* cDNA was cloned into pcDNA3.1 vector [12]. The L238F or R284G variant was introduced into the *PSEN2* cDNA and screened as described above. *PSEN2* WT and the pathogenic *PSEN2* N141I mutation were included as controls [13].

The full-length *APP* cDNA (isoform 695) was cloned into pcDNA3.1 [14]. The T719N variant was introduced into the APP cDNA and screened as described above. APP WT and the pathogenic APP KM670/671NL(Swe) mutation were included as controls.

Transient transfection
To assess novel *PSEN1* and *PSEN2* variants, we used neuroblastoma cells (N2A) stably expressing human APP WT (695 isoform; N2A695). To assess novel *APP* variants, we used N2A. N2A cells were maintained in equal amounts of DMEM and Opti-MEM, supplemented with 5% FBS, 2 mM L-glutamine, 100 μg/ml penicillin/streptomycin, and, for stable cells, 200 μg/ml G418 (Life Technologies). Upon reaching confluence, cells were transiently transfected with Lipofectamine 2000 reagent (Life Technologies). Culture media were replaced after 24 hours, and cells were incubated for another 24 hours prior to analysis. Four independent transfections were performed for each construct and used for subsequent analyses.

Aβ enzyme-linked immunosorbent assay
Conditioned medium was collected and centrifuged at $3000 \times g$ at 4 °C for 10 minutes to remove cell debris. The levels of $A\beta_{40}$ and $A\beta_{42}$ were measured in cell culture media by sandwich enzyme-linked immunosorbent assay (ELISA) as described by the manufacturer (Life Technologies). To account for variability in transfection efficiency between experiments, ELISA values were obtained (pg/ml) and corrected for total intracellular protein (μg/ml). Statistical difference was measured using an unpaired Student's t test.

Results and discussion
PSEN1 M84V
The proband was identified in a family with three generations of early-onset AD and with a mean age at onset of 59 years (Fig. 1; pedigree not shown to avoid

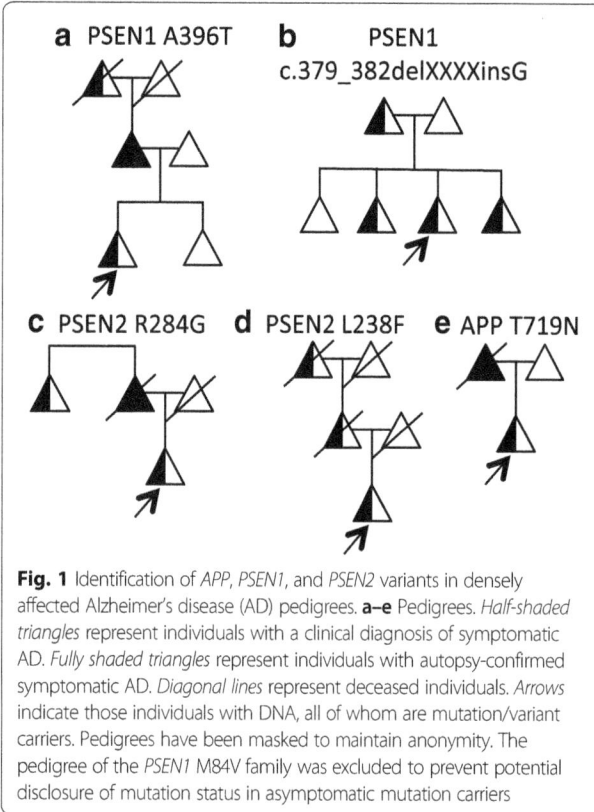

Fig. 1 Identification of *APP*, *PSEN1*, and *PSEN2* variants in densely affected Alzheimer's disease (AD) pedigrees. **a–e** Pedigrees. *Half-shaded triangles* represent individuals with a clinical diagnosis of symptomatic AD. *Fully shaded triangles* represent individuals with autopsy-confirmed symptomatic AD. *Diagonal lines* represent deceased individuals. *Arrows* indicate those individuals with DNA, all of whom are mutation/variant carriers. Pedigrees have been masked to maintain anonymity. The pedigree of the *PSEN1* M84V family was excluded to prevent potential disclosure of mutation status in asymptomatic mutation carriers

disclosing mutation status to asymptomatic proband and other family members). Sequencing of the proband revealed a single base substitution (ATG to GTG) at codon 84 in exon 4 of *PSEN1*, resulting in a methionine-to-valine change (M84V). *PSEN1* M84V was also identified in a family-based sequencing study of AD (National Institute of Mental Health Alzheimer's Disease Genetics Initiative Study) [15]. Two *PSEN1* M84V carriers were confirmed to have had AD at autopsy with ages at symptomatic onset of 70 and 72 years. The third carrier was cognitively normal at age 67 years [15].

To determine whether *PSEN1* M84V represents a rare polymorphism, we examined two population-based exome sequencing databases (Table 1). *PSEN1* M84V was absent from both EVS and ExAC. *PSEN1* M84L was identified in one individual in the ExAC browser. *PSEN1* M84V was also absent in more than 1700 AD and control samples with whole-exome sequencing.

CSF Aβ, total tau, and phosphorylated tau were measured in the *PSEN1* M84V carrier, who was cognitively normal at the time of lumbar puncture. CSF Aβ (361.5 pg/ml), total tau (84.93 pg/ml), and p-tau$_{181}$ (22.02 pg/ml) at 11 years prior to the parental age at symptomatic onset was consistent with other presymptomatic pathogenic mutation carriers but not completely distinct from noncarriers [3, 6]. The *PSEN1* M84V carrier produced a mean cortical PiB SUVR value of 1.132 at 15 years prior to the

parental age at symptomatic onset and 1.209 at 11 years prior to parent age of disease onset (Fig. 2). A related noncarrier was imaged at 16 years prior to the parent age of disease onset and produced mean cortical PiB SUVR values of 1.086 and 1.039 at 13 years prior to age at disease onset in the parent (Fig. 2). Thus, fluid and imaging biomarkers were consistent with those observed in presymptomatic ADAD mutation carriers.

We next sought to determine whether the *PSEN1* M84V variant alters Aβ isoform levels in a manner consistent with previously reported pathogenic *PSEN1* mutations. We expressed vectors containing *PSEN1* WT, A79V (a known pathogenic mutation), and M84V in N2A695 cells. We found that cells expressing *PSEN1* M84V produced significantly more Aβ$_{42}$ than cells expressing *PSEN1* WT (Fig. 3a–c). We also observed a significant increase in the Aβ$_{42}$/Aβ$_{40}$ ratio in cells expressing *PSEN1* M84V or the pathogenic *PSEN1* A79V-compared with *PSEN1* WT-expressing cells (Fig. 3c).

Thus, we can apply a pathogenicity algorithm, modified from Guerreiro and colleagues [4], to assess the pathogenicity of *PSEN1* M84V (Fig. 4). *PSEN1* M84V occurs within exon 4 and the first transmembrane domain. This residue is highly conserved between *PSEN1* and *PSEN2* [16]. Additionally, a pathogenic mutation has been reported at this site: ΔI83/M84 [17, 18]. In a cell model, Aβ levels were consistent with pathogenic mutations (Fig. 3a–c, g). Thus, *PSEN1* M84V satisfies all criteria for pathogenicity based on residue and Aβ levels [4]. Taken together, we propose that *PSEN1* M84V represents a pathogenic mutation.

PSEN1 A396T

The proband was identified in a family with three generations of early-onset AD (Fig. 1a). The proband had an age at symptomatic onset of 50 years. The parent of the proband had an age at symptomatic onset of 57 years, with AD confirmed at autopsy at age 67 years. Sequencing of the proband (Fig. 1a) revealed a single base substitution (GCG to ACG) at codon 396 in exon 11 of *PSEN1*, resulting in an alanine-to-threonine change (A396T). This variant was reported previously in one individual with sporadic AD [19]. *PSEN1* A396T was absent in the EVS and ExAC databases (Table 1). We found that cells expressing *PSEN1* A396T produced significantly more Aβ$_{42}$ than cells expressing *PSEN1* WT (Fig. 3a–c). Thus, applying the algorithm for assessing pathogenicity (Fig. 4), we propose that the *PSEN1* A396T represents a probable pathogenic mutation.

PSEN1 c.379_382delXXXXinsG

The proband had an age at symptomatic onset of 50 years, with an average age at symptomatic onset in family members aged 43 years (Fig. 1b). Sequencing of

Table 1 Bioinformatic analysis of *APP*, *PSEN1*, and *PSEN2* variants of unknown pathogenicity

Gene	Variant	EVS[a]	ExAC[b]	PolyPhen	SIFT	Variant previously reported	Location	PSEN1-PSEN2 conservation
APP	T719N	0	0	Probably damaging	Damaging	Yes	Exon 17	N/A
PSEN1	M84V	0	0	Probably damaging	Tolerated	Yes	Exon 4 (TM-1)	Yes
PSEN1	c.379_382delXXXXinsG	0	0	N/A	Tolerated	No	Exon 5 (HL1)	Yes
PSEN1	A396T	0	0	Probably damaging	Tolerated	Yes	Exon 11 (HL8)	No
PSEN2	L238F	2	2	Probably damaging	Damaging	Yes	Exon 7 (TM-V)	Yes
PSEN2	R284G	0	0	Probably damaging	Damaging	No	Exon 8	Yes

Abbreviations: PolyPhen Polymorphism phenotype, *SIFT* Sorting Intolerant From Tolerant, *EVS* Exome Variant Server, *ExAC* Exome Aggregation Consortium, *PSEN* Presenilin, *APP* Amyloid precursor protein
[a]Represents sequence data from 4300 unrelated European Americans (8598 alleles)
[b]Represents sequence data from 60,706 unrelated European Americans (121,204 alleles)

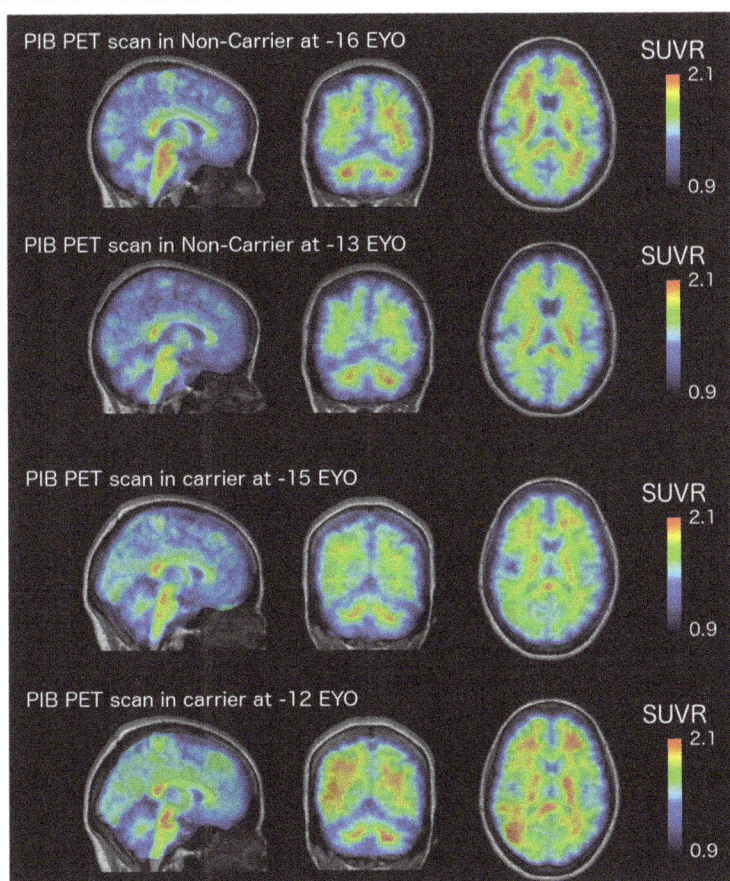

Fig. 2 Pittsburgh compound B (PiB) uptake in the brain of a presymptomatic *PSEN1* M84V carrier is consistent with presymptomatic autosomal dominant Alzheimer's disease mutation carriers. ^{11}C-PiB positron emission tomographic scans were performed longitudinally in a *PSEN1* M84V noncarrier and carrier. The color scale for standardized uptake values (SUV) indicate red (high), yellow (medium), and blue (low) PiB retention. *EYO* Estimated years of onset

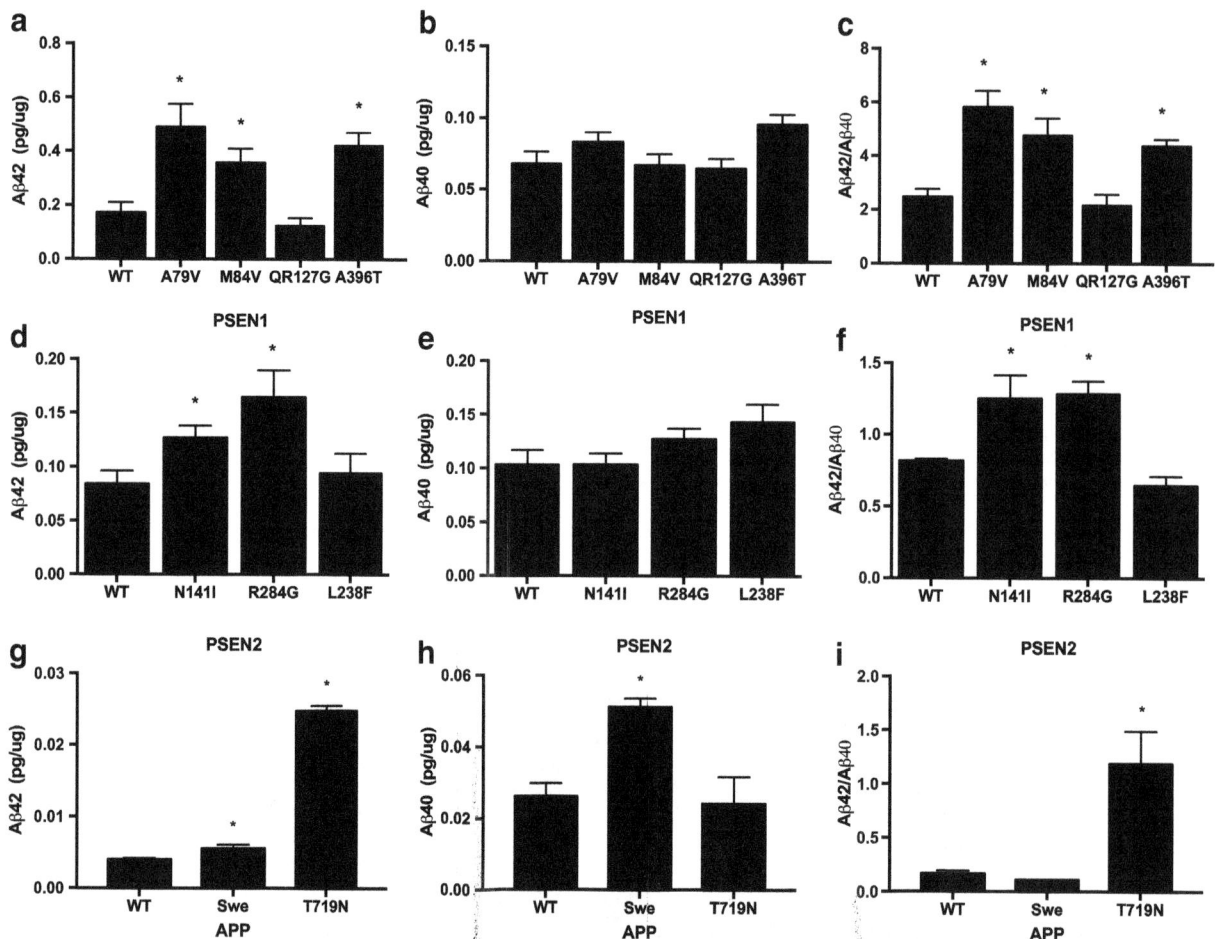

Fig. 3 Amyloid-β 1–42 peptide ($A\beta_{42}$) and $A\beta_{40}$ in cells expressing *APP*, *PSEN1*, and *PSEN2* variants of unknown pathogenicity. N2A695 cells were transfected with vectors expressing presenilin 1 or 2. Media was replaced 24 hours posttransfection and incubated for an additional 24 hours. Media were collected, and $A\beta_{42}$ and $A\beta_{40}$ were measured by enzyme-linked immunosorbent assay (ELISA) (pg/ml). Total intracellular protein was measured by bicinchoninic acid assay and used to normalize to ELISA Aβ values, resulting in a value represented as pg/μg (*see* the Methods section of text). **a–c** PSEN1 wild type (WT), pathogenic mutation A79V, and variants with unknown pathogenicity. **a** $A\beta_{42}$. **b** $A\beta_{40}$. **c** $A\beta_{42}/A\beta_{40}$ ratio. **d–f** PSEN2 WT, pathogenic mutation N141I, and variants with unknown pathogenicity. **d** $A\beta_{42}$. **e** $A\beta_{40}$. **f** $A\beta_{42}/A\beta_{40}$ ratio. **g–i** APP WT, pathogenic mutation KM670/671NL(Swe), and APP T719N. Graphs represent the mean (±SEM) of four replicate experiments. * $p < 0.05$. *PSEN1* QR127G is the amino acid representation for *PSEN1* c.379_382delXXXXinsG

the proband (Fig. 1b) revealed a 4-bp deletion and insertion of G at codon 127 in exon 5 of *PSEN1*, resulting in the deletion of glutamine and arginine and insertion of glycine (c.379_382delXXXXinsG). This is a novel variant and was absent from the EVS and ExAC databases (Table 1). N2A695 expressing *PSEN1* c.379_382delXXX-XinsG produced $A\beta_{42}$ and $A\beta_{40}$ levels similar to *PSEN1* WT (Fig. 3a–c). Thus, we propose that *PSEN1* c.379_382delXXXXinsG is an AD risk factor or benign polymorphism.

PSEN2 R284G

The proband had an age at symptomatic onset of 58 years, with average age at symptomatic onset in the family of 56 years (Fig. 1c). Sequencing of the proband

(Fig. 1c) revealed a single base pair substitution (CGG to GGG) at codon 284 in exon 8 of *PSEN2*, resulting in an arginine-to-glycine change (R284G). This is a novel variant and was absent from the EVS and ExAC databases (Table 1).

To assess the effects of *PSEN2* variants on Aβ isoform levels, we expressed vectors containing *PSEN2* WT, N141I, and R284G in N2A695 cells. Cells expressing *PSEN2* N141I and R284G produced significantly more $A\beta_{42}$ than cells expressing *PSEN2* WT (Fig. 3d and e). The $A\beta_{42}/A\beta_{40}$ ratio was also significantly higher in cells expressing *PSEN2* N141I and R284G (Fig. 3f). Thus, applying the algorithm for assessing pathogenicity (Fig. 4), we propose that the *PSEN2* R284G represents a probable pathogenic mutation.

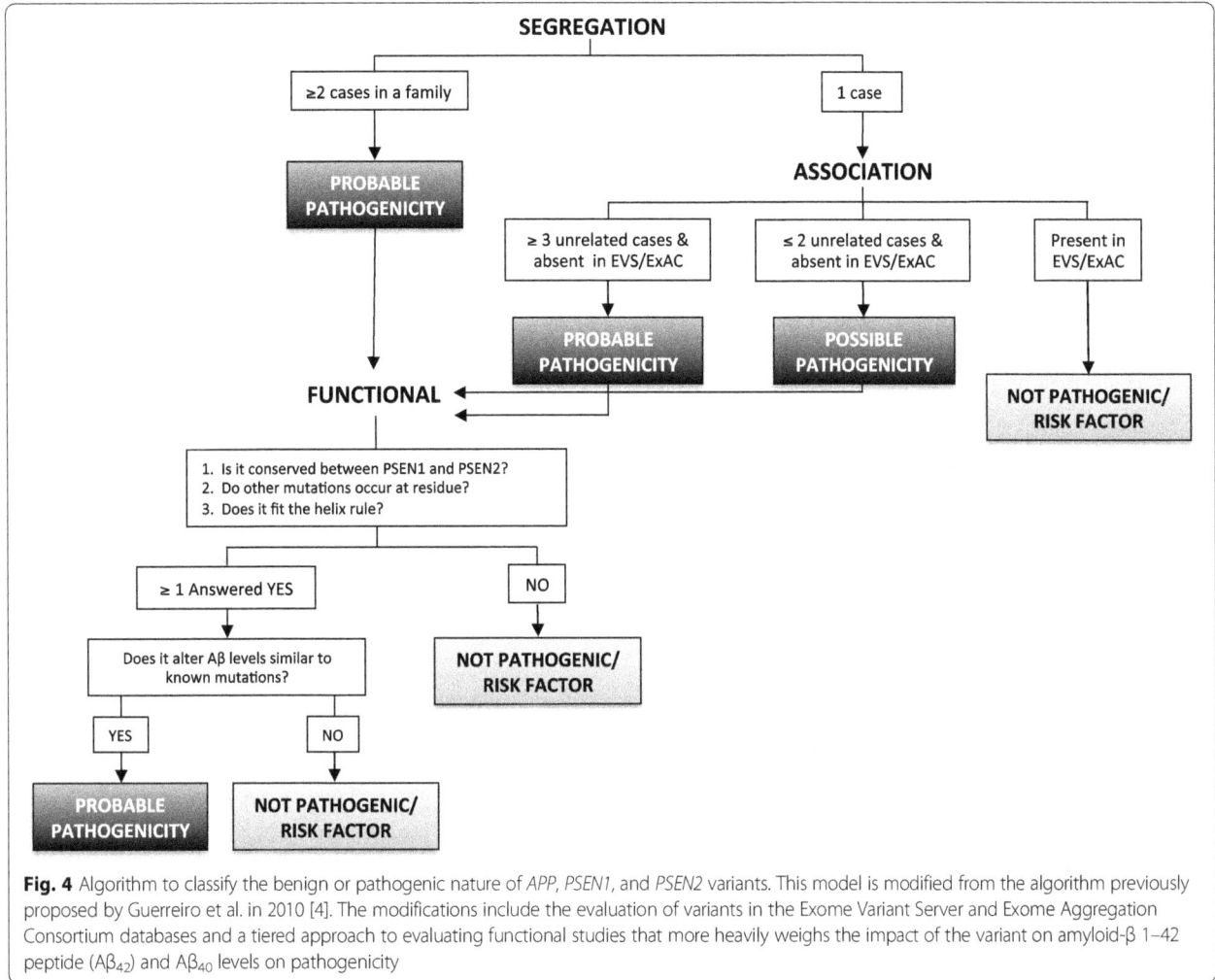

Fig. 4 Algorithm to classify the benign or pathogenic nature of *APP*, *PSEN1*, and *PSEN2* variants. This model is modified from the algorithm previously proposed by Guerreiro et al. in 2010 [4]. The modifications include the evaluation of variants in the Exome Variant Server and Exome Aggregation Consortium databases and a tiered approach to evaluating functional studies that more heavily weighs the impact of the variant on amyloid-β 1–42 peptide ($A\beta_{42}$) and $A\beta_{40}$ levels on pathogenicity

PSEN2 L238F

The proband was identified in a family with three generations of early-onset AD (Fig. 1d). The proband had an age at symptomatic onset of 49. The parent of the proband was diagnosed with AD at 57 years of age and died at age 77. Sequencing of the proband (Fig. 1d) revealed a single base pair substitution (CTT to TTT) at codon 238 in exon 7 of *PSEN2*, resulting in a leucine-to-phenylalanine change (L238F). *PSEN2* L238F was also identified in two alleles in EVS, in two alleles in ExAC, and in one individual with sporadic AD (Table 1; [20]). CSF Aβ, total tau, and phosphorylated tau were measured in a *PSEN2* L238F carrier related to the proband, who was cognitively normal at the time of lumbar puncture. CSF Aβ (506.54 pg/ml), total tau (38.75 pg/ml), and p-tau$_{181}$ (21.33 pg/ml) at 17 years prior to the parental age at symptomatic onset was consistent with biomarker levels in normal controls [3, 6]. Cells expressing *PSEN2* L238F produced $A\beta_{42}$ and $A\beta_{40}$ levels similar to *PSEN2* WT (Fig. 3d–f). Thus, we propose that *PSEN2* L238F represents an AD risk factor or benign polymorphism.

App T719N

The proband was identified in a family with two generations of early-onset AD (Fig. 1e). The proband had an age at symptomatic onset of 45 years. The parent of the proband was diagnosed at 45 years of age. Sequencing of the proband (Fig. 1e) revealed a single base pair substitution (ACC to AAC) at codon 719 in exon 17 of *APP*, resulting in a threonine-to-asparagine change (T719N). *APP* T719N was absent in the EVS and ExAC databases and was detected in one individual with early-onset AD (Table 1) [21]. Cells expressing *APP* T719N produced significantly elevated levels of $A\beta_{42}$ and $A\beta_{42}/A\beta_{40}$ relative to *APP* WT (Fig. 3g–i). Thus, we propose that *APP* T719N is a probable pathogenic mutation.

Conclusions

By applying genetic, bioinformatic, and functional data to an algorithm to assess pathogenicity, we propose that the *PSEN1* M84V, *PSEN1* A396T, *PSEN2* R284G, and *APP* T719N are likely pathogenic mutations resulting in ADAD, whereas *PSEN1* c.379_382delXXXXinsG and

PSEN2 L238F are likely benign polymorphisms. This algorithm was adapted and modified from a pathogenicity algorithm originally proposed by Guerreiro and colleagues [4]. We have expanded upon this algorithm in several important ways: (1) expanding the number of controls in the association analyses from 100 to 65,000 by exploiting the EVS and ExAC databases; (2) evaluating the bioinformatic functional findings (e.g., conservation between *PSEN1* and *PSEN2* and the presence of other mutations at the same residue) independent of the cell-based functional findings; and (3) incorporating cell-based assays to evaluate the impact of novel variants on Aβ levels. We propose that this modified approach to assessing pathogenicity provides an important pipeline for incorporating mutation data at several levels and that this algorithm may be adapted to impute pathogenicity when extensive genetic data are missing for affected families. Designation of a variant as pathogenic will allow individuals to enroll in observational and clinical trials for AD, with clear applications in clinical and research settings.

Acknowledgements
We gratefully acknowledge the altruism of the participants and their families and contributions of the DIAN research and support staff at each of the participating sites for their contributions to this study. The DIAN Expanded Registry welcomes contact from any families or treating clinicians interested in research about autosomal dominant familial Alzheimer's disease. This work was supported by access to equipment made possible by the Hope Center for Neurological Disorders and the departments of neurology and psychiatry at Washington University School of Medicine. This article was reviewed by DIAN Study investigators for scientific content and consistency of data interpretation with previous DIAN study publications. We acknowledge the altruism of the participants and their families and the contributions of the DIAN research and support staff at each of the participating sites for their contributions to this study. We thank the DIAN Steering Committee: Ricardo Allegri, Tammie Benzinger, Sarah Berman, Virginia Buckles, Nigel Cairns, Helena Chui, Maritza Ciliberto, Anne Fagan, Howard Feldman, Bernardino Ghetti, Neill Graff-Radford, David Holtzman, Rachel Huber, Mathias Jucker, Jae-Hong Lee, Johannes Levin, Daniel Marcus, Ralph Martins, Colin Masters, Hiroshi Mori, James Noble, Nick Fox, Stephen Salloway, Peter Schofield, Michael Weiner, and Chengjie Xiong.

Funding
Funding provided by the DIAN Expanded Registry (to RJB), National Institutes of Health grant K01 AG046374 (to CMK) and DIAN-TU Pharma Consortium (https://dian.wustl.edu/our-research/the-pharma-consortium/; to RJB, CC, AMG, CMK), Fidelity Biosciences Research Initiative (RJB, CC, and CMK), and the Gerald and Henrietta Rauenhorst Foundation (RJB, CC, and CMK). Data collection and sharing for this project were supported by The Dominantly Inherited Alzheimer's Network (DIAN; grant UF1AG032438) funded by the National Institute on Aging (NIA), the German Center for Neurodegenerative Diseases (DZNE), and the Institute for Neurological Research Dr. Raul Carrea (FLENI). Partial support was received through research and development grants for dementia from the Japan Agency for Medical Research and Development (AMED) and the Korea Health Technology R&D Project through the Korea Health Industry Development Institute (KHIDI). The funding bodies played no role in the design of the study; in the collection, analysis, and interpretation of data; or in the writing of the manuscript.

Authors' contributions
SH and CMK wrote the manuscript. CMK designed cell culture studies. SH, AL, and CMK performed cell culture experiments. JBN, DL, EZ, RL, GSD, EM, JC, JCM, and RJB recruited participants. BAG, RH, and TLSB performed and analyzed brain imaging. AMF analyzed CSF biomarker data. EZ, GSD, EM, AMG, CC, and RJB reviewed pedigrees. CMK performed bioinformatic analysis. All authors contributed to critical revision of the manuscript for intellectual content, and all authors read and approved the final manuscript.

Competing interests
AMG is a member of the scientific advisory board for Denali Therapeutics and serves on a genetic scientific advisory panel for Pfizer. RJB receives laboratory research funding from the National Institutes of Health, the Alzheimer's Association, the BrightFocus Foundation, the Rainwater Foundation Tau Consortium, the Association for Frontotemporal Degeneration, the Cure Alzheimer's Fund, and the tau SILK Consortium (AbbVie, Biogen, and Eli Lilly and Co.). Funding for clinical trials not related to this research include the National Institutes of Health, the Alzheimer's Association, Eli Lilly and Co., Hoffman La-Roche, Janssen, Avid Radiopharmaceuticals, the GHR Foundation, and an anonymous foundation. RJB also receives research funding from the DIAN Pharma Consortium (AbbVie, Amgen, AstraZeneca, Biogen, Eisai, Eli Lilly and Co., Hoffman La-Roche, Janssen, Pfizer, and Sanofi). RJB has received honoraria from Janssen and Pfizer as a speaker and from Merck and Pfizer as an advisory board member. Washington University, RJB, and DMH have equity ownership interest in C2N Diagnostics and receive royalty income based on technology (stable isotope labeling kinetics and blood plasma assay) licensed by Washington University to C2N Diagnostics. RJB receives income from C2N Diagnostics for serving on the scientific advisory board. Washington University, with RJB as coinventor, has submitted the U.S. nonprovisional patent application "Methods for measuring the metabolism of CNS derived biomolecules in vivo" and the provisional patent application "Plasma based methods for detecting CNS amyloid deposition." The remaining authors declare that they have no competing interests.

Author details
[1]Department of Psychiatry, Washington University School of Medicine, 425 S. Euclid Ave, Campus Box 8134, St. Louis, MO 63110, USA. [2]Department of Radiology, Washington University School of Medicine, St. Louis, MO, USA. [3]Department of Neurology, Washington University School of Medicine, St. Louis, MO, USA. [4]Clinique Interdisciplinaire de Mémoire du CHU de Québec, Département des Sciences Neurologiques, Faculté de Médecine, Université Laval, Québec City, Québec, Canada. [5]Massachusetts General Hospital/Martinos Center for Biomedical Imaging, 149 13th Street, Gerontology Research Room 2669, Charlestown, MA 02129, USA. [6]Mallinckrodt Institute of Radiology, Washington University School of Medicine, St. Louis, MO 63110, USA. [7]Department of Neuroscience, Mount Sinai School of Medicine, New York, NY, USA.

References
1. Karch CM, Cruchaga C, Goate AM. Alzheimer's disease genetics: from the bench to the clinic. Neuron. 2014;83:11–26.
2. Cruts M, Theuns J, Van Broeckhoven C. Locus-specific mutation databases for neurodegenerative brain diseases. Hum Mutat. 2012;33:1340–4.
3. Bateman RJ, Xiong C, Benzinger TL, Fagan AM, Goate A, Fox NC, Marcus DS, Cairns NJ, Xie X, Blazey TM, et al. Clinical and biomarker changes in dominantly inherited Alzheimer's disease. N Engl J Med. 2012;367:795–804.
4. Guerreiro RJ, Baquero M, Blesa R, Boada M, Brás JM, Bullido MJ, Calado A, Crook R, Ferreira C, Frank A, et al. Genetic screening of Alzheimer's disease genes in Iberian and African samples yields novel mutations in presenilins and APP. Neurobiol Aging. 2010;31:725–31.
5. Adzhubei IA, Schmidt S, Peshkin L, Ramensky VE, Gerasimova A, Bork P, Kondrashov AS, Sunyaev SR. A method and server for predicting damaging missense mutations. Nat Methods. 2010;7:248–9.

6. Fagan AM, Xiong C, Jasielec MS, Bateman RJ, Goate AM, Benzinger TL, Ghetti B, Martins RN, Masters CL, Mayeux R, et al. Longitudinal change in CSF biomarkers in autosomal-dominant Alzheimer's disease. Sci Transl Med. 2014;6:226ra230.

7. Jack CR Jr, Bernstein MA, Fox NC, Thompson P, Alexander G, Harvey D, Borowski B, Britson PJ, Whitwell JL, Ward C, et al. The Alzheimer's Disease Neuroimaging Initiative (ADNI): MRI methods. J Magn Reson Imaging. 2008; 27:685–91.

8. Jack CR Jr, Bernstein MA, Borowski BJ, Gunter JL, Fox NC, Thompson PM, Schuff N, Krueger G, Killiany RJ, Decarli CS, et al. Update on the magnetic resonance imaging core of the Alzheimer's disease neuroimaging initiative. Alzheimers Dement. 2010;6:212–20.

9. Su Y, D'Angelo GM, Vlassenko AG, Zhou G, Snyder AZ, Marcus DS, Blazey TM, Christensen JJ, Vora S, Morris JC, et al. Quantitative analysis of PiB-PET with FreeSurfer ROIs. PLoS One. 2013;8:e73377.

10. Su Y, Blazey TM, Owen CJ, Christensen JJ, Friedrichsen K, Joseph-Mathurin N, Wang Q, Hornbeck RC, Ances BM, Snyder AZ, et al. Quantitative amyloid imaging in autosomal dominant Alzheimer's disease: results from the DIAN study group. PLoS One. 2016;11:e0152082.

11. Brunkan AL, Martinez M, Walker ES, Goate AM. Presenilin endoproteolysis is an intramolecular cleavage. Mol Cell Neurosci. 2005;29:65–73.

12. Kovacs DM, Fausett HJ, Page KJ, Kim TW, Moir RD, Merriam DE, Hollister RD, Hallmark OG, Mancini R, Felsenstein KM, et al. Alzheimer-associated presenilins 1 and 2: neuronal expression in brain and localization to intracellular membranes in mammalian cells. Nat Med. 1996;2:224–9.

13. Walker ES, Martinez M, Brunkan AL, Goate A. Presenilin 2 familial Alzheimer's disease mutations result in partial loss of function and dramatic changes in Aβ42/40 ratios. J Neurochem. 2005;92:294–301.

14. Wang J, Brunkan AL, Hecimovic S, Walker E, Goate A. Conserved "PAL" sequence in presenilins is essential for gamma-secretase activity, but not required for formation or stabilization of gamma-secretase complexes. Neurobiol Dis. 2004;15:654–66.

15. Hooli BV, Kovacs-Vajna ZM, Mullin K, Blumenthal MA, Mattheisen M, Zhang C, Lange C, Mohapatra G, Bertram L, Tanzi RE. Rare autosomal copy number variations in early-onset familial Alzheimer's disease. Mol Psychiatry. 2014;19: 676–81.

16. Hardy J, Crook R. Presenilin mutations line up along transmembrane alpha-helices. Neurosci Lett. 2001;306:203–5.

17. Houlden H, Baker M, McGowan E, Lewis P, Hutton M, Crook R, Wood NW, Kumar-Singh S, Geddes J, Swash M, et al. Variant Alzheimer's disease with spastic paraparesis and cotton wool plaques is caused by PS-1 mutations that lead to exceptionally high amyloid-β concentrations. Ann Neurol. 2000; 48:806–8.

18. Steiner H, Revesz T, Neumann M, Romig H, Grim MG, Pesold B, Kretzschmar HA, Hardy J, Holton JL, Baumeister R, et al. A pathogenic presenilin-1 deletion causes abberrant Aβ42 production in the absence of congophilic amyloid plaques. J Biol Chem. 2001;276:7233–9.

19. Lohmann E, Guerreiro RJ, Erginel-Unaltuna N, Gurunlian N, Bilgic B, Gurvit H, Hanagasi HA, Luu N, Emre M, Singleton A. Identification of PSEN1 and PSEN2 gene mutations and variants in Turkish dementia patients. Neurobiol Aging. 2012;33(1850):e1817–27.

20. Sala Frigerio C, Lau P, Troakes C, Deramecourt V, Gele P, Van Loo P, Voet T, De Strooper B. On the identification of low allele frequency mosaic mutations in the brains of Alzheimer's disease patients. Alzheimers Dement. 2015;11:1265–76.

21. Scahill RI, Ridgway GR, Bartlett JW, Barnes J, Ryan NS, Mead S, Beck J, Clarkson MJ, Crutch SJ, Schott JM, et al. Genetic influences on atrophy patterns in familial Alzheimer's disease: a comparison of APP and PSEN1 mutations. J Alzheimers Dis. 2013;35:199–212.

MRI predictors of amyloid pathology: results from the EMIF-AD Multimodal Biomarker Discovery study

Mara ten Kate[1*†] (ID), Alberto Redolfi[2†], Enrico Peira[2], Isabelle Bos[3], Stephanie J. Vos[3], Rik Vandenberghe[4,5], Silvy Gabel[4,5], Jolien Schaeverbeke[4,5], Philip Scheltens[1], Olivier Blin[6], Jill C. Richardson[7], Regis Bordet[8], Anders Wallin[9], Carl Eckerstrom[9], José Luis Molinuevo[10], Sebastiaan Engelborghs[11,12], Christine Van Broeckhoven[13,14], Pablo Martinez-Lage[15], Julius Popp[16,17], Magdalini Tsolaki[18], Frans R. J. Verhey[3], Alison L. Baird[19], Cristina Legido-Quigley[20], Lars Bertram[21,22,23], Valerija Dobricic[21], Henrik Zetterberg[24,25,26,27], Simon Lovestone[19], Johannes Streffer[11,28], Silvia Bianchetti[2], Gerald P. Novak[29], Jerome Revillard[30], Mark F. Gordon[31,32], Zhiyong Xie[33], Viktor Wottschel[34], Giovanni Frisoni[2,35], Pieter Jelle Visser[1,3] and Frederik Barkhof[34,36]

Abstract

Background: With the shift of research focus towards the pre-dementia stage of Alzheimer's disease (AD), there is an urgent need for reliable, non-invasive biomarkers to predict amyloid pathology. The aim of this study was to assess whether easily obtainable measures from structural MRI, combined with demographic data, cognitive data and apolipoprotein E (*APOE*) ε4 genotype, can be used to predict amyloid pathology using machine-learning classification.

Methods: We examined 810 subjects with structural MRI data and amyloid markers from the European Medical Information Framework for Alzheimer's Disease Multimodal Biomarker Discovery study, including subjects with normal cognition (CN, $n = 337$, age 66.5 ± 7.2, 50% female, 27% amyloid positive), mild cognitive impairment (MCI, $n = 375$, age 69.1 ± 7.5, 53% female, 63% amyloid positive) and AD dementia ($n = 98$, age 67.0 ± 7.7, 48% female, 97% amyloid positive). Structural MRI scans were visually assessed and Freesurfer was used to obtain subcortical volumes, cortical thickness and surface area measures. We first assessed univariate associations between MRI measures and amyloid pathology using mixed models. Next, we developed and tested an automated classifier using demographic, cognitive, MRI and *APOE* ε4 information to predict amyloid pathology. A support vector machine (SVM) with nested 10-fold cross-validation was applied to identify a set of markers best discriminating between amyloid positive and amyloid negative subjects.

Results: In univariate associations, amyloid pathology was associated with lower subcortical volumes and thinner cortex in AD-signature regions in CN and MCI. The multi-variable SVM classifier provided an area under the curve (AUC) of 0.81 ± 0.07 in MCI and an AUC of 0.74 ± 0.08 in CN. In CN, selected features for the classifier included *APOE* ε4, age, memory scores and several MRI measures such as hippocampus, amygdala and accumbens volumes and cortical thickness in temporal and parahippocampal regions. In MCI, the classifier including demographic and *APOE* ε4 information did not improve after additionally adding imaging measures.

(Continued on next page)

* Correspondence: m.tenkate1@vumc.nl
†Mara ten Kate and Alberto Redolfi contributed equally to this work.
[1]Alzheimer Center & Department of Neurology, VU University Medical Center, PO Box 7057, 1007 MB Amsterdam, the Netherlands
Full list of author information is available at the end of the article

(Continued from previous page)

Conclusions: Amyloid pathology is associated with changes in structural MRI measures in CN and MCI. An automated classifier based on clinical, imaging and *APOE* ε4 data can identify the presence of amyloid pathology with a moderate level of accuracy. These results could be used in clinical trials to pre-screen subjects for anti-amyloid therapies.

Keywords: Alzheimer's disease, Mild cognitive impairment, Biomarkers, Magnetic resonance imaging, Amyloid, Machine learning, Support vector machine, European Medical Information Framework for Alzheimer's Disease

Background

Alzheimer's disease (AD) is characterized pathologically by beta-amyloid (Aβ) plaques and neurofibrillary tangles of misfolded tau protein [1]. As amyloid pathology may arise up to two decades before the onset of dementia, research focus has shifted towards the pre-dementia stage, which provides an opportunity for secondary prevention [2–4]. The design of clinical trials targeting the amyloid pathway in this early stage would be facilitated by the ability to recruit subjects with amyloid pathology. Amyloid pathology can be assessed in cerebrospinal fluid (CSF), obtainable by lumbar puncture, or on positron emission tomography (PET) scans. However, obtaining CSF is relatively invasive and PET scans are costly, invasive by exposing subjects to radiation and are not universally available. As the estimated prevalence of amyloid pathology between the ages of 60 and 80 ranges from 10 to 33% for cognitively normal (CN) subjects and from 37 to 60% for subjects with mild cognitive impairment (MCI) [5], assessing amyloid pathology with CSF or PET for screening purposes is likely inefficient. Finding minimally invasive biomarkers predicting amyloid pathology could reduce the number of invasive, costly and time-consuming measures in clinical trials.

Brain atrophy markers derived from structural magnetic resonance imaging (MRI) could serve as a potential biomarker for amyloid pathology [6–12]. In this study, we evaluate the use of easily obtainable MRI measures for the prediction of amyloid pathology. We included both visual rating scores, which can be easily performed in clinical settings, and quantitative measures of subcortical volumes, cortical thickness and surface area, which can be derived from freely available software and may be more sensitive than visual ratings. We first assessed univariate associations between MRI measures and amyloid pathology. Next, we used support vector machine (SVM) analysis to develop a multi-variable classifier for predicting brain amyloid pathology at a single subject level. Besides imaging measures, we also included other non-invasive measures relevant to AD in the classifier, including demographic information, cognitive testing and apolipoprotein E (*APOE*) ε4 genotype.

Methods
Participants
We included participants from the European Medical Information Framework for Alzheimer's Disease Multimodal

Biomarker Discovery (EMIF-AD MBD) study. The aim of this study was to discover novel diagnostic and prognostic markers for pre-dementia AD, by making use of existing data and samples [13]. The EMIF-AD MBD study pooled data of 494 CN, 526 MCI and 201 AD-dementia participants from three multicentre and eight single-centre studies. Inclusion criteria were: presence of normal cognition, MCI or a clinical diagnosis of AD-type dementia; availability of data on amyloid pathology, measured in CSF or on PET; age above 50 years; availability of MRI scans, plasma, DNA or CSF samples (at least two of the modalities); and absence of major neurological, psychiatric or somatic disorders that could cause cognitive impairment.

From the 1221 subjects included in the EMIF-AD MBD study, MRI scans of 873 subjects were contributed by the different studies (Fig. 1). Based on visual assessment, 863 MRI scans were of sufficient quality for visual rating, consisting of 365 CN, 398 MCI and 100 AD-dementia participants. Data were obtained from the following cohorts: DESCRIPA [14], EDAR [15], PharmaCog [16] and single-centre studies at VU University Medical Centre [17], San Sebastian GAP [18], University of Antwerp [19], Leuven [20], University of Lausanne [21], University of Gothenburg [22] and Barcelona IDIBAPS [23]. Each study was approved by the local medical ethics committee. Subjects had provided written informed consent at the time of inclusion in the MBD study for sharing of data, fluid samples and scans.

Clinical and cognitive data
From all parent cohorts, clinical information and neuropsychological tests were collected centrally, harmonized, pooled and stored in an online data platform as previously described [13]. In short, all parent cohorts administered the Mini-Mental State Examination (MMSE), and performed neuropsychological testing covering various cognitive domains, although the tests used varied across the different cohorts. For the cognitive domains memory, language, attention, executive functioning and visuo-construction, one priority test was selected from each cohort (Additional file 1: Table S1) and *z*-scores were computed based on local normative data when available, or published normative data from healthy controls otherwise.

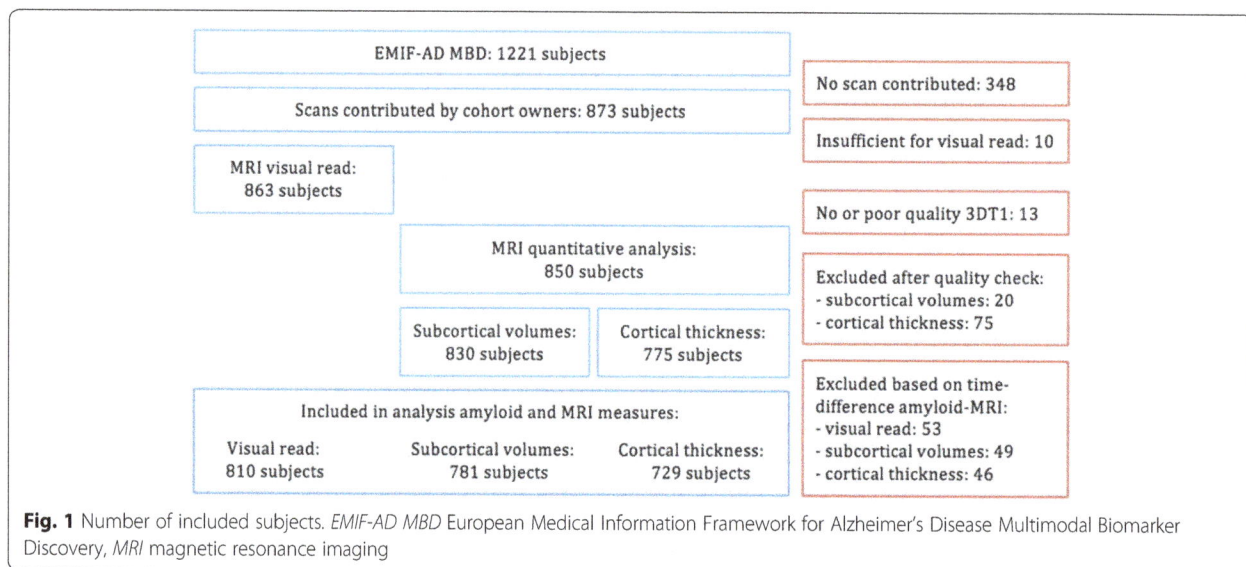

Fig. 1 Number of included subjects. *EMIF-AD MBD* European Medical Information Framework for Alzheimer's Disease Multimodal Biomarker Discovery, *MRI* magnetic resonance imaging

APOE genotyping

For the entire EMIF-AD MBD cohort, *APOE* genotyping data from the local genetic analyses were available for 1121 (91%) individuals. Central genetic analyses were performed at Lübeck University, Germany for 805 DNA and 148 whole blood samples. From the blood samples, DNA was extracted using the QIAamp® DNA Blood Mini Kit (QIA-GEN GmbH, Hilden, Germany) resulting in 953 DNA samples, of which 926 passed quality control. Genome-wide SNP genotyping was performed using the Infinium Global Screening Array (GSA) with Shared Custom Content (Illumina Inc.). *APOE* genotypes were determined either directly (rs7212) or by imputation (rs429358). For 80 samples for which no local *APOE* genotype was available, and for 45 mismatches between local and GSA-derived genotypes, the *APOE* genotype was determined using TaqMan assays (ThermoFisher Scientific, Foster City, CA, USA) on a QuantStudio-12 K-Flex system. TaqMan re-genotyping confirmed 23 GSA genotypes and 21 local genotypes. For one failed sample we retained the local genotype. We classified individuals as *APOE* ε4 carriers or non-carriers according to their genotype status at rs429358 (C-allele = ε4).

Amyloid classification

In the current selection ($n = 863$), amyloid status was defined by central analysis of CSF when available ($n = 510$), otherwise by local amyloid PET ($n = 174$) or local CSF ($n = 179$) measures. Central CSF analysis was performed at Gothenburg University, Sweden and included $A\beta_{1-40}$ and $A\beta_{1-42}$ measured using the V-PLEX Plus Aβ Peptide Panel 1 (6E10) Kit (Meso Scale Discovery, Rockville, MD, USA), as described by the manufacturer. The central cut-off value for Aβ positivity was an $A\beta_{42/40}$ ratio < 0.061. Amyloid PET was performed in one cohort using [^{18}F]flu-temetamol according to local standardized procedures,

with a standardized uptake value ratio (SUVR) cut-off value > 1.38 used for abnormality [24]. In short, SUVR images were computed from spatially normalized summed images with cerebellar grey matter as the reference region. The cut-off value was derived from an independent dataset [25] and based on the statistical difference between AD dementia patients and cognitively normal subjects [24]. Local CSF amyloid was determined according to local protocols with local cut-off values. The number of amyloid positive subjects per diagnosis per cohort is presented in Additional file 1: Table S2.

MRI acquisition

At each site, imaging was acquired according to local protocols. From each parent cohort, we centrally collected the T1-weighted images, and if available also fluid-attenuated inversion recovery (FLAIR) and susceptibility weighted images (SWI) or T2*, at the VU University Medical Center, where a visual quality check was performed. The acquired sequences and acquisition parameters for the T1-weighted scans for each cohort are presented in Additional file 1: Table S3. Usually, MRI was assessed at baseline together with baseline cognitive and amyloid measures. For 104 subjects there was more than a 1-year difference between MRI acquisition and amyloid assessment. In cases where amyloid was abnormal and acquired before MRI, this subject was included in the analysis ($n = 42$). In cases where amyloid was normal and acquired after MRI, this subject was included in the analysis ($n = 9$). All other cases were excluded ($n = 53$). For 99 subjects there was more than a 1-year difference between baseline cognitive assessment and MRI. For these cases, we did not use the cognitive data in the multi-variable analysis. Demographic differences between subjects who were included and excluded for differences in time between

MRI and amyloid or cognitive assessment are presented in Additional file 1: Tables S4 and S5.

MRI visual rating

MRI scans with sufficient quality ($n = 863$) were visually rated by a single experienced rater, blinded to demographic information during rating. Medial temporal lobe atrophy (MTA) was assessed on coronal reconstructions of the T1-weighted images using a 5-point scale ranging from no atrophy (0) to end-stage atrophy (4) [26]. The MTA results from the left and right hemisphere were averaged. Global cortical atrophy (GCA) was assessed on transversal FLAIR or T1 images using a 4-point scale [27]. Posterior atrophy was assessed using a 4-point scale [28] and averaged over hemispheres. White matter hyperintensities were visually assessed on FLAIR images ($n = 812$) using the 4-point Fazekas scale (none, punctate, early confluent, confluent) [29]. Microbleeds were assessed on SWI and/or T2* images ($n = 445$) and defined as rounded hypointense homogeneous foci of up to 10 mm in diameter in the brain parenchyma. Microbleeds were dichotomized as present (≥ 1 microbleeds) or absent (0 microbleeds).

MRI quantitative analysis

Good quality 3D T1 images ($n = 850$) were uploaded on the N4U platform (https://neugrid4you.eu/) for automated quantitative processing. Subcortical volumes, cortical thickness and surface area measures were estimated from 3D T1 MRI using Freesurfer (version 5.3.0, https://surfer.nmr.mgh.harvard.edu) as previously described [30]. All segmentations were visually inspected. We excluded data from 20 subjects for subcortical volumes (five due to complete failure of the algorithm and 15 due to segmentation errors) and from 75 subjects for cortical thickness and surface area (five due to complete failure of the algorithm, 66 due to segmentations errors of the cortical ribbon and four for other failures). Subcortical volumes were normalized by total intracranial volume (TIV). Cortical thickness and surface area were available for 68 regions according to the Desikan–Killiany atlas implemented in Freesurfer. Additionally, we computed two AD-signature meta-ROI measures that have previously been presented in the literature: one by Dickerson et al. [10] consisting of the average cortical thickness in angular, precuneus, supramarginal, superior frontal, superior parietal, temporal pole, inferior temporal, medial temporal and inferior frontal cortex; and one by Jack et al. [31] consisting of the surface-area weighted average mean cortical thickness in entorhinal, inferior temporal, middle temporal and fusiform regions.

Statistical methods

Univariate analysis

Univariate statistical analyses were performed in R (version 3.3.1). Comparisons of clinical characteristics between amyloid positive and negative subjects within each diagnostic group were performed using independent t tests or Mann–Whitney U tests for continuous variables and chi-square tests for categorical variables. Baseline comparisons in quantitative MRI measures between groups were performed with linear mixed models (continuous outcome measures) (lme4 package, version 1.1–12; lmerTest package 2.0–36), mixed effects ordered logistic regressions (ordinal outcome measures) (ordinal package, version 2015.6–28) and mixed effects logistic regressions (dichotomous outcome measures) (lme4 package). In each model, we entered amyloid status (negative, positive) and diagnosis (CN, MCI and AD) and their interaction as fixed effects. Age (centred on mean), gender and *APOE* ε4 status were added as covariates. Cohort was added as a random intercept. The analyses were corrected within diagnostic group (in total 22 tests: five visual ratings, 14 subcortical volumes, three cortical thickness summary measures) for multiple hypothesis testing with the p.adjust() function using the false discovery rate, and indicated as p_{FDR}.

Multi-variable analysis

To find the best multi-variable predictor of amyloid pathology, we used a supervised machine-learning approach based on SVM analysis. In SVM, two classes are separated by finding a hyperplane that maximizes the margin of separation between data points of each class in a high-dimensional feature space. SVMs are used extensively in neuroimaging as they have been shown to predict outcomes with high accuracy and possess the ability to model diverse and high-dimensional data [32]. We built a classifier to separate amyloid positive from amyloid negative subjects separately in the CN and MCI subgroups and, for the sake of completeness, also in the whole sample (including CN, MCI and AD-dementia patients). To address the imbalance between the number of amyloid positive and amyloid negative subjects in each diagnostic group, we adopted the re-weighting strategy [33]. That means we adjusted weights of each SVM feature inversely proportional to amyloid positive versus negative frequencies.

Machine-learning approach We used the python Scikit-learn library (version 0.19.1) to perform SVM classification [34]. To prevent overfitting (i.e. the classifier works perfectly on the training data, but is poorly generalizable to new data), we performed feature relevance evaluation and dimensionality reduction using a tree-based feature selection approach with a nested 10-fold cross-validation design [35, 36]. This was performed separately within each subgroup (CN, MCI and whole sample).

The nested cross-validation consists of an inner loop for model building and parameter estimation, and an outer loop for model testing. Consequently, the dataset was divided into two parts: a training plus validation subset and a test subset. In the inner loop, SVM models were trained with varying SVM hyper-parameters (i.e. cost parameters C and kernel function) based on a grid search, and a feature selection was performed using classification trees. The validation set was used to determine the SVM hyper-parameters over the grid of possible values. The performance of the resulting model, with optimized SVM hyper-parameters and features, was subsequently evaluated on the test set in the outer loop. For this outer loop, we used a 10-fold cross-validation scheme so that the data were divided into 10 equally sized parts. Nine of these were used as the training/validation set and one as the test set, and the 10 parts were permuted in each iteration of the outer loop so that each one was used for testing once. Finally, the SVM results were averaged over the 10 folds to estimate the predictive power of the proposed model on the whole dataset.

Feature selection As the input for the classifier, we used demographic information, neuropsychological information, *APOE* ε4 genotype and MRI measures (visual ratings, subcortical volumes, regional cortical thickness and regional surface area measures). To combine information measured on different scales, continuous demographic and MRI measures were normalized to *z*-scores. In the adopted tree-based feature selection strategy, the Gini index was used to measure the relevance of each feature [37]. Features with a Gini index above the mean were kept, others were discarded. The complete list of features considered and selected, in the whole dataset and for CN and MCI separately, is reported in Additional file 1: Table S8.

Performance evaluation To assess the performance of the classifier, we computed the averaged receiver operating characteristic (ROC) area under the curve (AUC), specificity, sensitivity and accuracy for the testing datasets. We initially maximized the Youden index, and then also explored the results when setting the sensitivity at 80%, 85%, 90%, 95% and 100%. To assess the added value of combining different sources of information, we also built classifiers including only demographic information and a single other biomarker type (neuropsychological tests, *APOE* ε4 genotype, MRI measures). Differences in AUC ROCs between classifiers were assessed with DeLong's test.

Results
Demographic and cognitive comparisons
We included 810 subjects divided over three diagnostic groups: CN ($n = 337$), MCI ($n = 375$) and AD dementia ($n = 98$). Within the CN group, 92 (27%) subjects were amyloid positive, in the MCI group 235 (63%) and in the AD-dementia group 95 (97%). Demographic and clinical data according to diagnosis and amyloid status are presented in Table 1. The amyloid positive MCI subjects

were older and had lower cognitive scores compared to the amyloid negative MCI subjects. In CN, there were no differences in age or cognition between amyloid positive and amyloid negative subjects. Amyloid positive subjects were more often *APOE* ε4 carriers in both the MCI and CN groups.

Univariate association between MRI measures and amyloid pathology
Within the MCI group, subjects with amyloid pathology had higher visual rating scores of medial temporal lobe atrophy, global cortical atrophy and parietal atrophy compared to amyloid negative subjects (Table 2). There were no differences in Fazekas score or presence of microbleeds. Amyloid positive MCI subjects had statistically significantly lower bilateral hippocampus, amygdala, thalamus, left caudate and right putamen volumes, and a trend towards lower right caudate ($p_{uncorrected} = 0.08$) and bilateral accumbens (both $p_{uncorrected} = 0.07$) volumes compared to amyloid negative MCI subjects (Table 3). Amyloid positive MCI subjects also had lower whole brain average cortical thickness, as well as in the two AD-signature meta-ROIs, compared to amyloid negative MCI subjects.

In the CN group, amyloid positive subjects had statistically significantly lower right hippocampus, left amygdala, left thalamus and bilateral accumbens volumes compared to amyloid negative subjects. The effect of amyloid pathology on hippocampal volume was stronger in MCI subjects compared to CN subjects (significant interaction diagnosis × amyloid status). Amyloid positive CN subjects had lower values in the Jack AD-signature meta-ROI ($p_{uncorrected} = 0.02$), but not in the Dickerson AD-signature meta-ROI ($p_{uncorrected} = 0.3$) or whole brain average cortical thickness ($p_{uncorrected} = 0.3$) compared to amyloid negative CN subjects. There were no differences in visual rating scores between amyloid positive and amyloid negative CN subjects. All individual cortical thickness and surface area regions are presented in Additional file 1: Tables S6 and S7.

Compared to amyloid positive CN subjects, amyloid positive MCI subjects had lower bilateral hippocampal and amygdala volumes (all $p < 0.001$) and lower whole brain average cortical thickness ($p = 0.001$), as well as in the two AD-signature meta-ROIs (both $p < 0.001$).

Multi-variable classifier results
The features selected by the classifier in CN subjects, MCI subjects and the whole sample are presented in Additional file 1: Table S8. Across diagnoses, *APOE* ε4 genotype was the most important feature. Other relevant features selected across samples were age, the neuropsychological memory scores and various MRI measures such as hippocampus

Table 1 Baseline characteristics by diagnosis and amyloid status

Characteristic	Cognitively normal		Mild cognitive impairment		Alzheimer-type dementia	
	Amyloid negative	Amyloid positive	Amyloid negative	Amyloid positive	Amyloid negative	Amyloid positive
N, % within diagnosis	245 (73)	92 (27)	140 (37)	235 (63)	3 (3)	95 (97)
Age (years)	66.1 ± 7.2	67.5 ± 7.2	67.3 ± 8.0	70.2 ± 7.0***	63.1 ± 8.0	67.1 ± 7.7
Male gender	120 (49)	47 (51)	73 (52)	105 (45)	3 (100)	48 (51)
Education (years)	13.2 ± 3.5	12.8 ± 3.8	10.8 ± 4.0	11.1 ± 3.7	10.3 ± 5.1	11.1 ± 3.3
MMSE	28.9 ± 1.2	28.8 ± 1.2	27.1 ± 2.2	26.0 ± 2.6***	27.7 ± 1.2	22.4 ± 4.0**
Memory immediate	0.10 ± 1.00	0.08 ± 1.10	− 0.64 ± 1.32	−1.22 ± 1.44***	−0.45 ± 0.91	−2.25 ± 1.06
Memory delayed	0.25 ± 1.01	0.30 ± 1.09	−0.90 ± 1.29	− 1.37 ± 1.41**	−0.96 ± 1.33	− 2.28 ± 1.04
Language	−0.21 ± 1.01	0.01 ± 1.04	−0.65 ± 1.30	−0.88 ± 1.27	−0.76 ± 0.38	−1.95 ± 1.02*
Attention	0.32 ± 1.03	0.26 ± 0.89	−0.74 ± 1.79	−0.81 ± 1.63	0.54 ± 0.52	− 2.03 ± 1.94*
Executive functioning	0.35 ± 1.09	0.12 ± 1.15	− 0.76 ± 1.89	−1.11 ± 1.98*	0.46 ± 0.32	−2.49 ± 2.46*
Visuo-construction	− 0.23 ± 1.36	− 0.19 ± 1.20	0.18 ± 1.46	−0.30 ± 1.66*	−0.59 ± 2.09	−1.30 ± 2.00
APOE ε4 genotype	89 (36)	53 (58)***	27 (19)	160 (66)***	2 (67)	66 (69)
Available markers						
Visual	245 (100)	92 (100)	140 (100)	235 (100)	3 (100)	95 (100)
Subcortical volumes	240 (98)	90 (98)	130 (93)	230 (98)*	2 (67)	89 (94)
Cortical thickness	232 (95)	88 (96)	119 (85)	200 (85)	2 (67)	88 (93)

Data presented as mean ± standard deviation or count (%). Demographic characteristics based on maximum available data (visual rating)
APOE apolipoprotein E, *MMSE* Mini-Mental State Examination
*p < 0.05, **p < 0.01, ***p < 0.001, difference between amyloid positive and negative within diagnostic group

and amygdala volumes, as well as cortical thickness in temporal and parahippocampal regions (Fig. 2).

Combining the informative selected features in the SVM resulted in AUC = 0.81 ± 0.06 in MCI subjects, AUC = 0.74 ± 0.08 in CN subjects and AUC = 0.85 ± 0.05 in the whole sample to classify amyloid positive versus amyloid negative subjects (Fig. 3; Additional file 2: Figure S1). In MCI, the combined classifier including information from all modalities performed statistically significantly better than the classifiers based on demographic information combined with neuropsychology or imaging measures alone. The classifier including demographic variables and *APOE* ε4 genotype did not improve after additionally adding imaging and cognitive variables in MCI. In CN, the combined classifier including information from all modalities (demographics, cognitive, genetics and imaging)

performed statistically significantly better than the classifiers including variables from only a subset of these modalities (Fig. 3; Additional file 2: Figure S2). The results from the SVM including only imaging variables are displayed in Additional file 2: Figure S3.

Table 4 presents the accuracy, sensitivity and specificity of the combined SVM in CN subjects, MCI subjects and the whole sample maximizing the Youden index, and at different levels of sensitivity. When optimizing both specificity and sensitivity, the positive predictive value for amyloid pathology was 0.84 in MCI (a 42% increase compared to the a priori probability (i.e. prevalence) of 0.59) and the negative predictive value was 0.62. In CN, the SVM obtained a positive predictive value of 0.41 (a 64% increase compared to the prevalence of 0.25) and a negative predictive value of 0.84.

Table 2 Visual rating scores according to diagnosis and amyloid status

Score	Cognitively normal		Mild cognitive impairment		Alzheimer-type dementia	
	Amyloid negative	Amyloid positive	Amyloid negative	Amyloid positive	Amyloid negative	Amyloid positive
MTA	0 (0–1)	0 (0–1)	0.5 (0–1)	1 (0.5–1.5)††	1 (0.5–2)	1 (1–2)
GCA	0 (0–1)	0 (0–1)	0 (0–1)	1 (0–1)††	1 (0–2)	1 (1–1)
Parietal	1 (0–1)	0.5 (0–1)	1 (0–1)	1 (0–1.63)†	2 (0–2)	1 (1–2)
Fazekas	1 (0–1)	1 (0–1)	1 (0–1)	1 (1–2)	1 (1–1)	1 (0–2)
Microbleeds present	6 (21%)	4 (20%)	29 (25%)	56 (29%)	1 (50%)	17 (22%)

Data presented as median (interquartile range) or count (%)
APOE apolipoprotein E, *FDR* false discovery rate, *GCA* global cortical atrophy, *MTA* medial temporal lobe atrophy
†p_{FDR} < 0.05, ††p_{FDR} < 0.01, difference between amyloid positive and negative within diagnostic group. Analyses corrected for age, gender, *APOE* ε4 genotype and cohort

Table 3 Quantitative MRI measures according to diagnosis and amyloid status

MRI measure	Cognitively normal		Mild cognitive impairment		Alzheimer-type dementia		F value		
	Amyloid negative	Amyloid positive	Amyloid negative	Amyloid positive	Amyloid negative	Amyloid positive	Diagnosis	Amyloid	Diagnosis × amyloid
Hippocampus left	3837 (39)	3752 (58)	3638 (46)	3353 (47)†††	3051 (340)	3124 (61)	32.0***	0.7	3.5*
Hippocampus right	3960 (53)	3830 (66)$^{#}$	3760 (57)	3389 (57)†††	3905 (337)	3172 (70)$^{#}$	19.7***	12.3***	5.4**
Amygdala left	1501 (36)	1439 (40)$^{#}$	1405 (37)	1294 (37)†††	1604 (171)	1188 (42)$^{#}$	9.2***	11.0**	2.5
Amygdala right	1567 (52)	1535 (55)	1522 (53)	1398 (53)†††	1612 (183)	1290 (57)	4.6**	6.7**	3.2*
Thalamus left	6834 (101)	6614 (119)$^{#}$	6951 (107)	6689 (108)†	6187 (564)	6787 (126)	1.1	0.04	1.1
Thalamus right	6388 (104)	6320 (113)	6419 (106)	6173 (107)†††	5600 (420)	6185 (117)	2.4	0.4	3.2*
Caudate left	3419 (67)	3336 (80)	3571 (71)	3407 (71)†	4151 (393)	3387 (85)	2.9	6.1*	1.7
Caudate right	3491 (88)	3396 (98)	3584 (91)	3463 (91)	4575 (407)	3413 (103)$^{#}$	3.7*	10.7**	3.4*
Putamen left	4831 (105)	4779 (117)	4689 (108)	4609 (109)	4692 (478)	4509 (122)	2.1	0.4	0.1
Putamen right	4627 (121)	4607 (130)	4659 (123)	4461 (124)†	4524 (444)	4302 (134)	0.6	0.9	1.5
Pallidum left	1366 (32)	1412 (37)	1370 (33)	1385 (33)	1488 (168)	1390 (39)	0.3	0.05	0.6
Pallidum right	1388 (26)	1382 (31)	1384 (28)	1379 (28)	1361 (148)	1392 (33)	0.02	0.01	0.03
Accumbens left	465 (23)	432 (24)$^{#}$	434 (23)	411 (23)	526 (79)	375 (25)	2.1	6.7**	1.5
Accumbens right	497 (22)	467 (23)$^{#}$	466 (22)	443 (22)	425 (78)	419 (24)	2.3	4.0*	0.6
Average CT	2.29 (0.02)	2.28 (0.02)	2.27 (0.02)	2.22 (0.02)†††	2.22 (0.07)	2.19 (0.02)	5.3**	1.6	1.5
CT Dickerson	2.54 (0.02)	2.52 (0.02)	2.50 (0.02)	2.45 (0.02)††	2.48 (0.09)	2.38 (0.02)	8.3***	3.5	1.6
CT Jack	2.68 (0.03)	2.63 (0.03)$^{#}$	2.63 (0.03)	2.56 (0.03)†††	2.67 (0.10)	2.47 (0.03)$^{#}$	6.7**	9.3**	1.7

Data presented as estimate (standard error). Estimates derived from linear mixed models including diagnosis × amyloid, age, gender and *APOE* ε4 genotype as covariates and cohort as random effect

APOE apolipoprotein E, *CT* cortical thickness, *FDR* false discovery rate, *MRI* magnetic resonance imaging

$^{†}p_{FDR} < 0.05$, $^{††}p_{FDR} < 0.01$, $^{†††}p_{FDR} < 0.001$, $^{#}p_{uncorrected} < 0.05$, compared to amyloid negative within diagnostic group

*p < 0.05, **p < 0.01, ***p < 0.001 for F statistic of main effect

Discussion

In this study, we found that amyloid pathology is associated with brain atrophy in CN and MCI subjects. Using machine-learning techniques, we built a classifier based on a combination of demographic, cognitive, *APOE* ε4 genotype and MRI data that could predict amyloid status at single subject level with a moderate level of accuracy. The performance of the classifier was higher in MCI subjects than in CN subjects. These results are of interest for clinical trial designers who wish to recruit amyloid positive subjects for inclusion.

Our results on the association between amyloid pathology and MRI measures in MCI are in line with previous studies that also found more cortical and subcortical atrophy in amyloid positive compared to amyloid negative MCI subjects [6, 7]. In CN, amyloid pathology has previously been associated with cortical atrophy [9–11], and lower hippocampal volume in some studies [8, 9], but not in all [11, 38]. To capture cortical changes associated with AD, two different AD-signature meta-ROIs have been proposed in the literature [10, 31]. In MCI, both AD-signature measures were related to amyloid pathology. In CN, only the AD-signature meta-ROI by Jack et al. [31] was associated with amyloid pathology in our study, suggesting that this one is more sensitive in the early disease stage. We also

found an effect of amyloid pathology on nucleus accumbens volume, which was most pronounced in CN subjects. Although nucleus accumbens volumes are not often measured in AD-related studies, it has been hypothesized that this structure could show secondary neurodegeneration in AD in response to reduced input from connections to medial-temporal lobe structures [39]. It should be noted, however, that the nucleus accumbens is a small structure, which is difficult to segment automatically. These results require further validation in future studies.

The optimal features selected in the SVM by the tree-based approach included some, but not all, of the variables that showed differences between amyloid positive and amyloid negative subjects in the univariate analyses. Similarly, some of the features selected did not show statistically significant univariate group differences, although for many a trend towards lower values in amyloid positive subjects compared to amyloid negative subjects was observed. By combining the selected features derived from demographic information, neuropsychological examination, MRI measures and *APOE* ε4 genotype, we were able to classify MCI and CN subjects as amyloid positive or negative with a moderate level of accuracy.

The AUC for prediction of amyloid pathology was slightly higher in the MCI group compared to the CN

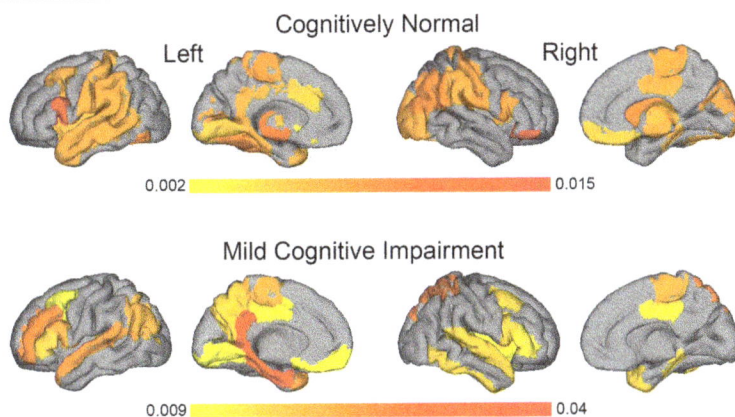

Fig. 2 Freesurfer regions selected as features for the classifier in cognitively normal (top row) and mild cognitive impairment (bottom row). Colour bars represent averaged feature weight

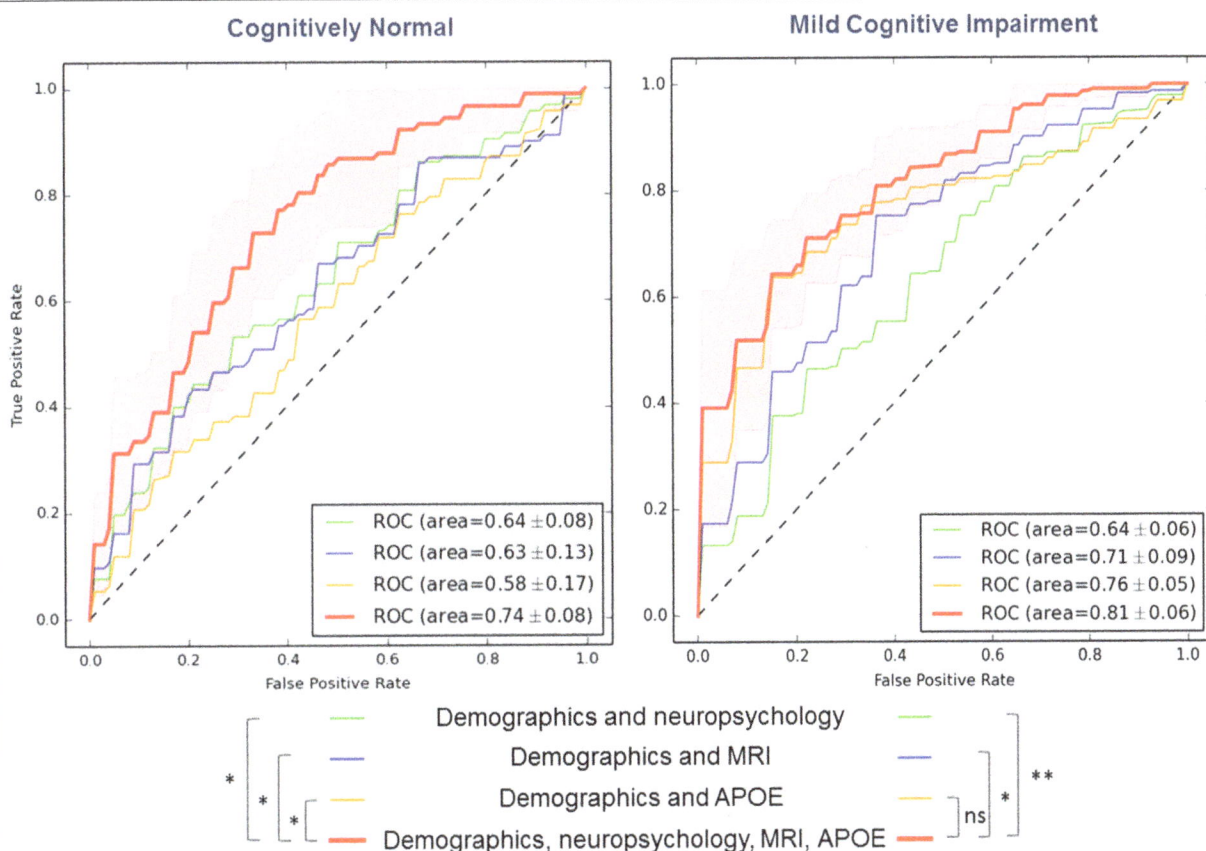

Fig. 3 Classifier results. Receiver operating characteristic (ROC) curves of support vector machine classifier to predict amyloid pathology in cognitively normal (left panel) and mild cognitive impairment (right panel) subjects. Red: results from the combined classifier, including demographic information, neuropsychological tests, MRI measures and *APOE* ε4 genotype. Specific features selected presented in Additional file 1: Table S8. Classifier results from demographic information combined with only neuropsychology (green), or MRI measures (blue) or *APOE* ε4 genotype (yellow). ROC significant differences assessed with DeLong's test. *p < 0.05, **p < 0.001, ns not significant. *APOE*, apolipoprotein E, MRI magnetic resonance imaging

Table 4 Sensitivity, specificity, accuracy, PPV and NPV of the SVM classifier

Group	Sensitivity	Specificity	Accuracy	PPV	NPV	Threshold SVM
Optimized sensitivity and specificity						
Cognitively normal	0.61	0.71	0.68	0.41	0.84	0.70
Mild cognitive impairment	0.71	0.77	0.74	0.84	0.62	0.33
Whole sample	0.75	0.79	0.77	0.80	0.74	0.48
80% sensitivity						
Cognitively normal	0.80	0.55	0.62	0.41	0.88	0.77
Mild cognitive impairment	0.80	0.64	0.74	0.79	0.66	0.47
Whole sample	0.80	0.69	0.75	0.74	0.76	0.56
85% sensitivity						
Cognitively normal	0.85	0.46	0.57	0.38	0.89	0.80
Mild cognitive impairment	0.85	0.54	0.73	0.75	0.68	0.53
Whole sample	0.85	0.59	0.73	0.69	0.78	0.64
90% sensitivity						
Cognitively normal	0.90	0.36	0.51	0.35	0.91	0.84
Mild cognitive impairment	0.90	0.46	0.73	0.73	0.74	0.60
Whole sample	0.90	0.51	0.71	0.67	0.83	0.70
95% sensitivity						
Cognitively normal	0.95	0.24	0.44	0.32	0.92	0.87
Mild cognitive impairment	0.95	0.37	0.73	0.71	0.83	0.70
Whole sample	0.95	0.40	0.69	0.63	0.88	0.79
100% sensitivity						
Cognitively normal	1.00	0.11	0.36	0.30	1.00	0.91
Mild cognitive impairment	1.00	0.08	0.66	0.64	1.00	0.87
Whole sample	1.00	0.04	0.54	0.53	1.00	0.95

Results from combined classifier, including demographic information, neuropsychological tests, MRI measures and *APOE* ε4 genotype. Specific features selected presented in Additional file 1: Table S8. Values averaged across 10-fold cross-validation. Youden's *J* statistic employed

APOE apolipoprotein E, *MRI* magnetic resonance imaging, *NPV* negative predictive value, *PPV* positive predictive value, *SVM* support vector machine

group, and in line with a previous study in MCI [40]. In that study, a SVM classifier to predict amyloid pathology in subjects with MCI was also developed. Using cognitive data, hippocampal volume, *APOE* ε4 genotype and peripheral blood protein markers from the Alzheimer's Disease Neuroimaging Initiative (ADNI) dataset, they obtained AUC = 0.80 for predicting amyloid pathology in subjects with MCI. In contrast to a previous study [12], we did not find that combining MRI markers with *APOE* ε4 genotype improved prediction of amyloid pathology in MCI over only including *APOE* ε4.

Our results in CN are comparable to the result from a similar study using data from the ADNI and a monocentric cohort [41]. In that study, a machine-learning-based classifier including demographic variables, *APOE* ε4 genotype, cognitive testing and structural MRI data reached an AUC of around 0.6 in CN subjects to predict amyloid positivity. Other studies have used combinations of demographic information, *APOE* ε4 genotype and cognitive testing (without imaging measures) to predict amyloid positivity in CN

[42, 43]. They obtained positive predictive values of 0.65 and 0.63 for amyloid positivity, which was a 43–59% increase compared to the baseline prevalence in the cohort (0.41 and 0.44 respectively). In comparison, in our study we obtained a positive predictive value of 0.41 for amyloid pathology in CN, with a baseline prevalence of 0.25 in our cohort, which is a 64% increase in predictive value. To recruit 1000 CN subjects with amyloid pathology, using the classifier could reduce the number of subjects needing to undergo amyloid assessment from 3925 to 2439, which is a 38% decrease. Assuming a cost of €850 for the pre-screening (including MRI, *APOE* genotyping and cognitive testing) and €3500 for an amyloid PET scan, using the classifier for pre-screening could reduce the total screening costs by nearly €2 million in this CN population. This example is based on an optimized sum of sensitivity and specificity (Youden index). For clinical trial design, it might be more interesting to optimize the sensitivity of the classifier, which would minimize the proportion of falsely excluded amyloid positive subjects, at the cost of the positive predictive value.

As can be seen in Table 4, with increasing sensitivity (and higher negative predictive value), the positive predictive value of the classifier becomes lower, which would lead to increasing costs of pre-screening.

We chose SVM as a classification method for several reasons. First, it is based on a robust strategy (i.e. maximum-margin hyper-plane), which is considered to be one of the best to reduce the prediction error in a classification task [44, 45]. Second, only few parameters need to be tuned in order to make it fully operational, making SVM relatively easy to set up and use. Finally, it is particularly well suited for the separation of two classes (in this case, amyloid positive and amyloid negative).

A strength of our study is that, unlike previous studies [40–42], we performed our study in a heterogeneous cohort, in which data acquisition protocols were not standardized and different MR scanners and acquisition parameters were used. In this heterogeneous cohort, we showed a similar predictive accuracy compared to prospective research cohorts, which used standardized data acquisition protocols. This highlights the robustness of our approach and suggests that the results may also be generalizable to other cohorts. This will need to be tested in future studies. Our results may be of interest for studies recruiting subjects from parent cohorts to be included in (secondary) prevention studies targeting anti-amyloid therapeutics [4]. Our findings suggest that for individuals with MCI, screening for amyloid positivity can best be done by age and *APOE* ε4 genotype, with limited added value of MRI. In CN, MRI measures have an added value above the other markers.

This study has some limitations. First, we used data acquired at various centres, which had different inclusion criteria for subjects and used different protocols for data collection. However, as already discussed, this also increased generalizability. Second, not everyone had the same measure of amyloid pathology. When possible, we used centralized analysis of the CSF Aβ$_{42/40}$ ratio to identify amyloid positivity, which has been shown to correlate highly with PET measures of amyloid pathology [46, 47]. For data from one cohort, we only had amyloid PET data available. Although CSF and PET measures are usually in good agreement, some studies have suggested that CSF values might become abnormal earlier than PET [48, 49]. Finally, the same dataset was used to train and test the SVM classifier. Although nested *k*-fold cross-validation grants good generalizability of the SVM model [36], studies in independent datasets are needed to further validate our results.

Conclusions

Amyloid pathology is associated with structural MRI changes in AD typical regions in CN subjects and in subjects with MCI. We developed a classifier that can predict amyloid pathology at a single subject level using a combination of easily obtainable, non-invasive measures. Our results are of interest for trial designers who intend to recruit a large number of amyloid positive subjects. Implementing pre-screening procedures consisting of simple, non-invasive tests could substantially reduce screening failure rates. In future studies, the classifier might be improved by adding data from other minimally invasive tests, such as blood proteins and genetic markers [40]. In the EMIF-AD MBD study, plasma proteomics and metabolomics, and genomics and epigenomics, will also be analysed.

Abbreviations

AD: Alzheimer's disease; *APOE*: Apolipoprotein E; CN: Cognitively normal; CSF: Cerebrospinal fluid; EMIF-AD MBD: European Medical Information Framework for Alzheimer's Disease Multimodal Biomarker Discovery; GCA: Global cortical atrophy visual rating; MCI: Mild cognitive impairment; MMSE: Mini-Mental State Examination; MRI: Magnetic resonance imaging; MTA: Medial temporal lobe atrophy visual rating; PET: Positron emission tomography; SVM: Support vector machine; TIV: Total intracranial volume

Acknowledgements

The authors acknowledge the contribution of the personnel of the Genomic Service Facility at the VIB-U Antwerp Center for Molecular Neurology.

Funding

The present study was conducted as part of the EMIF-AD project which has received support from the Innovative Medicines Initiative Joint Undertaking under EMIF grant agreement n° 115372, resources of which are composed of a financial contribution from the European Union's Seventh Framework Programme (FP7/2007–2013) and an EFPIA companies' in-kind contribution. The DESCRIPA study was funded by the European Commission within the Fifth Framework Programme (QLRT-2001-2455). The EDAR study was funded by the European Commission within the Fifth Framework Programme (contract # 37670). The VUmc Alzheimer Center is supported by Stichting Alzheimer Nederland and Stichting VUmc fonds, and the clinical database structure was developed with funding from Stichting Dioraphte. The Leuven cohort was funded by the Stichting voor Alzheimer Onderzoek (grant numbers #11020, #13007 and #15005). The GAP study is supported by grants from the Department of Economic Promotion, Rural Areas and Territorial Balance of the Provincial Government of Gipuzkoa (124/16), the Department of Health of the Basque Government (2016111096), the Carlos III Institute of Health (PI15/00919, PN de I + D + I 2013–2016), Obra Social Kutxa-Fundazioa and anonymous private donors. The Gothenburg MCI study was supported by the Sahlgrenska University Hospital, Gothenburg, Sweden. The Lausanne cohort study was supported by a grant from the Swiss National Research Foundation to JP (SNF 320030_141179). The research at VIB-CMN is funded in part by the University of Antwerp Research Fund. RV is a senior clinical investigator of the Flemish Research Foundation (FWO). CVB is partly supported by the Flemish government-initiated Flanders Impulse Program on Networks for Dementia Research (VIND) and the Methusalem Excellence Program, the Research Foundation Flanders (FWO) and the University of Antwerp Research Fund, Belgium. FB is supported by the NIHR UCLH Biomedical Research Centre. HZ is supported by the Dementia Research Institute at UCL and is a Wallenberg Academy Fellow. SJV receives research support from ZonMw. VW has received funding from the European Union's Horizon 2020 Research and Innovation Programme under grant agreement no. 666992.

Authors' contributions

MtK and AR provided data analyses, statistical analysis and data interpretation, and wrote the manuscript. EP provided data analyses. IB and SJV provided data management. RV, SG, JS, PS OB, JCR, RB, AW, CE, JLM, SE, CVB, PM-L, JP, MT and FRJV provided data and sample collection. ALB was responsible for plasma proteomics in EMIF-AD MBD. CL-Q was responsible for plasma metabolomics in EMIF-AD MBD. LB was responsible for genetic analyses in EMIF-AD MBD. VD was responsible for APOE analyses in EMIF-AD MBD. HZ was responsible for CSF analysis in EMIF-AD MBD. SL and JS provided study design and study coordination. SB provided data analyses. GPN is a member of the EMIF-AD MBD imaging workgroup and provided data interpretation. JR provided MRI data management. MFG and ZX are members of the EMIF-AD MBD imaging workgroup and provided data interpretation. VW provided critical revision of the manuscript. GF provided data and sample collection, and supervision of the project. PJV provided study design, study coordination and supervision of the project, and is a member of the EMIF-AD MBD imaging workgroup. FB provided study design, study coordination and supervision of the project, and is head of the EMIF-AD MBD imaging workgroup. All authors revised the manuscript and approved the final version.

Consent for publication

Not applicable.

Competing interests

The authors declare that they have no competing interests. HZ has served on scientific advisory boards of Eli Lilly and Roche Diagnostics, has received travel support from Teva and is a co-founder of Brain Biomarker Solutions in Gothenburg AB, a GU Ventures-based platform company at the University of Gothenburg. MFG's current employer is Teva Pharmaceuticals, Inc., Malvern, PA, USA; his former employer was Boehringer Ingelheim Pharmaceuticals, Inc., Ridgefield, CT, USA. Any views expressed in this publication represent the personal opinions of the authors and not those of their respective employer. JCR is a full-time employee of GlaxoSmithkline. PM-L reports personal fees from Lilly, Axon, General Electric and Nutricia for advisory boards, and lecturing fees from Lilly, Nutricia, Piramal. RV was principal investigator of the phase 1 and 2 [18F]flutemetamol trials. RV's institution has clinical trial agreements (RV as PI) with AbbVie, Biogen, EliLilly, Merck and Novartis, and consultancy agreements (RV as PI) with Novartis and Cytox Ltd. SL has done consultancy for Eaisi, EIP Pharma, SomaLogic, Merck and Optum Labs.

Author details

[1]Alzheimer Center & Department of Neurology, VU University Medical Center, PO Box 7057, 1007 MB Amsterdam, the Netherlands. [2]Laboratory of Epidemiology & Neuroimaging, IRCCS San Giovanni di Dio Fatebenefratelli, Brescia, Italy. [3]Alzheimer Centrum Limburg, Department of Psychiatry and Neuropsychology, Maastricht University, Maastricht, the Netherlands. [4]University Hospital Leuven, Leuven, Belgium. [5]Laboratory for Cognitive Neurology, Department of Neurosciences, KU Leuven, Leuven, Belgium. [6]AP-HM, CHU Timone, CIC CPCET, Service de Pharmacologie Clinique et Pharmacovigilance, Marseille, France. [7]Neurosciences Therapeutic Area Unit, GlaxoSmithKline R&D, Stevenage, UK. [8]U1171 Inserm, CHU Lille, Degenerative and Vascular Cognitive Disorders, University of Lille, Lille, France. [9]Sahlgrenska Academy, Institute of Neuroscience and Physiology, Section for Psychiatry and Neurochemistry, University of Gothenburg, Gothenburg, Sweden. [10]Barcelona βeta Brain Research Center, Pasqual Maragall Foundation, Barcelona, Spain. [11]Reference Center for Biological Markers of Dementia (BIODEM), Institute Born-Bunge, University of Antwerp, Antwerp, Belgium. [12]Department of Neurology and Memory Clinic, Hospital Network Antwerp (ZNA) Middelheim and Hoge Beuken, Antwerp, Belgium. [13]Neurodegenerative Brain Diseases, Center for Molecular Neurology, VIB, Antwerp, Belgium. [14]Laboratory of Neurogenetics, Institute Born-Bunge, University of Antwerp, Antwerp, Belgium. [15]Department of Neurology, Center for Research and Advanced Therapies, CITA-Alzheimer Foundation, San Sebastian, Spain. [16]Department of Psychiatry, University Hospital of Lausanne, Lausanne, Switzerland. [17]Geriatric Psychiatry, Department of Mental Health and Psychiatry, Geneva University Hospitals, Geneva, Switzerland. [18]Memory and Dementia Center, 3rd Department of Neurology, "G Papanicolau" General Hospital, Aristotle University of Thessaloniki, Thessaloniki, Greece. [19]University of Oxford, Oxford, UK. [20]King's College London, London, UK. [21]Lübeck Interdisciplinary Platform for Genome Analytics, University of Lübeck, Lubeck, Germany. [22]School of Public Health, Imperial College London, London, UK. [23]Department of Psychology, University of Oslo, Oslo, Norway. [24]Department of Psychiatry and Neurochemistry, University of Gothenburg, Mölndal, Sweden. [25]Department of Molecular Neuroscience, UCL Institute of Neurology, Queen Square, London, UK. [26]UK Dementia Research Institute at UCL, London, UK. [27]Clinical Neurochemistry Laboratory, Sahlgrenska University Hospital, Mölndal, Sweden. [28]UCB Biopharma SPRL, Braine-l'Alleud, Belgium. [29]Janssen Pharmaceutical Research and Development, Titusville, NJ, USA. [30]MAAT, Archamps, France. [31]Teva Pharmaceuticals, Inc., Malvern, PA, USA. [32]Boehringer Ingelheim Pharmaceuticals, Inc., Ridgefield, CT, USA. [33]Worldwide Research and Development, Pfizer Inc, Cambridge, MA, USA. [34]Department of Radiology and Nuclear Medicine, VUMC, Amsterdam, the Netherlands. [35]University of Geneva, Geneva, Switzerland. [36]Institutes of Neurology and Healthcare Engineering, UCL, London, UK.

References

1. Scheltens P, Blennow K, Breteler MMB, de Strooper B, Frisoni GB, Salloway S, et al. Alzheimer's disease. Lancet. 2016;388:505–17.
2. Reiman EM, Langbaum JBS, Fleisher AS, Caselli RJ, Chen K, Ayutyanont N, et al. Alzheimer's Prevention Initiative: a plan to accelerate the evaluation of presymptomatic treatments. J Alzheimers Dis. 2011;26(Suppl 3):321–9.
3. Sperling RA, Rentz DM, Johnson KA, Karlawish J, Donohue M, Salmon DP, et al. The A4 study: stopping AD before symptoms begin? Sci Transl Med. 2014;6:228fs13.
4. Ritchie CW, Molinuevo JL, Truyen L, Satlin A, Van der Geyten S, Lovestone S, et al. Development of interventions for the secondary prevention of Alzheimer's dementia: the European Prevention of Alzheimer's Dementia (EPAD) project. Lancet Psychiatry. 2016;3:179–86.
5. Jansen WJ, Ossenkoppele R, Knol DL, Tijms BM, Scheltens P, Verhey FRJ, et al. Prevalence of cerebral amyloid pathology in persons without dementia: a meta-analysis. JAMA. 2015;313:1924–38.
6. Ten Kate M, Barkhof F, Visser PJ, Teunissen CE, Scheltens P, van der Flier WM, et al. Amyloid-independent atrophy patterns predict time to progression to dementia in mild cognitive impairment. Alzheimers Res Ther. 2017;9:73.
7. Huijbers W, Mormino EC, Schultz AP, Wigman S, Ward AM, Larvie M, et al. Amyloid-β deposition in mild cognitive impairment is associated with increased hippocampal activity, atrophy and clinical progression. Brain. 2015;138:1023–35.
8. Hedden T, Dijk KRAV, Becker JA, Mehta A, Sperling RA, Johnson KA, et al. Disruption of functional connectivity in clinically normal older adults harboring amyloid burden. J Neurosci. 2009;29:12686–94.
9. Storandt M, Mintun M, Head D, Morris J. Cognitive decline and brain volume loss as signatures of cerebral amyloid-β peptide deposition identified with Pittsburgh compound b: cognitive decline associated with Aβ deposition. Arch Neurol. 2009;66:1476–81.
10. Dickerson BC, Bakkour A, Salat DH, Feczko E, Pacheco J, Greve DN, et al. The cortical signature of Alzheimer's disease: regionally specific cortical thinning relates to symptom severity in very mild to mild AD dementia and is detectable in asymptomatic amyloid-positive individuals. Cereb Cortex. 2009;19:497–510.
11. Becker JA, Hedden T, Carmasin J, Maye J, Rentz DM, Putcha D, et al. Amyloid-β associated cortical thinning in clinically normal elderly. Ann Neurol. 2011;69:1032–42.
12. Tosun D, Joshi S, Weiner MW. Alzheimer's Disease Neuroimaging Initiative. Neuroimaging predictors of brain amyloidosis in mild cognitive impairment. Ann Neurol. 2013;74:188–98.

13. Bos I, Vos S, Vandenberghe R, Scheltens P, Engelborghs S, Frisoni G, et al. The EMIF-AD Multimodal Biomarker Discovery study: design, methods and cohort characteristics. Alzheimers Res Ther. 2018;10:64.

14. Visser PJ, Verhey FRJ, Boada M, Bullock R, Deyn PPD, Frisoni GB, et al. Development of screening guidelines and clinical criteria for predementia Alzheimer's disease. NED. 2008;30:254–65.

15. Reijs BLR, Ramakers IHGB, Köhler S, Teunissen CE, Koel-Simmelink M, Nathan PJ, et al. Memory correlates of Alzheimer's disease cerebrospinal fluid markers: a longitudinal cohort study. J Alzheimers Dis. 2017;60:1119–28.

16. Galluzzi S, Marizzoni M, Babiloni C, Albani D, Antelmi L, Bagnoli C, et al. Clinical and biomarker profiling of prodromal Alzheimer's disease in workpackage 5 of the Innovative Medicines Initiative PharmaCog project: a 'European ADNI study'. J Intern Med. 2016;279:576–91.

17. van der Flier WM, Pijnenburg YAL, Prins N, Lemstra AW, Bouwman FH, Teunissen CE, et al. Optimizing patient care and research: the Amsterdam Dementia Cohort. J Alzheimers Dis. 2014;41:313–27.

18. Ten Kate M, Sanz-Arigita EJ, Tijms BM, Wink AM, Clerigue M, Garcia-Sebastian M, et al. Impact of APOE-ε4 and family history of dementia on gray matter atrophy in cognitively healthy middle-aged adults. Neurobiol Aging. 2016;38:14–20.

19. Somers C, Struyfs H, Goossens J, Niemantsverdriet E, Luyckx J, De Roeck N, et al. A decade of cerebrospinal fluid biomarkers for Alzheimer's disease in Belgium. J Alzheimers Dis. 2016;54:383–95.

20. Adamczuk K, De Weer A-S, Nelissen N, Dupont P, Sunaert S, Bettens K, et al. Functional changes in the language network in response to increased amyloid β deposition in cognitively intact older adults. Cereb Cortex. 2017; 27:3879.

21. Oikonomidi A, Tautvydaitė D, Gholamrezaee MM, Henry H, Bacher M, Popp J. Macrophage migration inhibitory factor is associated with biomarkers of Alzheimer's disease pathology and predicts cognitive decline in mild cognitive impairment and mild dementia. J Alzheimers Dis. 2017;60:273–81.

22. Wallin A, Nordlund A, Jonsson M, Lind K, Edman Å, Göthlin M, et al. The Gothenburg MCI study: design and distribution of Alzheimer's disease and subcortical vascular disease diagnoses from baseline to 6-year follow-up. J Cereb Blood Flow Metab. 2016;36:114–31.

23. Fortea J, Sala-Llonch R, Bartrés-Faz D, Bosch B, Lladó A, Bargalló N, et al. Increased cortical thickness and caudate volume precede atrophy in PSEN1 mutation carriers. J Alzheimers Dis. 2010;22:909–22.

24. Adamczuk K, Schaeverbeke J, Nelissen N, Neyens V, Vandenbulcke M, Goffin K, et al. Amyloid imaging in cognitively normal older adults: comparison between (18)F-flutemetamol and (11)C-Pittsburgh compound B. Eur J Nucl Med Mol Imaging. 2016;43:142–51.

25. Vandenberghe R, Van Laere K, Ivanoiu A, Salmon E, Bastin C, Triau E, et al. 18F-flutemetamol amyloid imaging in Alzheimer disease and mild cognitive impairment: a phase 2 trial. Ann Neurol. 2010;68:319–29.

26. Scheltens P, Leys D, Barkhof F, Huglo D, Weinstein HC, Vermersch P, et al. Atrophy of medial temporal lobes on MRI in "probable" Alzheimer's disease and normal ageing: diagnostic value and neuropsychological correlates. J Neurol Neurosurg Psychiatry. 1992;55:967–72.

27. Pasquier F, Leys D, Weerts JG, Mounier-Vehier F, Barkhof F, Scheltens P. Inter- and intraobserver reproducibility of cerebral atrophy assessment on MRI scans with hemispheric infarcts. Eur Neurol. 1996;36:268–72.

28. Koedam ELGE, Lehmann M, van der Flier WM, Scheltens P, YAL P, Fox N, et al. Visual assessment of posterior atrophy development of a MRI rating scale. Eur Radiol. 2011;21:2618–25.

29. Fazekas F, Chawluk JB, Alavi A, Hurtig HI, Zimmerman RA. MR signal abnormalities at 1.5 T in Alzheimer's dementia and normal aging. Am J Neuroradiol. 1987;8:421–6.

30. Fischl B. FreeSurfer. Neuroimage. 2012;62:774–81.

31. Jack CR, Wiste HJ, Weigand SD, Therneau TM, Lowe VJ, Knopman DS, et al. Defining imaging biomarker cut points for brain aging and Alzheimer's disease. Alzheimers Dement. 2017;13:205–16.

32. Orrù G, Petterson-Yeo W, Marquand AF, Sartori G, Mechelli A. Using support vector machine to identify imaging biomarkers of neurological and psychiatric disease: a critical review. Neurosci Biobehav Rev. 2012;36:1140–52.

33. Chang C-C, Lin C-J. LIBSVM: A Library for Support Vector Machines. ACM Trans Intell Syst Technol. 2011;2:27 1–27:27.

34. Pedregosa F, Varoquaux G, Gramfort A, Michel V, Thirion B, Grisel O, et al. Scikit-learn: Machine Learning in Python. J Mach Learn Res. 2011;12:2825–30.

35. Ambroise C, McLachlan GJ. Selection bias in gene extraction on the basis of microarray gene-expression data. Proc Natl Acad Sci U S A. 2002;99:6562–6.

36. Cawley GC, Talbot NLC. On over-fitting in model selection and subsequent selection bias in performance evaluation. J Mach Learn Res. 2010;11:2079–107.

37. Cutler A, Cutler DR, Stevens JR. Random Forests. In: Zhang C, Ma Y, editors. Ensemble Machine Learning: Methods and Applications [Internet]. Boston: Springer US; 2012. p. 157–75. Available from: https://doi.org/10.1007/978-1-4419-9326-7_5.

38. Mattsson N, Insel PS, Nosheny R, Tosun D, Trojanowski JQ, Shaw LM, et al. Emerging β-amyloid pathology and accelerated cortical atrophy. JAMA Neurol. 2014;71:725–34.

39. Pievani M, Bocchetta M, Boccardi M, Cavedo E, Bonetti M, Thompson PM, et al. Striatal morphology in early-onset and late-onset Alzheimer's disease: a preliminary study. Neurobiol Aging. 2013;34:1728–39.

40. Apostolova LG, Hwang KS, Avila D, Elashoff D, Kohannim O, Teng E, et al. Brain amyloidosis ascertainment from cognitive, imaging, and peripheral blood protein measures. Neurology. 2015;84:729–37.

41. Ansart M, Epelbaum S, Gagliardi G, Colliot O, Dormont D, Dubois B, et al. Prediction of Amyloidosis from Neuropsychological and MRI Data for Cost Effective Inclusion of Pre-symptomatic Subjects in Clinical Trials. Deep Learning in Medical Image Analysis and Multimodal Learning for Clinical Decision Support [Internet]. Cham: Springer; 2017. p. 357–64. [cited 2018 Jan 11] Available from: https://link.springer.com/chapter/10.1007/978-3-319-67558-9_41

42. Insel PS, Palmqvist S, Mackin RS, Nosheny RL, Hansson O, Weiner MW, et al. Assessing risk for preclinical β-amyloid pathology with APOE, cognitive, and demographic information. Alzheimers Dement. 2016;4:76–84.

43. Mielke MM, Wiste HJ, Weigand SD, Knopman DS, Lowe VJ, Roberts RO, et al. Indicators of amyloid burden in a population-based study of cognitively normal elderly. Neurology. 2012;79:1570–7.

44. Burges CJC. A tutorial on support vector machines for pattern recognition. Data Min Knowl Disc. 1998;2:121–67.

45. Kounelakis M, Zervakis M, Kotsiakis X. Chapter 13—the impact of microarray technology in brain cancer. In: AFG T, Fisher AC, editors. Outcome Prediction in Cancer [Internet]. Amsterdam: Elsevier; 2007. p. 339–88. [cited 2018 Aug 1] Available from: http://www.sciencedirect.com/science/article/pii/B9780444528551500155.

46. Janelidze S, Pannee J, Mikulskis A, Chiao P, Zetterberg H, Blennow K, et al. Concordance between different amyloid immunoassays and visual amyloid positron emission tomographic assessment. JAMA Neurol. 2017;74:1492–501.

47. Lewczuk P, Matzen A, Blennow K, Parnetti L, Molinuevo JL, Eusebi P, et al. Cerebrospinal fluid Aβ42/40 corresponds better than Aβ42 to amyloid PET in Alzheimer's disease. J Alzheimers Dis. 2017;55:813–22.

48. Mattsson N, Insel PS, Donohue M, Landau S, Jagust WJ, Shaw LM, et al. Independent information from cerebrospinal fluid amyloid-β and florbetapir imaging in Alzheimer's disease. Brain. 2015;138:772–83.

49. Palmqvist S, Mattsson N, Hansson O. Alzheimer's Disease Neuroimaging Initiative. Cerebrospinal fluid analysis detects cerebral amyloid-β accumulation earlier than positron emission tomography. Brain. 2016;139: 1226–36.

Single-word comprehension deficits in the nonfluent variant of primary progressive aphasia

Jolien Schaeverbeke[1,2] ⓘ, Silvy Gabel[1,2], Karen Meersmans[1], Rose Bruffaerts[1,2,3], Antonietta Gabriella Liuzzi[1], Charlotte Evenepoel[1,2], Eva Dries[3], Karen Van Bouwel[3], Anne Sieben[4,5,6], Yolande Pijnenburg[7,8], Ronald Peeters[9], Guy Bormans[10,11], Koen Van Laere[2,11], Michel Koole[11], Patrick Dupont[1,2] and Rik Vandenberghe[1,2,3*]

Abstract

Background: A subset of patients with the nonfluent variant of primary progressive aphasia (PPA) exhibit concomitant single-word comprehension problems, constituting a 'mixed variant' phenotype. This phenotype is rare and currently not fully characterized. The aim of this study was twofold: to assess the prevalence and nature of single-word comprehension problems in the nonfluent variant and to study multimodal imaging characteristics of atrophy, tau, and amyloid burden associated with this mixed phenotype.

Methods: A consecutive memory-clinic recruited series of 20 PPA patients (12 nonfluent, five semantic, and three logopenic variants) were studied on neurolinguistic and neuropsychological domains relative to 64 cognitively intact healthy older control subjects. The neuroimaging battery included high-resolution volumetric magnetic resonance imaging processed with voxel-based morphometry, and positron emission tomography with the tau-tracer [^{18}F]-THK5351 and amyloid-tracer [^{11}C]-Pittsburgh Compound B.

Results: Seven out of 12 subjects who had been classified a priori with nonfluent variant PPA showed deficits on conventional single-word comprehension tasks along with speech apraxia and agrammatism, corresponding to a mixed variant phenotype. These mixed variant cases included three females and four males, with a mean age at onset of 65 years (range 44–77 years). Object knowledge and object recognition were additionally affected, although less severely compared with the semantic variant. The mixed variant was characterized by a distributed atrophy pattern in frontal and temporoparietal regions. A more focal pattern of elevated [^{18}F]-THK5351 binding was present in the supplementary motor area, the left premotor cortex, midbrain, and basal ganglia. This pattern was closely similar to that seen in pure nonfluent variant PPA. At the individual patient level, elevated [^{18}F]-THK5351 binding in the supplementary motor area and premotor cortex was present in six out of seven mixed variant cases and in five and four of these cases, respectively, in the thalamus and midbrain. Amyloid biomarker positivity was present in two out of seven mixed variant cases, compared with none of the five pure nonfluent cases.

Conclusions: A substantial proportion of PPA patients with speech apraxia and agrammatism also have single-word comprehension deficits. At the neurobiological level, the mixed variant shows a high degree of similarity with the pure nonfluent variant of PPA.

(Continued on next page)

---

* Correspondence: rik.vandenberghe@uzleuven.be;
rik.vandenberghe@uz.kuleuven.ac.be
[1]Laboratory for Cognitive Neurology, Department of Neurosciences, KU Leuven, Herestraat 49, 3000 Leuven, Belgium
[2]Alzheimer Research Centre KU Leuven, Leuven Research Institute for Neuroscience & Disease, KU Leuven, Herestraat 49, 3000 Leuven, Belgium
Full list of author information is available at the end of the article

(Continued from previous page)

Keywords: [^{18}F]-THK5351, Mixed variant, Primary progressive aphasia, Frontotemporal dementia, Alzheimer's disease, Tau, Positron emission tomography, Semantic, Amyloid

Background

Primary progressive aphasia (PPA) is a neurodegenerative syndrome characterized by an isolated language impairment with relative sparing of other cognitive domains [1]. Current consensus recommendations describe clinical criteria for three subtypes: a nonfluent/agrammatic variant (NFV), a semantic variant (SV), and a logopenic variant (LV) [1]. NFV PPA patients present with speech apraxia and/or agrammatism [1, 2], whereas SV PPA patients have single-word comprehension deficits and/or object recognition problems [1, 3, 4]. LV PPA patients experience word retrieval difficulties in spontaneous speech and are deficient on repetition tasks that have a high short-term phonological memory load [5, 6]. Even with the most careful clinical phenotyping, the link between the clinical phenotype and the underlying neuropathology remains probabilistic: 43–83% of NFV have underlying frontotemporal lobar degeneration (FTLD) tauopathy [7, 8] and 67%–88% of SV cases have FTLD transactive response DNA binding protein 43 kDa (TDP-43) type C pathology [7, 8]. Of the LV cases, 56–100% show underlying Alzheimer's disease pathology [7–10].

The clinical diagnosis of NFV PPA is based on the presence of two core clinical features, namely speech apraxia and/or agrammatism, and at least two of the following three features: impaired comprehension of syntactically complex sentences indicative of agrammatism; spared single-word comprehension; or spared object knowledge [1]. Cases who have purely speech apraxia without clear agrammatism are sometimes classified as primary progressive apraxia of speech [11, 12], a disorder which has been set apart from PPA [12–14]. The phenotype of NFV PPA has been associated with loss of structural integrity of the dorsal language stream [15], implicated in speech production and grammatical processes [16, 17], while ventral language stream functions [18], such as single-word comprehension and object knowledge, remain relatively intact. However, a subset of NFV cases exhibit single-word comprehension deficits in addition to motor speech problems and/or agrammatism [7, 19, 20]. This has been proposed to constitute a fourth, 'mixed' variant (MV) of PPA [7, 19–21]. This variant is not formally recognized in the current diagnostic classification of PPA [1]. The current classification guidelines might be reconsidered since some studies report that 16–41% of PPA patients remain unclassified as they fit criteria for more than one PPA variant [20, 22–26]. Moreover, data-driven mathematical analyses of neurolinguistic and neuropsychological data of PPA patients confirm the existence of a separate, mixed variant [26]. Inclusion of a mixed phenotype into the list of variants raises the comprehensiveness of the classification from 80% to nearly 90% of PPA cases [20]. The mixed phenotype can emerge as a distinct clinical form in mild or early disease and is not merely due to a more advanced disease stage [20]. To date, limited neuroimaging data in small case series of MV PPA indicate left frontotemporal atrophy on structural magnetic resonance imaging (MRI) [20, 27]. In vivo amyloid positron emission tomography (PET) imaging in four MV cases showed amyloid-positivity in three out of four cases [10]. However, the distribution pattern of the other Alzheimer's disease hallmark protein, i.e., tau, remains to be investigated on tau-PET. At pathological examination, in a series of six MV cases, four had underlying Alzheimer's disease pathology [7] and, in another series, three out of four had FTLD tauopathy [27].

The presence of single-word comprehension problems together with speech apraxia or agrammatism is intriguing. Word comprehension relies on a distributed network [28]. The underlying mechanism and anatomical basis of the single-word comprehension problems may differ between PPA subtypes. In SV, word comprehension deficits have been related to damage to the anterior temporal cortex [29], while in LV the occurrence of word comprehension problems may be due to extension of damage into the posterior third of the superior temporal sulcus and into the middle temporal gyrus [30, 31]. Neuropsychological evidence of a role of inferior frontal and premotor cortex, the regions most prominently affected in NFV, in word comprehension is relatively scarce [32]. Functional imaging studies, however, in healthy subjects have revealed consistent evidence for the contribution of the pars triangularis [33], the inferior frontal sulcus, and the anterior inferior frontal gyrus [34] to the processing of word meaning. The left pars triangularis codes for the representation of the meaning of written and auditory words [33]. The dorsal part of the pars triangularis has also been implicated in semantic working memory [35], semantic selection [36], and semantic control [37]. Disintegration of the inferior frontal cortex in NFV may also alter predictive coding during speech perception [32]. The mechanisms for the word comprehension deficits in MV may therefore be fundamentally different from those underlying the word comprehension problems in SV or LV.

The primary objectives of this study were to assess the prevalence and nature of single-word comprehension problems in individual PPA patients with speech apraxia and/or agrammatism and to study their characteristics on multimodal imaging including high-resolution volumetric MRI, tau PET with $[^{18}F]$-THK5351 [38], and amyloid PET with $[^{11}C]$-Pittsburgh Compound B ($[^{11}C]$-PIB) [39]. $[^{18}F]$-THK5351 has high binding affinity and selectivity for tau aggregates [38], although some studies have revealed displacement of $[^{18}F]$-THK5351 binding by selegiline, indicative of monoamine oxidase-B (MAO-B) binding [40]. Increased MAO-B expression is observed in reactive astrogliosis [41] and can therefore also have a neurobiological meaning. The purpose of amyloid PET was to ascertain fibrillary amyloid plaque load. A negative amyloid PET scan in a patient virtually excludes Alzheimer's disease as the underlying cause [39]. As a secondary objective, performance on domains apart from single-word comprehension, grammatical processing, and motor speech was assessed and compared between other PPA variants.

Methods
Subjects
Patients
A consecutive series of 21 patients who fulfilled the international consensus criteria for PPA [1] enrolled. Eighteen patients were recruited through the memory clinic University Hospitals Leuven, case 3 was referred by the Free University Amsterdam, and cases 17 and 20 by the University Hospitals Ghent (Table 1). One case (case 15) had to be excluded due to a subarachnoidal cyst anterior to the left temporal lobe. Classification of patients relied on the clinical evaluation by an experienced neurologist in combination with the results from the clinical MRI and 2-$[^{18}F]$-fluoro-2-deoxy-D-glucose PET scan. None of the cases could be considered as primary progressive apraxia of speech [11, 12, 42] since agrammatism was present in all patients who concomitantly exhibited speech apraxia (Table 1). The presence of clinical signs and symptoms on neurological-clinical examination was documented for hypomimetic facies, dysarthria, limb dystonia, extrapyramidal signs, alien limb, nuchal rigidity, diminished postural reflexes, falls, tremor, myoclonus, pyramidal signs, dysphagia, pseudobulbar affect, ideomotor apraxia, and apraxia of eyelid closure (Table 2). A subset of PPA patients ($n = 13$) underwent a cerebrospinal fluid (CSF) Alzheimer's disease biomarker measurement (Innotest enzyme-linked immunosorbent assay (ELISA) for amyloid-β_{1-42} (Aβ_{1-42}; cut-off = 853 pg/ml [43]), total-tau (t-tau; Aβ_{1-42}/t-tau cut-off = 2.258), and phospho$_{181}$-tau (p$_{181}$-tau); Fujirebio Europe, Ghent, Belgium), which was performed at the Laboratory

of Medical analysis (Medicine Department of UZ Leuven, Leuven, Belgium) as part of the clinical work-up (Table 1). Two cases (case 9 and 14) received $[^{11}C]$-PIB PET as part of the prior clinical work-up [44] (Table 1). In PPA patients who had not previously received an amyloid biomarker measurement, $[^{11}C]$-PIB PET was acquired for the current study.

Control subjects
For normative reasons, data of four groups of cognitively intact older healthy controls were used (Additional file 1: Table S1). Inclusion criteria for controls were Mini-Mental State Examination (MMSE) [45] score ≥ 27, a Clinical Dementia Rating (DCR) scale [46] global score of zero, and no history of neurological or psychiatric disease or brain lesions on structural MRI [44, 47–49]. The neuropsychological data of the first group of 64 healthy controls were used to calculate whether neuropsychological and language performance of an individual PPA patient was within normal limits (Additional file 1: Table S1). Of these 64 control subjects, 20 also underwent $[^{18}F]$-THK5351 PET in the context of the current study, 22 underwent high resolution T$_1$-weighted structural MRI on the same scanner as patients, and 14 of these 20 subjects (six had to be excluded due to claustrophobia or movement) also underwent $[^{11}C]$-PIB PET as part of the current study protocol. Of these 64 control subjects, 16 additional subjects had also received an amyloid PET scan for other studies which was negative on visual assessment [47].

For the purpose of comparing gray matter volume in PPA patients with healthy controls, 19 additional high-resolution T$_1$-weighted structural MRI scans of a second healthy control group were selected, resulting in a total control group of 41 MRI scans for gray matter volumetric analyses (Additional file 1: Table S1). These 41 cognitively intact older controls were amyloid-negative based on visual assessment.

For the purpose of comparing $[^{11}C]$-PIB binding, $[^{11}C]$-PIB scans of a group of 19 additional amyloid-negative healthy controls were used [48], leaving a total group of 33 $[^{11}C]$-PIB scans (Additional file 1: Table S1). Amyloid-negativity of these controls was assured visually and using a semiquantitative cut-off as described previously [48].

Neuropsychological and neurolinguistic protocol
General cognitive functioning was assessed by CDR and MMSE [45]. Colored Progressive Matrices (CPM) were used to assess nonverbal fluid intelligence. Confrontation naming was assessed by means of the Boston Naming Test (BNT) [50], a 60-item standardized test in which items are administered in order of decreasing frequency of occurrence in the language. Category verbal

Table 1 Demographics, neurolinguistic, and neuropsychological assessment

	Case																			
	2	4	13	16	17	18	21	3	12	14	19	20	1	5	6	8	10	7	9	11
PPA variant	MV	MV	MV	MV	MV	MV	MV	NFV	NFV	NFV	NFV	NFV	SV	SV	SV	SV	SV	LV	LV	LV
Age (years)	80	62	76	70	65	49	76	57	68	66	63	70	73	71	63	52	55	77	63	74
Gender	M	F	M	M	M	F	F	F	F	F	M	M	F	F	F	F	M	M	F	M
Education (years)	17	12	12	12	15	12	12	16	10	15	10	10	14	8	13	13	14	10	12	18
Handedness	R	L	R	R	R	R	R	R	R	R	R	R	R	R	R	R	R	R	R	R
Symptom duration (months)	33	16	37	39	40	53	24	43	60	74	29	45	19	44	11	131	6	59	95	48
[11C]-PIB SUVR	–	1.26	2.1	1.35	1.57	–	–	–	–	1.16	1.37	–	–	–	1.12	1.14	1.2	–	1.81	–
CSF $A\beta_{1-42}$ (pg/ml)	816	–	477	–	759	1077	1144	1057	832	–	–	887	1558	733	–	–	–	564	664	321
CSF t-tau (pg/ml)	195	–	442	–	744	231	265	247	320	–	–	270	428	262	–	–	–	407	–	858
CSF $A\beta_{1-42}$/t-tau	4.18	–	1.08	–	1.02	4.66	4.32	4.28	2.60	–	–	3.29	3.64	2.80	–	–	–	1.39	–	0.37
CSF p_{181}-tau (pg/ml)	42	–	59.6	–	87.1	31	39.9	34	43	–	–	48	52	36.3	–	–	–	65.7	–	95
CDR	1	0.5	0.5	0.5	1	–	0.50	0.5	0.5	0	0.5	0.5	1	0.5	0.5	0.5	0.5	1	0	0.5
MMSE (/30)[c]	28	28	24	23	5	–	18	24	18	30	26	26	26	25	29	23	30	26	29	24
CPM (/36)[a]	26	31	29	29	24	–	17	–	29	26	25	26	28	27	34	36	34	32	32	12
BNT (/60)[b]	52	46	43	41	4	17	48	7	30	47	53	53	11	14	17	9	33	46	57	24
AVF (1 min)[b]	8	12	7	9	2	–	5	7	2	13	16	4	7	11	13	6	16	7	23	8
AAT sum single-word comprehension (/60)[c]	41	49	41	42	37	27	47	56	55	51	53	51	31	32	39	35	58	53	54	50
PALPA auditory word-picture matching (/40)[c]	40	39	39	39	38	–	36	37	39	38	40	40	26	27	26	21	39	38	39	38
PALPA verbal assoc.-sem. HI (/15)[c]	11	15	12	14	11	–	14	15	10	14	13	10	9	15	12	5	14	15	15	15
PALPA verbal assoc.-sem. LI (/15)[c]	12	11	14	11	7	–	5	14	7	12	11	9	3	7	10	6	14	13	14	12
PPT (/52)[c]	46	47	47	47	47	–	45	47	48	48	49	48	31	31	38	34	47	49	52	45
BORB easy B (/32)[c]	28	25	29	28	29	–	27	31	30	28	30	28	22	19	22	18	25	28	30	26
BORB hard A (/32)[c]	25	19	22	24	20	–	20	31	22	26	21	30	17	19	22	17	26	23	26	21
WEZT verb comprehension (/60)[b]	56	45	55	52	42	–	49	60	40	42	58	55	43	32	51	48	58	57	57	53
WEZT auditory sentence comprehension (/40)[c]	36	36	33	31	12	–	23	29	26	35	33	32	37	33	38	38	39	27	40	37
WEZT active sentence anagram (/10)[c]	10	10	9	10	5	–	10	10	9	10	10	10	10	10	10	10	10	10	10	10
WEZT passive sentence anagram (/10)[c]	10	9	9	5	5	–	5	10	6	10	10	3	10	9	10	9	10	10	10	10
AAT phoneme repetition (/30)[b]	24	28	22	20	–	14	29	27	27	30	27	26	30	29	30	30	30	30	30	29
AAT monosyllabic word repetition (/30)[b]	28	30	19	30	–	19	30	29	30	30	24	28	29	28	27	30	30	30	30	29
AAT cognate word repetition (/30)[b]	29	30	16	29	–	5	30	28	30	30	29	27	30	30	28	30	30	30	29	29
AAT concatenated word repetition (/30)[b]	27	29	23	29	–	1	30	15	29	30	26	25	30	29	28	26	30	15	29	30
AAT sentence repetition (/30)[c]	27	28	28	28	–	0	27	17	24	28	25	23	29	29	30	27	30	13	26	24
PALPA single-word repetition (/80)[a]	77	80	55	77	–	–	80	76	79	80	49	76	79	77	77	80	79	79	80	80
PALPA pseudoword repetition (/80)[a]	21	72	11	57	–	–	53	63	72	78	20	59	77	69	67	79	77	66	74	56

Table 1 Demographics, neurolinguistic, and neuropsychological assessment *(Continued)*

	Case																			
	2	4	13	16	17	18	21	3	12	14	19	20	1	5	6	8	10	7	9	11
DIAS diadochokinesis[c]	103	**50**	**42**	115	75	–	**32**	**24**	**51**	77	79	**18**	**50**	70	147	125	80	77	114	117
DIAS consonant and vowel repetition (/30)[c]	**28**	**24**	**12**	**27**	**11**	–	**28**	**28**	**20**	30	30	**25**	**27**	**24**	30	30	30	30	30	**29**

Data in bold are abnormal based on a Crawford and Garthwaite [64] regression method, correcting for education[a] or correcting for age[b] or depending on the outcome of a Crawford and Howell [52] modified t test[c]

AAT Aachen Aphasia Test, *assoc.-sem* associative semantic, $A\beta_{1-42}$ amyloid-β_{1-42}, *AVF* Animal Verbal Fluency, *BNT* Boston Naming Test, *BORB* Birmingham Object Recognition Battery, *CDR* Clinical Dementia Rating, *[^{11}C]-PIB* [^{11}C]-Pittsburgh Compound B, *CPM* Colored Progressive Matrices, *CSF* cerebrospinal fluid, *DIAS* Diagnostisch Instrument voor Apraxie van de Spraak, *F* female, *HI* high imageability, *L* left-handed, *LI* low imageability, *LV* logopenic variant, *M* male, *MMSE* Mini-Mental State Examination, *MV* mixed variant, *NFV* nonfluent variant, *PALPA* Psycholinguistic Assessment of Language Processing in Aphasia, *PPA* primary progressive aphasia, *PPT* Pyramids and Palm trees Test, *p181-tau* phospho181-tau, *R* right-handed, *SUVR* standardized uptake value ratio in a composite cortical volume of interest, *SV* semantic variant, *t-tau* total-tau, *WEZT* Werkwoorden En Zinnen test
– no data collected.

fluency was assessed by the 1-min Animal Verbal Fluency (AVF) test.

The main aim was to study single-word comprehension problems in patients with speech apraxia and/or agrammatism. Single-word comprehension was assessed using the Dutch version of the Aachen Aphasia Test (AAT) [51]. Performance on auditory and written single-word comprehension was considered as one 'sum' score (Tables 1 and 3). In both the auditory and written single-word comprehension subtests of the AAT, 10 words are presented per modality. One target picture and three distracter pictures are presented simultaneously, and subjects have to indicate the picture that corresponds to the word. One distracter picture is semantically related to the target picture. Interpretation of an individual patient's performance on the sum of the AAT auditory and written single-word comprehension test was statistically compared with the healthy control group (Additional file 1: Table S1) based on a modified t test [52] (see Statistical analyses).

The Dutch version of the Psycholinguistic Assessment of Language Processing in Aphasia (PALPA) [53] auditory word-picture matching task (PALPA subtest 45) was additionally used to assess single-word comprehension deficits. In this task (40 trials), a concrete noun is presented auditorily together with a target picture and four distractors. Two distractors are semantically

Table 2 Clinical signs and symptoms in primary progressive aphasia (PPA)

Case	2	4	13	16	17	18	21	3	12	14	19	20	1	5	6	8	10	7	9	11
PPA variant	MV	MV	MV	MV	MV	MV	MV	NFV	NFV	NFV	NFV	NFV	SV	SV	SV	SV	SV	LV	LV	LV
Hypomimetic facies	–	+	–	–	–	–	–	–	+	–	–	–	–	–	–	–	–	–	–	–
Dysarthria	–	+	–	–	–	–	+	–	+	–	–	–	–	–	–	–	–	–	–	–
Right-sided limb dystonia	–	+	–	–	–	–	–	–	–	–	–	–	–	–	–	–	–	–	–	–
Right-sided extrapyramidal signs	–	+	+	–	–	–	–	–	+	+	+	+	–	–	–	–	–	–	–	–
Alien limb	–	–	–	–	–	–	–	–	+	–	–	–	–	–	–	–	–	–	–	–
Nuchal rigidity	–	+	+	–	–	–	+	–	–	–	–	–	–	–	–	–	–	–	–	–
Reduced postural reflexes	–	+	–	–	–	–	–	–	–	–	–	–	–	–	–	–	–	–	–	–
Falls	+	+	–	–	–	–	–	–	+	–	–	–	–	–	–	–	–	–	–	–
Tremor	–	–	+	–	–	–	–	–	+	–	–	–	–	–	–	–	–	–	–	–
Myoclonus	–	–	–	–	–	–	–	–	–	–	–	–	–	–	–	–	–	–	–	–
Vertical gaze slowing or palsy	–	+	+	+	–	–	+	–	+	+	–	+	–	–	–	–	–	–	–	–
Decrease in vertical optokinetic nystagmus	+	+	+	+	–	–	+	–	+	+	–	+	–	–	–	–	–	–	–	–
Pyramidal signs	–	–	–	–	–	–	–	+	+	–	–	–	–	–	–	–	–	–	–	–
Dysphagia	+	+	–	–	–	–	–	–	–	–	–	–	–	–	–	–	–	–	–	–
Pseudobulbar affect	+	–	–	–	–	–	–	–	–	–	–	–	–	–	–	–	–	–	–	–
Ideomotor apraxia	–	–	–	–	–	–	–	–	–	–	–	–	–	–	–	–	–	–	–	–
Apraxia of eyelid closure	–	–	–	–	–	–	–	–	–	–	–	–	–	–	–	–	–	–	–	–

LV logopenic variant, *MV* mixed variant, *NFV* nonfluent variant, *SV* semantic variant

Table 3 Statistical group comparisons of neurolinguistic and neuropsychological data

Variables	Group					N HC	$p^{a,b}$	MV comparisons[c]				Other comparisons[c]			
	MV	NFV	SV	LV	HC			MV-HC	MV-NFV	MV-SV	MV-LV	NFV-HC	NFV-SV	SV-HC	LV-HC
Age (years)	70 (49–80)	66 (57–70)	63 (52–73)	74 (63–77)	67.5 (53–89)	64	0.50[a]	–	–	–	–	–	–	–	–
Gender (female/male)	3/4	3/2	4/1	1/2	34/30	64	0.68[b]	–	–	–	–	–	–	–	–
Education (years)	12 (12–17)	10 (10–16)	13 (8–14)	12 (10–18)	13 (8–22)	64	0.76[a]	–	–	–	–	–	–	–	–
Symptom duration (months)	37 (16–53)	45 (29–74)	19 (6–131)	59 (48–95)	–	–	0.11[a]	–	–	–	–	–	–	–	–
CDR	0.5 (0.5–1)	0.5 (0–0.5)	0.5 (0.5–1)	0.5 (0–1)	0 (0)	64	<0.001[a]	<0.001	0.064	0.43	0.45	<0.001	0.18	<0.001	<0.001
MMSE (/30)	23.5 (5–28)	26 (18–30)	26 (23–30)	26 (24–29)	29 (27–30)	64	0.002[a]	0.001	0.46	0.17	0.24	0.015	0.67	0.07	0.04
CPM (/36)	27.5 (17–31)	26 (25–29)	34 (27–36)	32 (12–32)	33 (24–36)	62	0.001[a]	0.001	0.83	0.099	0.44	0.003	0.048	0.70	0.15
BNT (/60)	43 (4–52)	47 (7–53)	14 (9–33)	46 (24–57)	56 (44–60)	64	<0.001[a]	<0.001	0.46	0.074	0.49	0.005	0.17	<0.001	0.16
AVF (1 min)	7.5 (2–12)	7 (2–16)	11 (6–16)	8 (7–23)	22.0 (14–30)	35	<0.001[a]	<0.001	0.85	0.23	0.44	0.001	0.53	0.001	0.087
AAT sum single-word comprehension (/60)	41 (27–49)	53 (51–56)	35 (31–58)	53 (50–54)	58 (48–60)	62	0.001[a]	<0.001	0.004	0.37	0.016	0.011	0.12	0.003	0.023
PALPA auditory word-picture matching (/40)	39 (36–40)	39 (37–40)	26 (21–39)	38 (38–39)	40 (38–40)	49	<0.001[a]	0.001	0.71	0.031	0.49	0.030	0.035	<0.001	0.001
PALPA verbal assoc.-sem. HI (/15)	13 (11–15)	13 (10–15)	12 (5–15)	15 (15–15)	15 (10–15)	51	0.004[a]	0.02	0.64	0.58	0.041	0.025	0.60	0.018	0.17
PALPA verbal assoc.-sem. LI (/15)	11 (5–14)	11 (7–14)	7 (3–14)	13 (12–14)	13 (11–15)	51	<0.001[a]	0.003	0.78	0.36	0.12	0.009	0.25	0.006	0.46
PPT (/52)	47 (45–47)	48 (47–49)	34 (31–49)	49 (45–52)	51 (45–52)	60	<0.001[a]	<0.001	0.012	0.035	0.34	<0.001	0.011	<0.001	0.23
BORB easy B (/32)	28 (25–29)	30 (28–31)	22 (18–25)	28 (26–30)	30 (25–32)	62	<0.001[a]	0.017	0.091	0.008	0.79	0.68	0.008	<0.001	0.17
BORB hard A (/32)	21 (19–25)	26 (21–31)	19 (17–26)	23 (21–26)	27 (20–31)	62	<0.001[a]	<0.001	0.081	0.36	0.30	0.79	0.073	0.001	0.034
WEZT verb comprehension (/60)	50.5 (42–56)	55 (40–60)	48 (32–58)	57 (53–57)	59 (56–60)	21	<0.001[a]	<0.001	0.71	0.58	0.070	0.037	0.53	0.001	0.013
WEZT auditory sentence comprehension (/40)	32 (12–36)	32 (26–35)	38 (33–39)	37 (27–40)	40 (36–40)	23	<0.001[a]	<0.001	0.93	0.022	0.20	<0.001	0.021	0.001	0.097
WEZT active sentence anagram (/10)	10 (5–10)	10 (9–10)	10 (10–10)	10 (10–10)	10 (10–10)	23	0.046[a]	0.005	0.56	0.18	0.29	0.032	0.32	1	1

Table 3 Statistical group comparisons of neurolinguistic and neuropsychological data (Continued)

Variables	Group MV	NFV	SV	LV	HC	N HC	$p^{a,b}$	MV comparisons[c] MV-HC	MV-NFV	MV-SV	MV-LV	Other comparisons[c] NFV-HC	NFV-SV	SV-HC	LV-HC
WEZT passive sentence anagram (/10)	7 (5–10)	10 (3–10)	10 (9–10)	10 (10–10)	10 (10–10)	23	**<0.001**[a]	**<0.001**	0.40	0.066	**0.038**	**0.002**	0.64	**0.002**	1
AAT phoneme repetition (/30)	23 (14–29)	27 (26–30)	30 (29–30)	30 (29–30)	30 (28–30)	49	**<0.001**[a]	**<0.001**	0.20	**0.007**	**0.027**	**<0.001**	**0.032**	0.93	0.55
AAT monosyllabic word repetition (/30)	29 (19–30)	29 (24–30)	29 (27–30)	30 (29–30)	30 (27–30)	49	0.076[a]	–	–	–	–	–	–	–	–
AAT cognate word repetition (/30)	29 (5–30)	29 (27–30)	30 (28–30)	30 (29–30)	30 (27–30)	49	**0.002**[a]	**<0.001**	0.71	0.16	0.27	**0.002**	0.24	0.46	0.24
AAT concatenated word repetition (/30)	28 (1–30)	26 (15–30)	29 (26–30)	29 (15–30)	30 (28–30)	49	**0.001**[a]	**0.001**	0.93	0.35	0.69	**0.002**	0.24	0.058	0.088
AAT sentence repetition (/30)	27.5 (0–28)	24 (17–28)	29 (27–30)	24 (13–26)	30 (26–30)	49	**<0.001**[a]	**<0.001**	0.22	**0.04**	0.11	**<0.001**	**0.016**	0.33	**0.001**
PALPA single-word repetition (/80)	77 (55–80)	76 (49–80)	79 (77–80)	80 (79–80)	80 (73–80)	50	0.10[a]	–	–	–	–	–	–	–	–
PALPA pseudoword repetition (/80)	53 (11–72)	63 (20–78)	77 (67–79)	66 (56–74)	77 (45–80)	50	**0.001**[a]	**0.001**	0.21	**0.028**	0.18	**0.022**	0.17	0.53	**0.035**
DIAS diadochokinesis	62.5 (32–115)	51 (18–79)	80 (50–147)	114 (77–117)	126 (56–192)	23	**0.001**[a]	**0.003**	0.47	0.23	0.12	**0.001**	0.12	0.093	0.10
DIAS consonant and vowel repetition (/30)	25.5 (11–28)	28 (20–30)	30 (24–30)	30 (29–30)	30 (29–30)	23	**<0.001**[a]	**<0.001**	0.20	0.10	**0.019**	**0.008**	0.58	0.096	0.37

Data are shown as median and range (minimum–maximum)

AAT Aachen Aphasia Test, assoc.-sem associative semantic, AVF Animal Verbal Fluency, BNT Boston Naming Test, BORB Birmingham Object Recognition Battery, CDR Clinical Dementia Rating, CPM Colored Progressive Matrices, DIAS Diagnostisch Instrument voor Apraxie van de Spraak, HI high imageability, LI low imageability, LV logopenic variant, MMSE Mini-Mental State Examination, MV mixed variant, NFV nonfluent variant, PALPA Psycholinguistic Assessment of Language Processing in Aphasia, PPT Pyramids and Palm trees Test, SV semantic variant, WEZT Werkwoorden En Zinnen test

– Data not available

[a]Kruskal-Wallis statistical analyses were performed to assess between-group differences (HC, MV, NFV, SV and LV) for continuous variables and [b]chi-square tests for categorical variables. Pair-wise post-hoc comparisons were performed with Mann-Whitney U tests[c]. P values are not corrected for multiple comparisons. P values in bold are significantly different between groups

related to the target, a third is perceptually similar, and the fourth picture is unrelated. Subjects were asked to point to the target picture.

In the PALPA associative-semantic task (PALPA subtest 49), a noun is presented visually together with four choice noun stimuli (a target noun, a noun that is semantically related to the target, and two unrelated nouns). Subjects have to underline or circle the noun that matches the sample stimulus most closely in meaning, for a total of a 15-word series with high imageability and 15 with low imageability. Associative-semantic memory was also assessed by the picture-version of the Pyramids and Palm trees Test (PPT) (52 trials) [54] which relies on the capability to make semantic associations between two pictures. The Birmingham Object Recognition Battery (BORB) (easy (B) and hard (A), 32 trials each) [55] was used as a measure of object identification. In this task, subjects have to indicate whether an animal or tool depicted in a line drawing is real or unreal.

Verb comprehension and grammaticality were assessed by the Werkwoorden En Zinnen Test (WEZT) [56]. Grammaticality was quantified using both the WEZT auditory sentence comprehension test (40 trials) as well as the WEZT sentence anagram test (20 trials). During administration of the WEZT sentence anagram test, the patient is asked to manually put together single words which are each printed on separate cards into a syntactic structure that describes the action depicted in the target picture. Sentences can occur in the active or passive tense, of which half represent reversible actions and half represent irreversible actions.

In the AAT repetition task, the examiner pronounces 10 phonemes, 10 monosyllabic words, 10 cognate (foreign) words, 10 composed (concatenated) words, and 10 sentences of increasing length which the subject has to repeat. In the PALPA word repetition task (PALPA subtest 9), the examiner who is sitting in front of the subject pronounces 80 nouns and 80 pseudowords which the subject has to repeat.

The Diagnostisch Instrument voor Apraxie van de Spraak (DIAS) [57] was used to assess consonant and vowel repetition (15 trials each), of which the sum is considered the 'DIAS severity score'. Diadochokinesis, which is the ability to make antagonistic movements using different parts of the mouth, tongue, and soft palate in quick succession, was also assessed using DIAS. During this DIAS diadochokinesis task, the examiner first reads three successive sounds or tokens aloud, e.g., the alternating task 'pa ta ka' or the sequential task 'pa pa pa', and asks the patient to repeat these once. If the patient was able to repeat this sequence correctly, he/she was asked to repeat it as many times as possible during a period of s-8. In

total, the patient has to repeat six alternating and six sequential sounds, for which the total number of repetitions was scored (Tables 1 and 3).

[^{18}F]-THK5351 PET acquisition and analysis

[^{18}F]-THK5351 PET scans were acquired on a 16-slice Siemens Biograph PET/computed tomography (CT) scanner (Siemens Medical Solutions, Erlangen, Germany) in 20 patients and in 20 healthy control subjects (Additional file 1: Table S1). After bolus injection of [^{18}F]-THK5351 (mean dose = 185.2 MBq, range 178.7–191.0 MBq) in an antecubital vein, five healthy control subjects were scanned dynamically with arterial sampling between 0 and 100 min postinjection to assess the optimal PET imaging window. The remaining healthy controls and all PPA patients were scanned between 50 and 80 min postinjection with [^{18}F]-THK5351 (controls: mean dose = 184.1 MBq, range 165.8–196.0 MBq; patients: mean dose = 181.8 MBq, range 164.9–192.3 MBq). A low-dose CT scan was acquired for attenuation correction prior to PET scan acquisition. PET emission images were acquired in 3D mode and subsequently reconstructed using ordered subsets expectation maximization (4 iterations × 16 subsets). Individual [^{18}F]-THK5351 PET emission frames were realigned to correct for head-motion, summed, and rigidly coregistered to the subject's T$_1$-weighted MRI scan using Statistical Parametric Mapping software (SPM12, Wellcome Trust Centre for Neuroimaging, London, UK) implemented in Matlab R2014b (Mathworks, Natick, USA). Summed PET images as well as the T$_1$-weighted MRI segmentations were warped to Montreal Neurological Institute (MNI) template space. The normalized [^{18}F]-THK5351 PET scans were subsequently corrected for partial volume effects using the modified Müller-Gärtner method [58]. Partial volume corrected (PVC) standardized uptake value ratio (SUVR) images with the subject-specific cerebellar gray matter as reference region were created. For voxel-based statistical analyses, PVC [^{18}F]-THK5351 SUVR images were smoothed with an isotropic 8-mm full-width half-maximum (FWHM) Gaussian kernel. The [^{18}F]-THK5351 PET data were obtained within 2–182 days from the [^{11}C]-PIB PET scan (mean 82 days in controls, mean 19 days in PPA patients).

Volumetric MRI acquisition and analysis

All subjects received MRI scanning on the same day as the neuropsychological testing. The high-resolution T$_1$-weighted structural MRI scan was acquired on a 3-Tesla Philips Achieva dstream equipped with a 32-channel head volume coil (Philips, Best, The Netherlands), using a 3D turbo field echo sequence (coronal inversion recovery prepared 3D gradient-echo images, inversion time (TI) 900 ms, shot interval = 3000 ms, echo time (TE) = 4.6 ms, repetition time (TR) = 9.6 ms, flip angle 8 degrees, field of view (FoV) = 250 × 250 mm,

182 slices, slice thickness = 1.2 mm, voxel size = 0.98 × 1.2 × 0.98 mm^3).

All T_1-weighted images underwent preprocessing with voxel-based morphometry (VBM8) [59] as previously described [60, 61]. This included corrections for gradient nonlinearity and intensity inhomogeneity in the MRI. The resulting modulated gray matter volumes were adjusted for overall brain size (total intracranial volume) by using the 'nonlinear-only' component in the spatial normalization process for modulation of gray matter voxel intensities [62]. For voxel-based statistical analyses, modulated gray matter maps were smoothed with an 8-mm FWHM Gaussian 3D kernel.

Amyloid biomarker measurement and analysis

[^{11}C]-PIB PET scans were acquired on a GE Signa 3-T PET/MRI scanner (GE Healthcare, Chicago, USA) operating in 3D mode to estimate amyloid burden in eight patients and 14 healthy control subjects. [^{11}C]-PIB was injected intravenously as a bolus in an antecubital vein (controls: mean dose = 267.8 MBq, range 197.5–364.9 MBq; patients: mean dose = 270.5 MBq, range 230.6–316.4 MBq). Dynamic [^{11}C]-PIB images were acquired during a 70-min period and reconstructed with atlas-based attenuation correction using the manufacturer's software. Two patients received a 30-min [^{11}C]-PIB PET scan between 40 and 70-min postinjection on a Siemens Biograph PET/CT scanner (Siemens Medical Solutions, Erlangen, Germany) in a clinical context (See Subjects section). For the purpose of comparing [^{11}C]-PIB binding in these two patients, [^{11}C]-PIB scans acquired on the same Siemens Biograph PET/CT scanner in 19 older amyloid-negative cognitively intact control subjects were used (Additional file 1: Table S1) [48]. Processing of [^{11}C]-PIB PET images was performed in SPM12 using the same MRI-based method as previously described [48]. [^{11}C]-PIB PET images were corrected for partial volume effects using a modified Müller-Gärtner method [58]. The mean [^{11}C]-PIB PET SUVR value was calculated in a neocortical composite region [63] and considered positive if this value was significantly elevated compared with healthy controls based on a modified t test [52]. For voxel-based statistical analyses, PVC [^{11}C]-PIB SUVR images were smoothed with an isotropic 6-mm FWHM Gaussian kernel.

Statistical analyses
Neuropsychological and neurolinguistic data analyses

Standard statistical analyses were performed in Statistics Software Package for the Social Sciences (version 24, IBM Statistics, Armonk, USA). The significance was set at $P < 0.05$ for all standard statistical analyses. Demographic data were statistically compared using Kruskal-Wallis for continuous variables and using Pearson chi-squared tests for categorical variables.

A first objective was to assess the prevalence of single-word comprehension deficits in individual PPA patients with speech apraxia and/or agrammatism. The neuropsychological test scores of individuals were statistically contrasted with scores derived from 64 healthy controls (Additional file 1: Table S1) following the procedure developed by Crawford and Garthwaite [64]. As a first step, a hierarchical multiple linear regression analysis was performed in the healthy control group for each task, with the neuropsychological test scores as outcome variable and age and education as predictor variables. Variables that had a significant effect (i.e. $\alpha < 0.05$) on any of the test scores in the healthy controls were included as predictor variables in the regression equation for that test.

There was a statistically significant positive effect of education on performance on the CPM task (R^2 adjusted = 0.069, $P = 0.022$) and on PALPA repetition of words (R^2 adjusted = 0.11, $P = 0.009$) and pseudowords (R^2 adjusted = 0.11, $P = 0.013$). Age had a significant negative effect on performance on the BNT (R^2 adjusted = 0.047, $P = 0.046$), AVF (R^2 adjusted = 0.19, $P = 0.005$), WEZT verb comprehension (R^2 adjusted = 0.15, $P = 0.045$), AAT repetition of phonemes (R^2 adjusted = 0.068, $P = 0.039$), of single words (R^2 adjusted = 0.065, $P = 0.043$), cognates (R^2 adjusted = 0.15, $P = 0.003$), and concatenated words (R^2 adjusted = 0.11, $P = 0.011$). Consequently, education or age, respectively, were entered in the regression equation as predictor variables and the test score of the individual patient as a dependent variable in order to obtain a predicted score for that individual patient. The discrepancy between the predicted score and the observed score was expressed as a Z score. Individual performance on the other tasks was statistically compared with the healthy control group based on a modified t test [52]. The corresponding P values were converted to a Z score. For all tests, Z scores were considered abnormal at 1.96 standard deviations [65] (Table 1).

The nature of the single-word comprehension deficit in MV PPA was subsequently analyzed in detail by assessing the influence of word frequency and the effect of the number of phonemes contained in a word (phonemic length). Word frequency was retrieved using the SUBTLEX-NL database for the dominant meaning of words [66]. In 11 out of 20 trials of the AAT auditory and written single-word comprehension test, the nondominant meaning of a word with multiple meanings (i.e., a homonym) is targeted. For instance, in case the word 'star' is presented to the subject, the target picture depicts a 'popstar' and the distractor picture depicts a 'sun', which is semantically related to the dominant meaning but not to the non-dominant meaning of 'star'. To estimate the relative meaning frequencies of each meaning of a homonym, we made use of lexical associations as described in Armstrong et al. [67]. Associations of the words used in the AAT single-word comprehension task were taken from the Small World of Words Project [68]. The estimated frequency of the nondominant meaning of a word was calculated by multiplying the relative frequency with the frequency retrieved from the SUBTLEX-NL database. The frequency of the words assessed in the PALPA word-picture matching task (PALPA subtest 45) were directly taken from the SUBTLEX-NL database, as only the dominant meaning of words was targeted in this test. In total, we were able to retrieve word frequency for 53 out of 60 words from the pooled AAT and PALPA single-word comprehension tasks. For these 53 words, phonemic length was calculated by counting the numbers of phonemes contained in a word. The effects of word frequency and phonemic length on single-word comprehension was assessed by calculating a logistic regression equation for each patient with the patient's response (correct/not correct) as a dependent variable and word frequency and phonemic length as independent variables [69]. The individual β coefficients derived from this regression equation were compared between MV and SV PPA using two-tailed Mann-Whitney U tests with significance set at α < 0.05. The effect of 'meaning dominance' on single-word comprehension was calculated by dividing the errors made on trials targeting the nondominant meaning of a word by the total number of errors and this proportion was compared between MV and SV PPA using two-tailed Mann-Whitney U tests with significance set at α < 0.05.

As a secondary objective, neuropsychological performance in domains apart from the defining domains of single-word comprehension, grammatical processing, and motor speech was compared to healthy controls, NFV pure, SV, and LV PPA using Kruskal-Wallis, followed by two-tailed Mann-Whitney U post-hoc tests with significance set at $P < 0.05$.

Imaging-based analyses
At the group-level, gray matter volume images, [^{18}F]-THK5351, and [^{11}C]-PIB PET PVC SUVR images of MV PPA patients were compared with healthy control subjects, NFV pure, SV, and LV PPA patients (between-subjects factor) using separate whole-brain voxel-wise analyses of variance (ANOVA) with two-tailed post-hoc t tests in SPM12 running on Matlab R2014b (Mathworks, Natick, USA) with age and gender as nuisance variables. For the ANOVA

with [^{11}C]-PIB PET SUVR images, scanner type was additionally added as a nuisance variable. The default significance threshold was set at voxel-level uncorrected $P < 0.001$, with a cluster-level family wise error (FWE)-corrected threshold of $P < 0.05$ [70]. At the individual patient level, imaging data were statistically contrasted with the healthy control group for each imaging modality using a voxel-wise modified t test [52] at a voxel-level uncorrected $P < 0.001$.

Results
Groups were matched for age, education, and gender (Table 3), and PPA patients did not differ in symptom duration (Table 3).

Neuropsychological, neurolinguistic, and clinical-neurological profile of individual MV PPA patients
Significant deficits at the individual patient level are shown in bold in Table 1. Twelve cases fulfilled a priori diagnostic criteria for NFV PPA encompassing agrammatism in language production and/or apraxia of speech presenting as effortful, halting speech with inconsistent speech sound errors and distortions [1] as measured by the repetition tests of AAT and PALPA subtest 9 along with the DIAS and WEZT (Table 1). In these NFV PPA patients, syntactic comprehension measured with the WEZT auditory sentence comprehension test was additionally affected, and object identification measured with the BORB object recognition task was preserved (i.e., fulfilling two out of three ancillary features) [1]. In one NFV case (case 14) agrammatism was the most prominent clinical abnormality without features of apraxia of speech. Seven out of the 12 cases classified a priori as NFV PPA had concomitant single-word comprehension problems as measured with the sum of the AAT auditory and written single-word comprehension test (Table 1). Hence, these patients did not strictly fulfill criteria for NFV pure nor for any of the other PPA variants [1]. This phenotype was in accordance with a diagnosis of MV PPA [19, 20]. These MV PPA cases included three females and four males, with a mean age of onset of 65 years (range 44–77 years).

At the time of testing, mild right-sided extrapyramidal signs were present in two of the MV cases (cases 4 and 13) and in four of the pure NFV cases (cases 12, 14, 19, and 20) (Table 2). Five of the MV cases (cases 2, 4, 13, 16, and 21) and three of the NFV cases (cases 12, 14, and 20) showed mild vertical eye movement abnormalities (Table 2).

Detailed assessment of single-word comprehension problems
In none of the individual MV or SV cases was a significant effect of word frequency or phonemic length on

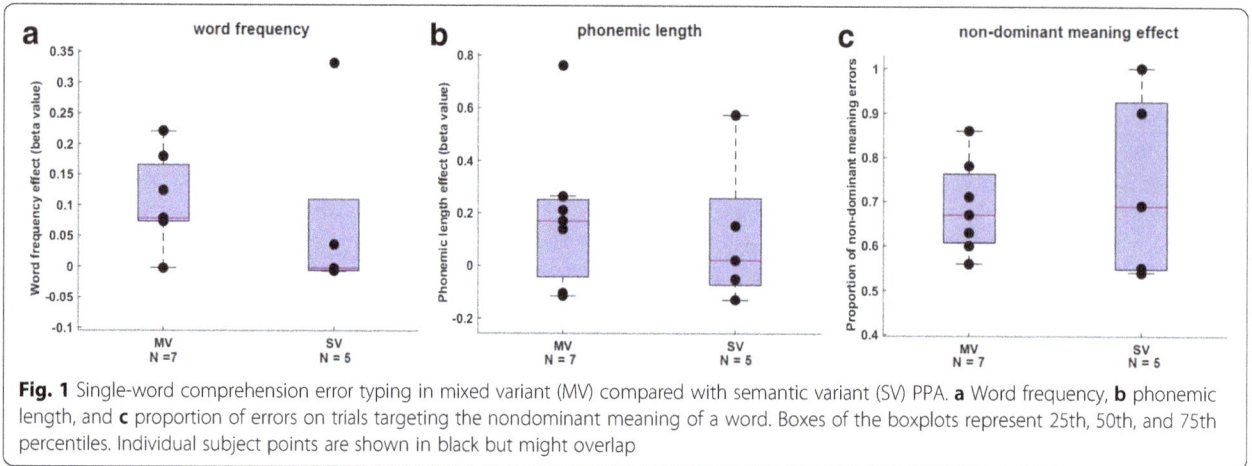

Fig. 1 Single-word comprehension error typing in mixed variant (MV) compared with semantic variant (SV) PPA. **a** Word frequency, **b** phonemic length, and **c** proportion of errors on trials targeting the nondominant meaning of a word. Boxes of the boxplots represent 25th, 50th, and 75th percentiles. Individual subject points are shown in black but might overlap

single-word comprehension present. Word frequency effects on single-word comprehension in MV were not significantly different compared with SV PPA ($U = 8.5$, $P = 0.14$) (Fig. 1a), nor did effects of phonemic length on single-word comprehension differ between MV and SV PPA ($U = 13$, $P = 0.47$) (Fig. 1b). A detailed assessment of the type of single-word comprehension deficits in MV PPA patients revealed that 69% of errors were made on trials assessing the nondominant meaning of a homonym (Fig. 1c). In these trials, patients were not able to retrieve the nondominant meaning of a word but pointed to the

distracter picture, which was semantically related to the dominant meaning of that word. The proportion of errors on trials targeting the nondominant meaning of a word did not significantly differ between MV and SV PPA ($U = 17$, $P = 0.94$) (Fig. 1c).

Group-based deficits of MV PPA for additional neuropsychological domains

Deficits in MV PPA were present in other neuropsychological domains apart from grammatical, motor speech, or

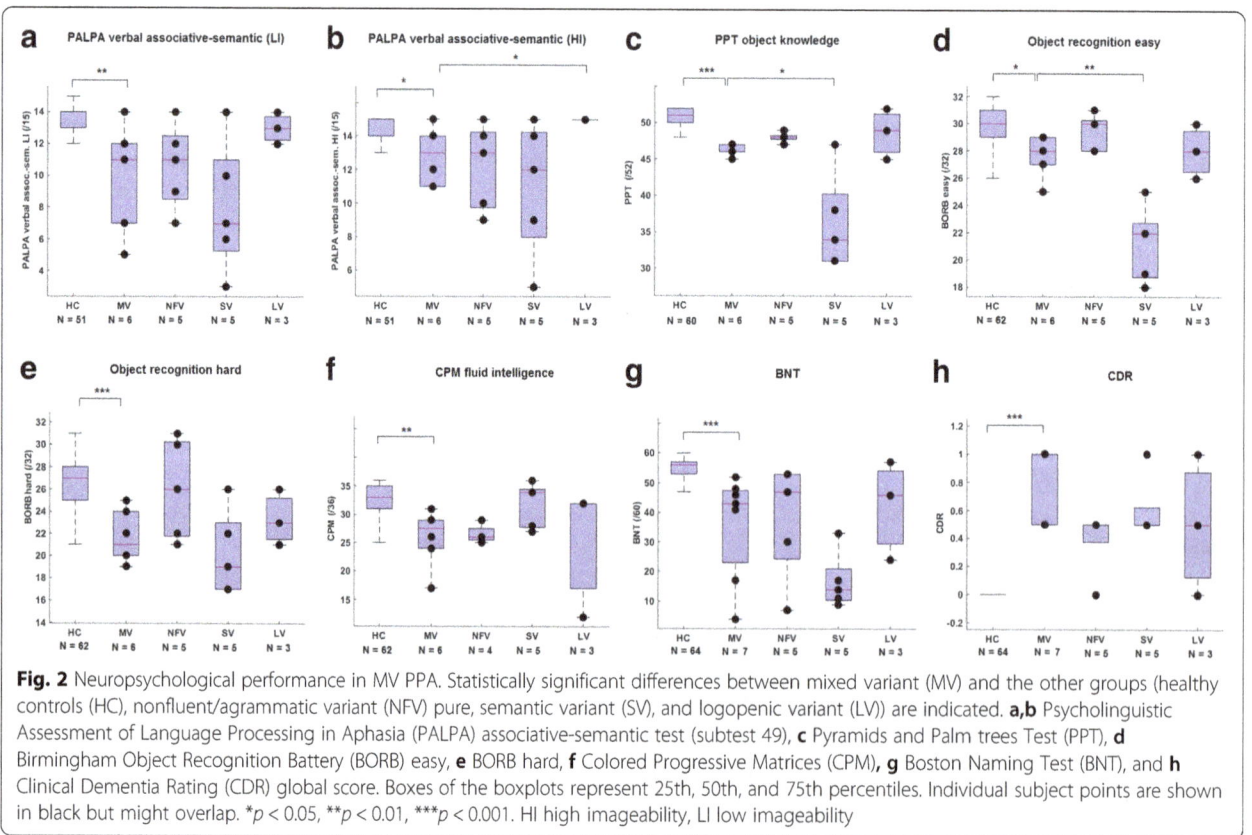

Fig. 2 Neuropsychological performance in MV PPA. Statistically significant differences between mixed variant (MV) and the other groups (healthy controls (HC), nonfluent/agrammatic variant (NFV) pure, semantic variant (SV), and logopenic variant (LV)) are indicated. **a,b** Psycholinguistic Assessment of Language Processing in Aphasia (PALPA) associative-semantic test (subtest 49), **c** Pyramids and Palm trees Test (PPT), **d** Birmingham Object Recognition Battery (BORB) easy, **e** BORB hard, **f** Colored Progressive Matrices (CPM), **g** Boston Naming Test (BNT), and **h** Clinical Dementia Rating (CDR) global score. Boxes of the boxplots represent 25th, 50th, and 75th percentiles. Individual subject points are shown in black but might overlap. *$p < 0.05$, **$p < 0.01$, ***$p < 0.001$. HI high imageability, LI low imageability

single-word comprehension tasks (Fig. 2) (Table 3). The full statistical results for all tasks are shown in Table 3.

Scores on the PALPA verbal associative-semantic task were significantly lower in the MV PPA group compared with healthy controls for words with low ($U = 40.5$, $P = 0.003$) as well as high imageability ($U = 72$, $P = 0.020$) (Fig. 2a, b). These scores were lower in MV compared with LV for the high imageability task ($U = 1.5$, $P = 0.041$) (Fig. 2b). Scores on the picture-version of the PPT were significantly lower in MV PPA compared with healthy controls ($U = 5.5$, $P < 0.001$) and were significantly higher compared with SV PPA ($U = 4.0$, $P = 0.035$) (Fig. 2c). Scores on the BORB object recognition task were significantly lower in MV PPA compared with healthy controls for the easy task ($U = 77$, $P = 0.017$) and for the hard task ($U = 26$, $P < 0.001$) (Fig. 2d, e). However, MV patients scored better than SV on the easy BORB object recognition task ($U = 0.5$, $P = 0.008$) (Fig. 2d), but not on the hard BORB object recognition task ($P = 0.36$) (Fig. 2e). No differences were found between MV and NFV pure and between MV and LV on the BORB object recognition tasks ($P > 0.081$) (Fig. 2d, e) (Table 3).

Compared with healthy controls, MV patients had significantly lower scores on nonverbal fluid intelligence measured by the CPM ($U = 38.5$, $P = 0.001$). No differences were found compared with other variants ($P > 0.099$) (Fig. 2f) (Table 3).

Scores on the BNT were significantly lower in MV PPA compared with healthy controls ($U = 22.5$, $P < 0.001$), but did not differ compared with the other variants ($P > 0.074$) (Fig. 2g) (Table 3).

The global CDR score was significantly higher in MV PPA compared with healthy controls ($U = 0$, $P < 0.001$), with no differences in global CDR score compared with the other PPA variants ($P > 0.064$) (Fig. 2h) (Table 3). Despite the single-word comprehension deficit measured on AAT in MV, performance on the PALPA auditory word-picture matching was less affected in MV compared with SV (Table 3).

Anatomy of atrophy
Atrophy in the MV PPA group was relatively widespread and comprised mainly frontal and temporoparietal regions with left-sided predominance (Fig. 3a). The highest degree of atrophy was observed in the premotor cortex, supplementary motor area, pars triangularis and pars opercularis, inferior parietal lobule, insula, precuneus, and in the cingulum bilaterally (Fig. 3a). The superior temporal gyrus and sulcus, left putamen, hippocampus, and perirhinal cortex were also atrophic compared with the healthy control group (Fig. 3a). NFV pure showed atrophy in the left dorsal premotor cortex compared with healthy controls (Fig.

3b). There were no significant differences in gray matter volume between MV and NFV pure at the preset threshold (Fig. 3c, d). MV had significantly more atrophy compared with SV in the left premotor cortex and left inferior frontal sulcus (Fig. 3e). SV in turn had lower gray matter volume in the anterior temporal lobes bilaterally and in the right ventromedial frontal cortex compared with MV (Fig. 3f) and compared with controls (Fig. 3g). MV PPA showed more atrophy in the caudate nuclei bilaterally compared with LV (Fig. 3i). In the current study, LV PPA did not have lower gray matter volume compared with controls (Fig. 3h) or compared with MV (Fig. 3j).

Individual T maps of reduced gray matter volume in MV compared with healthy controls are shown in Fig. 4a–g (shown in red). Atrophy was present in the left inferior frontal gyrus and dorsal premotor cortex in five MV cases (Fig. 4b–e, g; shown in red) and in posterior temporal regions in six MV cases (Fig. 4b–g; shown in red). Three MV cases showed atrophy in the pons (Fig. 4a, b, e; shown in red).

[^{18}F]-THK5351 binding pattern
[^{18}F]-THK5351 binding in MV PPA was significantly higher in the supplementary motor area bilaterally and in the left dorsal premotor cortex, left pars triangularis, and pars opercularis extending medially into the insula, basal ganglia, thalamus, subthalamic nucleus, red nucleus, and substantia nigra compared with healthy controls (Fig. 5a). When a more lenient threshold was applied (voxel-level uncorrected $P < 0.005$), additional elevated [^{18}F]-THK5351 binding in the superior temporal gyrus and in the lateral temporal lobe was present in MV. An almost identical pattern of [^{18}F]-THK5351 binding was present when MV was compared with SV PPA (Fig. 5e). In NFV pure, elevated [^{18}F]-THK5351 binding compared with controls was observed in the left supplementary motor area and in the basal ganglia, thalamus, subthalamic nucleus, red nucleus, and substantia nigra (Fig. 5b). MV and NFV pure did not differ in [^{18}F]-THK5351 binding at the preset significance threshold (Fig. 5c, d). SV showed elevated [^{18}F]-THK5351 binding compared with MV in the right inferior lateral temporal gyrus and in the right ventromedial frontal gyrus (Fig. 5f). MV had increased [^{18}F]-THK5351 binding compared with LV in the left substantia nigra, thalamus, and subthalamic nucleus (Fig. 5g), while LV patients had elevated [^{18}F]-THK5351 binding compared with MV in the right temporooccipital lobe (Fig. 5h).

Individual T maps of elevated [^{18}F]-THK5351 binding of all MV PPA patients are shown in Fig. 4a–g (shown in blue). All MV PPA cases showed elevated [^{18}F]-THK5351 binding in the medial frontal cortex. More specifically, elevated [^{18}F]-THK5351 binding was present in six out of

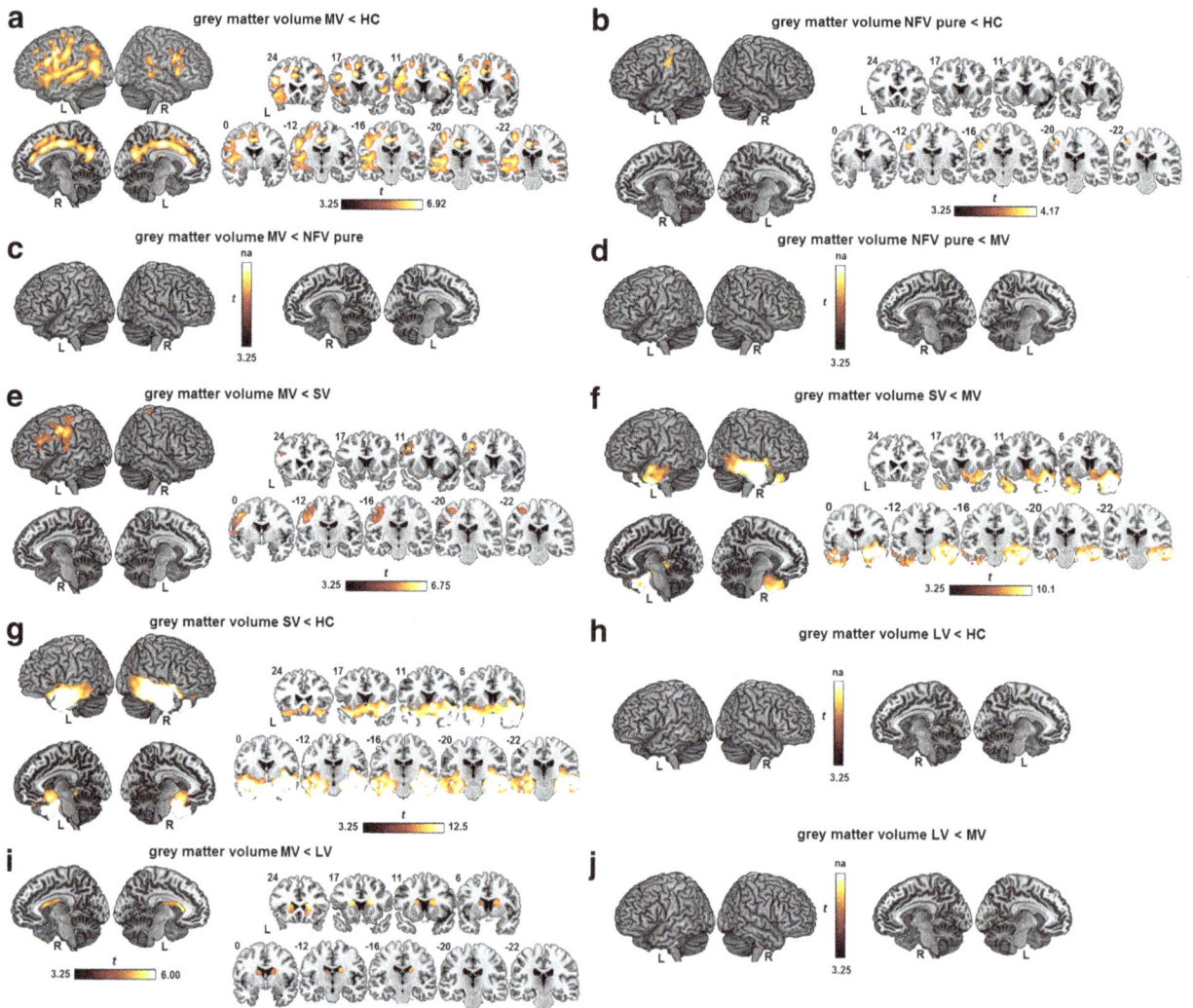

Fig. 3 Reduced gray matter volume. Reduced gray matter volume based on a voxel-wise ANOVA with age and gender as covariates, depicted by a one-sided t contrast on an MNI template brain rendering and on coronal slices in **a** mixed variant (MV) PPA compared with healthy controls (HC), **b** nonfluent/agrammatic variant (NFV) pure PPA compared with HC, **c** MV compared with NFV pure, **d** NFV pure compared with MV, **e** MV compared with semantic variant (SV), **f** SV compared with MV, **g** SV compared with HC, **h** logopenic variant (LV) compared with HC, **i** MV compared with LV, and **j** LV compared with MV. The significance threshold was set at voxel-level uncorrected $P < 0.001$ with cluster-level family wise error (FWE)-corrected threshold $P < 0.05$. L left, R right

seven cases in the supplementary motor area bilaterally and in the left dorsal premotor cortex (Fig. 4b–g; shown in blue). Five of these six cases showed elevated [18F]-THK5351 binding in the thalamus (Fig. 4b–e, g; shown in blue), three in the midbrain including the substantia nigra (Fig. 4b, d, g; shown in blue) and two of these six cases also showed elevated binding in the basal ganglia (Fig. 4e, g; shown in blue). In one case (case 2; Fig. 4a; shown in blue), binding in the basal ganglia, thalamus, cingulum, and midbrain without supplementary motor area/premotor cortical involvement was present. Another case (case 18) showed only elevated [18F]-THK5351 binding in cortical regions but not in subcortical regions (Fig. 4f; shown in blue). The latter case, together with case 17

(Fig. 4e; shown in blue) showed extensive [18F]-THK5351 binding encompassing almost the entire temporal lobe with a left-hemispheric predominance. This pattern overlapped with the atrophy pattern (red) in these patients (Fig. 4e–f; overlap shown in violet).

Amyloid biomarker positivity

As a group, MV PPA patients showed significantly elevated [11C]-PIB binding in the orbitofrontal cortex, the anterior cingulate cortex, and in the precuneus/posterior cingulate cortex bilaterally compared with healthy controls (Additional file 2: Figure S1). At the individual patient level, two out of seven MV PPA

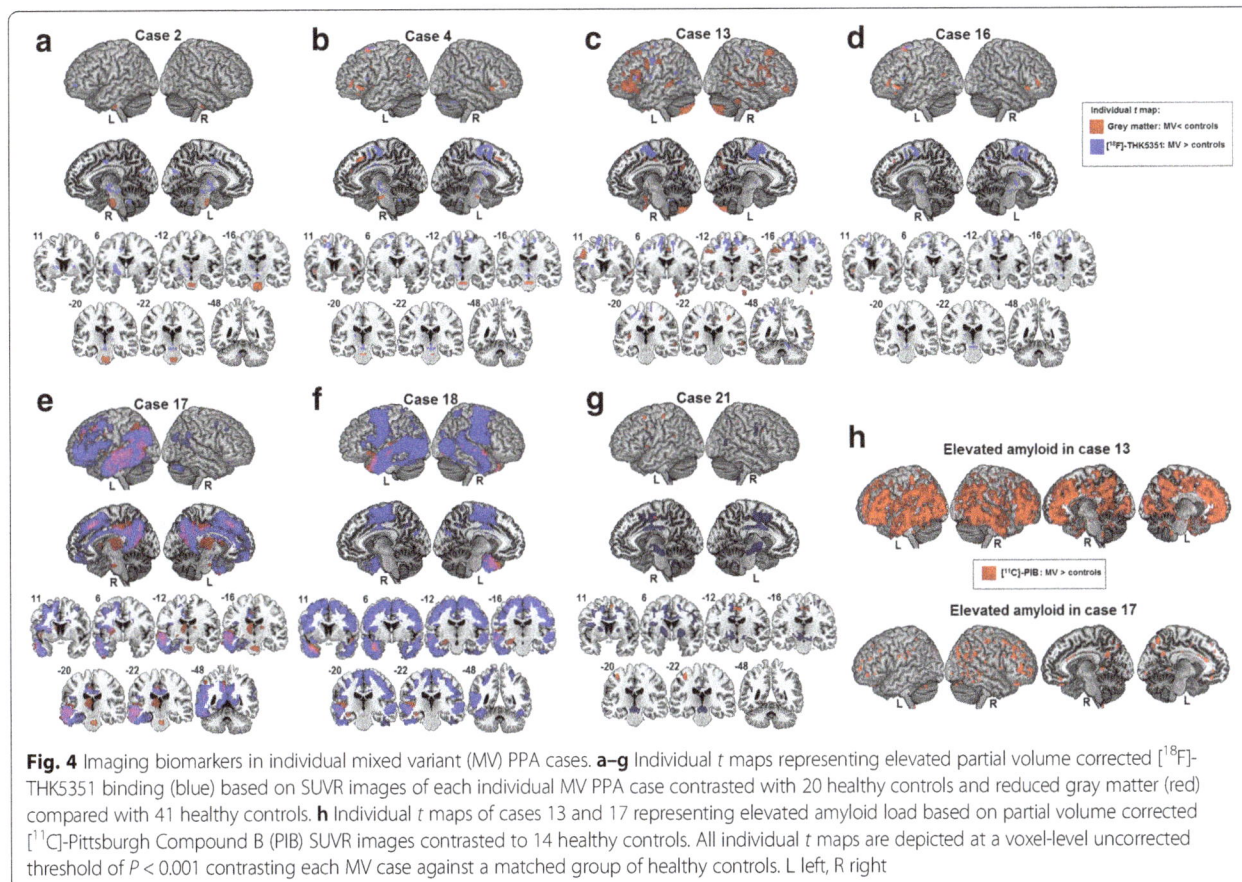

Fig. 4 Imaging biomarkers in individual mixed variant (MV) PPA cases. **a–g** Individual t maps representing elevated partial volume corrected [^{18}F]-THK5351 binding (blue) based on SUVR images of each individual MV PPA case contrasted with 20 healthy controls and reduced gray matter (red) compared with 41 healthy controls. **h** Individual t maps of cases 13 and 17 representing elevated amyloid load based on partial volume corrected [^{11}C]-Pittsburgh Compound B (PIB) SUVR images contrasted to 14 healthy controls. All individual t maps are depicted at a voxel-level uncorrected threshold of $P < 0.001$ contrasting each MV case against a matched group of healthy controls. L left, R right

cases (case 13 (76 years old) and case 17 (65 years old)) were amyloid-positive based on either neocortical [^{11}C]-PIB PET SUVR values (Fig. 4h) (Table 1) or on CSF Aβ_{42} values (Table 1). MV case 4 and case 16 did not show any elevated [^{11}C]-PIB binding, and neither did MV cases 2, 18, and 21 show positivity on CSF Aβ_{42} or CSF Aβ_{42}/t-tau (Table 1). In the LV group, all three cases were amyloid-positive (Table 1). In contrast, none of the NFV pure or SV cases were amyloid-positive (Table 1).

Discussion

This study provides a comprehensive analysis of the prevalence and nature of single-word comprehension problems in PPA, which occurred in a substantial number of cases with speech apraxia and/or agrammatism. These patients were classified as MV PPA and showed additional deficits on object knowledge and object recognition.

We demonstrated for the first time a focal pattern of elevated [^{18}F]-THK5351 binding which was narrowly circumscribed and highly similar to NFV pure PPA.

At a clinical level, data-driven mathematical analyses of neurolinguistic and neuropsychological data of PPA patients suggest the existence of a mixed phenotype [25, 26].

In the first study reporting on MV PPA [19], single-word comprehension was assessed by a selected subset of 36 moderately difficult items of the Peabody Picture Vocabulary Test (PPVT) [71]. The proposed cut-off to define cases with MV PPA was a PPVT score and a Northwestern anagram test score < 60% [19]. In the current study, we did not use percentiles to define abnormality of performance but used a regression equation correcting for age or education effects and a modified t test assessing each individual case against a healthy control group [52, 64]. To date, no consensus exists, however, on which neuropsychological tests or which cut-offs to apply and thus considerable variation can arise when assigning a diagnosis of PPA. In this series of MV cases, the cut-off for single-word comprehension deficits was a priori defined based on the sum score of the AAT, in which words are presented in the auditory or written modality and need to be matched to a picture [51]. Three MV patients who showed object recognition problems measured with BORB (Table 1) also showed deficits on a purely verbal associative-semantic task (PALPA subtest 49), suggesting that both visual and verbal modalities of semantic representations are affected.

A detailed assessment of the single-word comprehension errors revealed that retrieving the nondominant

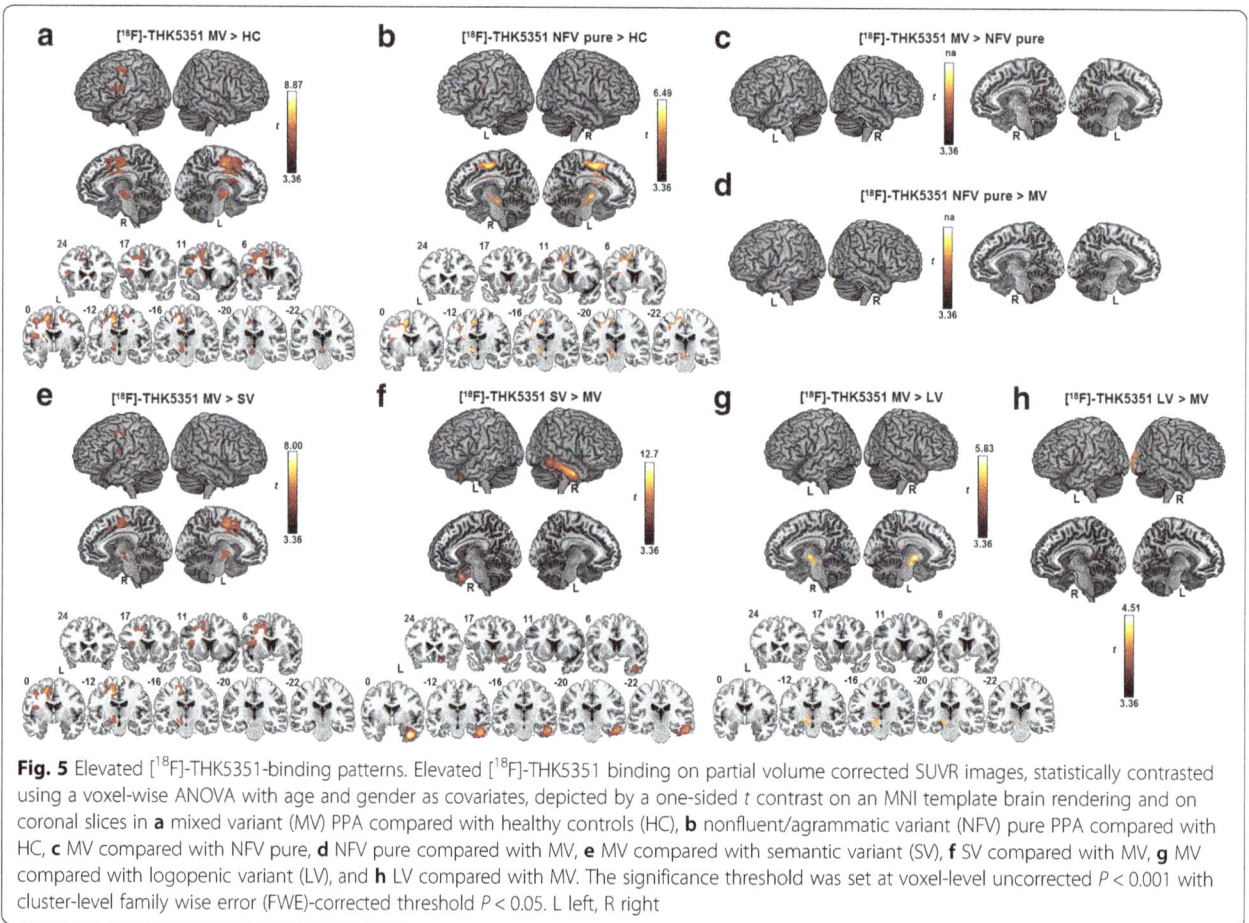

Fig. 5 Elevated [^{18}F]-THK5351-binding patterns. Elevated [^{18}F]-THK5351 binding on partial volume corrected SUVR images, statistically contrasted using a voxel-wise ANOVA with age and gender as covariates, depicted by a one-sided t contrast on an MNI template brain rendering and on coronal slices in **a** mixed variant (MV) PPA compared with healthy controls (HC), **b** nonfluent/agrammatic variant (NFV) pure PPA compared with HC, **c** MV compared with NFV pure, **d** NFV pure compared with MV, **e** MV compared with semantic variant (SV), **f** SV compared with MV, **g** MV compared with logopenic variant (LV), and **h** LV compared with MV. The significance threshold was set at voxel-level uncorrected $P < 0.001$ with cluster-level family wise error (FWE)-corrected threshold $P < 0.05$. L left, R right

meaning of a word was particularly problematic in MV PPA. This finding might relate to disturbances in top-down semantic control mechanisms [37, 72, 73]. In SV PPA, word comprehension problems are associated with atrophy of the anterior temporal lobes [29, 74, 75]. This has engendered the hub-and-spoke theory, which considers the anterior temporal pole as a hub region that binds together the distributed representations of the meaning of a word [28, 76]. The mechanism for the single-word comprehension deficits in MV probably differs fundamentally from that postulated in SV and also from the mechanism that may occur in LV. In LV, there is evidence for a phonological short-term memory deficit that may contribute to the hesitancy during spontaneous speech [77, 6]. This is related to atrophy of the temporo-parietal junction [77, 6]. The presence of word comprehension deficits in some LV cases may reflect expansion of atrophy to the posterior superior temporal sulcus and might be due to impaired lexical-semantic retrieval [30, 31]. We postulate that the single-word comprehension deficits in MV relate to the role of the inferior frontal cortex in the processing of word meaning [34]. The pars triangularis and the inferior frontal sulcus have been implicated in a variety of semantic processes, including

semantic working memory, dynamic uploading of semantic representations, semantic selection, and semantic control [33, 34, 36, 37, 73, 78]. The prominent meaning dominance effect in MV may suggest dysfunctional semantic control processes. Semantic control mechanisms in the pars triangularis would enable one to ignore the distracter picture, which was semantically related to the dominant meaning of that word, and select the less-frequent, nondominant meaning [73]. Meaning dominance effects have previously been located to left middle and superior temporal regions, but also to the right globus pallidus and putamen, based on task-based functional MRI studies in healthy controls [79]. A role of the basal ganglia has been demonstrated in suppressing irrelevant words [80]. Disturbance of frontal-subcortical systems influencing inhibitory semantic mechanisms has been linked to a circumscribed deficit in the selective attentional engagement of the semantic network on the basis of meaning frequency [81]. Meaning dominance effects on single-word comprehension deficits in MV PPA might possibly also relate to damage of white matter tracts connecting the main anterior temporal lobe with regions involved in cognitive semantic control such as the inferior frontal gyrus [34].

This hypothesis remains to be investigated using diffusion-weighted imaging which was not available in the current cohort. Deficits in semantic control have also been implied in the word comprehension deficits following left inferior frontal ischemic damage in stroke patients [72, 82]. Further empirical investigation is required to test these hypotheses and determine the origin of the single-word comprehension deficits in MV.

This study was the first to characterize MV PPA with [18F]-THK5351 PET. Elevated [18F]-THK5351 binding was present bilaterally in the supplementary motor area and left dorsal premotor cortex in both MV and NFV pure PPA (Fig. 5). These regions have been implicated previously in primary progressive apraxia of speech, a syndrome which shows underlying FTLD tauopathy at postmortem examination [12] and elevated retention of the tau PET tracer [18F]-AV1451 in the supplementary motor area, dorsal premotor cortex, and inferior frontal gyrus [11]. The supplementary motor area plays a crucial role in speech motor control [83], and premotor cortical involvement has been linked with the severity of speech apraxia [84]. Damage to the white matter tract connecting the supplementary motor area with the inferior frontal gyrus (i.e., the aslant tract) [16, 85, 86] affects the amount of distortion errors that NFV PPA patients make in spontaneous speech [86]. Apraxia of speech features in the current series of MV cases would be categorized as the 'phonetic type', dominated by sound distortions and distorted sound substitutions [12–14, 87, 88]. While apraxia of speech is not included in the proposed diagnostic criteria for MV PPA [20], all MV PPA cases in a previous case series also showed apraxia of speech accompanied by agrammatism and single-word comprehension deficits [27]. In that study, atrophy of the premotor cortex was observed in MV PPA, which could possibly be linked with their features of speech apraxia. We noticed that, by applying a more lenient statistical threshold, [18F]-THK5351 binding was also present in temporal regions in MV PPA but not in NFV PPA. The temporal lobe was also affected by atrophy in MV, which was consistent with previous MRI-based findings [20, 27]. Loss of the structural integrity of posterior temporal regions is associated with single word-comprehension problems [28, 30] and with prominent agrammatic features [84]. The left inferior frontal gyrus and middle frontal gyrus showed atrophy both in MV and in NFV PPA. These regions have been implicated in sentence comprehension as an index for agrammatism [89, 90].

Elevated [18F]-THK5351 binding in MV PPA did not only encompass cortical regions but also involved subcortical regions; i.e., the midbrain, thalamus, and basal ganglia. These regions are typically vulnerable to FTLD tauopathy corresponding to corticobasal degeneration (CBD) or progressive supranuclear palsy (PSP) pathology [91, 92], which can be visualized with the [18F]-THK5351 tracer [93, 94]. The striatum and subthalamic nucleus are involved early in the disease course of CBD, while the substantia nigra can be involved in later stages of the disease [92, 95]. A subset of MV and NFV cases in this study showed mild clinical signs and symptoms that may be indicative of underlying PSP or CBD pathology, including right-sided extrapyramidal signs or vertical eye movement abnormalities (Table 2). While the initial and most salient feature in these MV PPA cases was the language and speech impairment, these patients may develop a PSP- or CBD-like syndrome over time, similar to what has been reported to occur in patients with primary progressive apraxia of speech [42].

Besides binding to FTLD tauopathy, [18F]-THK5351 also binds to tau pathology of the Alzheimer's disease type [38]. At the individual patient level, the two amyloid-positive MV PPA cases showed elevated [18F]-THK5351 binding in the left temporoparietal junction but not in the midbrain (Fig. 4). This suggests that these MV cases have underlying Alzheimer's disease pathology. This would be in line with the positive amyloid PET result, indicative of an increased fibrillary amyloid load [39]. Amyloid PET positivity should, however, be cautiously interpreted in this age group, as it may also occur in the absence of cognitive deficits [43, 48, 63, 96]. However, numerically a proportion of two out of seven (29%) amyloid PET-positive cases exceeds the expected proportion based on studies in healthy controls of similar age (15%) [43, 48, 63]. The proportion of amyloid-positive MV cases in this study is lower than observed in a previous PPA study, which demonstrated amyloid-positivity in three out of four MV cases based on amyloid PET [10]. The latter study also demonstrated a higher prevalence of amyloid-positivity in MV compared with NFV pure cases [10]. This is consistent with our findings, but obviously must be considered preliminary given the low sample size. There were no differences in age between MV and NFV pure PPA and therefore age is unlikely to account for the higher prevalence of amyloid positivity in the MV cases. In one postmortem study, Alzheimer's disease pathology was present in four out of six MV cases [7]. In another series, the prevalence of Alzheimer's disease pathology was lower in MV PPA (25%, one out of four) and FTLD tauopathy was more prevalent (75%, three out of four) [27]. However, the negative amyloid PET in most MV patients virtually rules out Alzheimer's disease as the underlying cause of the cognitive deficits.

Implications for PPA classification

The current findings may have implications for possible revisions of the currently recommended PPA classification scheme [1]. In summary, the two most relevant points taken from the current study are the following. First, speech apraxia and agrammatism were relatively commonly associated with single-word comprehension deficits. In these patients, object knowledge was also mildly deficient according to standard neuropsychological tests. These deficits were, however, less pronounced than those seen in SV. Second, the underlying neurobiology did not appear fundamentally different between NFV pure and MV; [18F]-THK5351 binding patterns were comparable between MV and NFV pure, and structural MRI did not reveal a significant difference. Taken together, these two main observations do not justify the addition of a fourth subtype to the PPA classification scheme, principally given the close neurobiological similarity between MV and NFV pure as testified by the similarity in [18F]-THK5351 binding patterns. On the other hand, the exclusionary criteria of spared single-word comprehension and object knowledge for NFV might be questioned based on the current findings. Making these two exclusionary criteria less restrictive would provide for a proper classification of the cases we described as MV within the current three-variants scheme [1].

Study limitations

No firm conclusions regarding the underlying type of tauopathy can be drawn as this study is limited by the lack of postmortem confirmation. Furthermore, the total number of PPA patients included is rather small, which is partly inherent to the relatively low prevalence of the syndrome. A drawback of using [18F]-THK5351 PET is the nonspecific binding to an undefined molecular substrate in the basal ganglia [38, 40]. In-vivo experiments using selegiline displacement in patients with Alzheimer's disease and PSP indicate that [18F]-THK5351 may bind to MAO-B [40], suggesting that [18F]-THK5351 binds to astrogliosis. Nonetheless, elevated [18F]-THK5351 binding in the current study was highly focalized and colocalized with regions known to be associated with conditions in which a tauopathy is the underlying neuropathological cause [91, 92, 97, 98].

Conclusions

A PPA subtype characterized by speech apraxia and/or agrammatism with concomitant single-word comprehension problems in an early disease stage clearly exists. MV PPA showed focal [18F]-THK5351 PET binding in the supplementary motor area, premotor cortex, midbrain, and basal ganglia, highly similar to NFV pure. Given the high neurobiological similarity, the addition of a fourth subtype to the three currently used subtypes is not warranted based on the current data. However, the exclusionary criteria of spared single-word comprehension and object knowledge for NFV may need to be

reconsidered based on the current data. At a basic scientific level, the relatively frequent occurrence of single-word comprehension problems in NFV resonates with the increasing evidence for a role of the inferior frontal cortex in a variety of semantic processes.

Abbreviations

[11C]-PIB: [11C]-Pittsburgh Compound B; AAT: Aachen Aphasia Test; ANOVA: Analysis of variance; AVF: Animal Verbal Fluency; $A\beta_{1-42}$: Amyloid-β_{1-42}; BNT: Boston Naming Test; BORB: Birmingham Object Recognition Battery; CBD: Corticobasal degeneration; CDR: Clinical Dementia Rating; CPM: Colored Progressive Matrices; CSF: Cerebrospinal fluid; CT: Computed tomography; DIAS: Diagnostisch Instrument voor Apraxie van de Spraak; FTLD: Frontotemporal lobar degeneration; FWE: Family wise error; FWHM: Full-width half-maximum; LV: Logopenic variant; MAO-B: Monoamine oxidase-B; MMSE: Mini-Mental State Examination; MRI: Magnetic resonance imaging; MV: Mixed variant; NFV: Nonfluent/agrammatic variant; p_{181}-tau: Phospho$_{181}$-tau; PALPA: Psycholinguistic Assessment of Language Processing in Aphasia; PET: Positron emission tomography; PPA: Primary progressive aphasia; PPT: Pyramids and Palm trees Test; PPVT: Peabody Picture Vocabulary Test; PSP: Progressive supranuclear palsy; PVC: Partial volume corrected; SUVR: Standardized uptake value ratio; SV: Semantic variant; t-tau: Total tau; WEZT: Werkwoorden En Zinnen Test

Acknowledgements
The authors would like to thank the staff of Nuclear Medicine, Neurology and Radiology at the University Hospitals Leuven. Special thanks to Kwinten Porters, Jef Van Loock and Nathalie Mertens for assistance with the PET scanning procedure and to Dr. Lieven Declercq for establishing the synthesis procedure for the tau PET tracer. Also, many thanks to all patients, their family, and all volunteers who made this work possible.

Funding
[18F]-THK5351 precursors were provided through a material transfer agreement between KU Leuven Research & Development (LRD) and Tohoku University, Japan. RV and KVL are senior clinical investigators of the Flemish Research Foundation (FWO) and RB is a postdoctoral fellow of the FWO. Funded by the Stichting Alzheimer Onderzoek #15005 and the Flemish government (Vlaams Initiatief voor Netwerken voor Dementie Onderzoek (VIND)). No funders had a role in the design of the study, data collection, analysis or interpretation of the data, or in writing the manuscript.

Authors' contributions
All authors fulfill the criteria for authorship and no one else who fulfills these criteria has been excluded. RV, GB, and KVL designed the study. RV, AS, and YP clinically diagnosed patients prior to study entry. JS, SG, KM, RB, CE, ED, and KVB conducted neuropsychological and neurolinguistic assessments. JS, SG, KM, and AGL were involved in analyzing neuropsychological and neurolinguistic data. JS, SG, CE, and RP were involved in MRI data collection and/or analysis. GB was involved in PET tracer development. JS, KVL, MK, and PD were involved in PET data collection and/or analysis. All authors were involved in writing and critically revising the article, and all have approved the final submitted version. RV accepts full responsibility for the work and controlled the decision to publish.

Consent for publication

Not applicable.

Competing interests

The authors declare that they have no competing interests.

Author details

[1]Laboratory for Cognitive Neurology, Department of Neurosciences, KU Leuven, Herestraat 49, 3000 Leuven, Belgium. [2]Alzheimer Research Centre KU Leuven, Leuven Research Institute for Neuroscience & Disease, KU Leuven, Herestraat 49, 3000 Leuven, Belgium. [3]Neurology Department, University Hospitals Leuven, Herestraat 49 - box 7003, 3000 Leuven, Belgium. [4]Neurodegenerative Brain Diseases Group, Center for Molecular Neurology, VIB, Universiteitsplein 1, 2610 Antwerp, Belgium. [5]Institute Born-Bunge, Neuropathology and Laboratory of Neurochemistry and Behavior, University of Antwerp, Universiteitsplein 1, 2610 Antwerp, Belgium. [6]Neurology Department, University Hospitals Ghent, Corneel Heymanslaan 10, 9000 Ghent, Belgium. [7]Old Age Psychiatry Department, GGZinGeest, Van Hilligaertstraat 21, 1072 JX Amsterdam, The Netherlands. [8]Alzheimer Center & Department of Neurology, VU University Medical Center, De Boelelaan 1117, 1081 HV Amsterdam, The Netherlands. [9]Radiology Department, University Hospitals Leuven, Herestraat 49, Leuven 30000, Belgium. [10]Laboratory of Radiopharmaceutical Research, KU Leuven, Herestraat 49, 3000 Leuven, Belgium. [11]Nuclear Medicine and Molecular Imaging, University Hospitals Leuven, Herestraat 49, 3000 Leuven, Belgium.

References

1. Gorno-Tempini ML, Hillis a E, Weintraub S, Kertesz a MM, Cappa SF, et al. Classification of primary progressive aphasia and its variants. Neurology. 2011;76:1–10.
2. Ash S, McMillan C, Gunawardena D, Avants B, Morgan B, Khan A, et al. Speech errors in progressive non-fluent aphasia. Brain Lang. 2010;113:13–20.
3. Hodges JR, Patterson K, Oxbury S, Funnell E. Semantic dementia. Progressive fluent aphasia with temporal lobe atrophy. Brain. 1992;115:1783–806.
4. Bozeat S, Lambon Ralph MA, Patterson K, Garrard P, Hodges JR. Non-verbal semantic impairment in semantic dementia. Neuropsychologia. 2000;38:1207–15.
5. Leyton CE, Savage S, Irish M, Schubert S, Piguet O, Ballard KJ, et al. Verbal repetition in primary progressive aphasia and Alzheimer's disease. J Alzheimers Dis. 2014;41:575–85.
6. Henry ML, Wilson SM, Babiak MC, Mandelli ML, Beeson PM, Miller ZA, et al. Phonological processing in primary progressive aphasia. J Cogn Neurosci. 2015;1–13.
7. Mesulam M-M, Weintraub S, Rogalski EJ, Wieneke C, Geula C, Bigio EH. Asymmetry and heterogeneity of Alzheimer's and frontotemporal pathology in primary progressive aphasia. Brain. 2014;137:1176–92.
8. Leyton CE, Britton AK, Hodges JR, Halliday GM, Kril JJ. Distinctive pathological mechanisms involved in primary progressive aphasias. Neurobiol Aging. 2016;38:82–92.
9. Harris JM, Gall C, Thompson JC, Richardson AMT, Neary D, du Plessis D, et al. Classification and pathology of primary progressive aphasia. Neurology. 2013;81:1832–9.
10. Santos-Santos MA, Rabinovici GD, Iaccarino L, Ayakta N, Tammewar G, Lobach I, et al. Rates of amyloid imaging positivity in patients with primary progressive aphasia. JAMA Neurol. 2018;75:342–52.

11. Utianski RL, Whitwell JL, Schwarz CG, Senjem ML, Tosakulwong N, Duffy JR, et al. Tau-PET imaging with [18F]AV-1451 in primary progressive apraxia of speech. Cortex. 2018;99:358–74.
12. Josephs KA, Duffy JR, Strand EA, Whitwell JL, Layton KF, Parisi JE, et al. Clinicopathological and imaging correlates of progressive aphasia and apraxia of speech. Brain. 2006;129:1385–98.
13. Josephs KA, Duffy JR, Strand EA, Machulda MM, Senjem ML, Master AV, et al. Characterizing a neurodegenerative syndrome: primary progressive apraxia of speech. Brain. 2012;135:1522–36.
14. Josephs KA, Duffy JR, Strand EA, Machulda MM, Senjem ML, Lowe V, et al. Syndromes dominated by apraxia of speech show distinct characteristics from agrammatic PPA. Neurology. 2013;81:337–45.
15. Galantucci S, Tartaglia MC, Wilson SM, Henry ML, Filippi M, Agosta F, et al. White matter damage in primary progressive aphasias: a diffusion tensor tractography study. Brain. 2011;134:3011–29.
16. Mandelli ML, Vilaplana E, Brown JA, Hubbard HI, Binney RJ, Attygalle S, et al. Healthy brain connectivity predicts atrophy progression in non-fluent variant of primary progressive aphasia. Brain. 2016;139:2778–91.
17. Marcotte K, Graham NL, Fraser KC, Meltzer JA, Tang-Wai DF, Chow TW, et al. White matter disruption and connected speech in non-fluent and semantic variants of primary progressive aphasia. Dement Geriatr Cogn Dis Extra. 2017;7:52–73.
18. Hickok G, Poeppel D. Neural basis of speech perception. Handb Clin Neurol. 2015;129:149–60.
19. Mesulam M, Wieneke C, Rogalski E, Cobia D, Thompson C, Weintraub S. Quantitative template for subtyping primary progressive aphasia. Arch Neurol. 2009;66:1545–51.
20. Mesulam M-M, Wieneke C, Thompson C, Rogalski E, Weintraub S. Quantitative classification of primary progressive aphasia at early and mild impairment stages. Brain. 2012;135:1537–53.
21. Vandenberghe R. Classification of the primary progressive aphasias: principles and review of progress since 2011. Alzheimers Res Ther. 2016;8:16.
22. Martersteck A, Murphy C, Rademaker A, Wieneke C, Weintraub S, Chen K, et al. Is in vivo amyloid distribution asymmetric in primary progressive aphasia? Ann Neurol. 2016;79:496–501.
23. Giannini LAA, Irwin DJ, McMillan CT, Ash S, Rascovsky K, Wolk DA, et al. Clinical marker for Alzheimer disease pathology in logopenic primary progressive aphasia. Neurology. 2017;88:2276–84.
24. Sajjadi SA, Patterson K, Arnold RJ, Watson PC, Nestor PJ. Primary progressive aphasia: a tale of two syndromes and the rest. Neurology. 2012;78:1670–7.
25. Wicklund MR, Duffy JR, Strand EA, Machulda MM, Whitwell JL, Josephs KA. Quantitative application of the primary progressive aphasia consensus criteria. Neurology. 2014;82:1119–26.
26. Hoffman P, Sajjadi SA, Patterson K, Nestor PJ. Data-driven classification of patients with primary progressive aphasia. Brain Lang Academic Press. 2017; 174:86–93.
27. Spinelli EG, Mandelli ML, Miller ZA, Santos-Santos MA, Wilson SM, Agosta F, et al. Typical and atypical pathology in primary progressive aphasia variants. Ann Neurol. 2017;81:430–43.
28. Lambon-Ralph MA, Jefferies E, Patterson K, Rogers TT. The neural and computational bases of semantic cognition. Nat Rev Neurosci. 2017;18:42–55.
29. Mummery CJ, Patterson K, Wise RJ, Vandenberghe R, Vandenbergh R, Price CJ, et al. Disrupted temporal lobe connections in semantic dementia. Brain. 1999;122:61–73.
30. Vandenbulcke M, Peeters R, Dupont P, Van Hecke P, Vandenberghe R. Word reading and posterior temporal dysfunction in amnestic mild cognitive impairment. Cereb Cortex. 2007;17:542–51.
31. Nelissen N, Pazzaglia M, Vandenbulcke M, Sunaert S, Fannes K, Dupont P, et al. Gesture discrimination in primary progressive aphasia: the intersection between gesture and language processing pathways. J Neurosci. 2010;30:6334–41.
32. Cope TE, Sohoglu E, Sedley W, Patterson K, Jones PS, Wiggins J, et al. Evidence for causal top-down frontal contributions to predictive processes in speech perception. Nat Commun. 2017;8:2154.
33. Liuzzi AG, Bruffaerts R, Peeters R, Adamczuk K, Keuleers E, De Deyne S, et al. Cross-modal representation of spoken and written word meaning in left pars triangularis. NeuroImage. 2017;150:292–307.

34. Goldberg RF, Perfetti CA, Fiez JA, Schneider W. Selective retrieval of abstract semantic knowledge in left prefrontal cortex. J Neurosci. 2007;27:3790–8.

35. Demb JB, Desmond JE, Wagner AD, Vaidya CJ, Glover GH, Gabrieli JD. Semantic encoding and retrieval in the left inferior prefrontal cortex: a functional MRI study of task difficulty and process specificity. J Neurosci. 1995;15:5870–8.

36. Thompson-Schill SL, D'Esposito M, Aguirre GK, Farah MJ. Role of left inferior prefrontal cortex in retrieval of semantic knowledge: a reevaluation. Proc Natl Acad Sci U S A. 1997;94:14792–7.

37. Whitney C, Kirk M, O'Sullivan J, Lambon Ralph MA, Jefferies E. The neural organization of semantic control: TMS evidence for a distributed network in left inferior frontal and posterior middle temporal gyrus. Cereb Cortex. 2011;21:1066–75.

38. Harada R, Okamura N, Furumoto S, Furukawa K, Ishiki A, Tomita N, et al. [^{18}F]-THK5351: A Novel PET Radiotracer for Imaging Neurofibrillary Pathology in Alzheimer Disease. J Nucl Med. 2016;57:208–14.

39. Klunk WE, Engler H, Nordberg A, Wang Y, Blomqvist G, Holt DP, et al. Imaging brain amyloid in Alzheimer's disease with Pittsburgh compound-B. Ann Neurol. 2004;55:306–19.

40. Ng KP, Pascoal TA, Mathotaarachchi S, Therriault J, Kang MS, Shin M, et al. Monoamine oxidase B inhibitor, selegiline, reduces [18F]-THK5351 uptake in the human brain. Alzheimers Res Ther. 2017;9:25.

41. Saura J, Luque JM, Cesura AM, Da Prada M, Chan-Palay V, Huber G, et al. Increased monoamine oxidase B activity in plaque-associated astrocytes of Alzheimer brains revealed by quantitative enzyme radioautography. Neuroscience. 1994;62:15–30.

42. Josephs KA, Duffy JR, Strand EA, Machulda MM, Senjem ML, Gunter JL, et al. The evolution of primary progressive apraxia of speech. Brain. 2014;137:2783–95.

43. Adamczuk K, Schaeverbeke J, Vandenberghe HMJ, Lilja J, Nelissen N, Van Laere K, et al. Diagnostic value of cerebrospinal fluid Abeta ratios in preclinical Alzheimer's disease. Alzheimers Res Ther. 2015;7:75.

44. Grube M, Bruffaerts R, Schaeverbeke J, Neyens V, De Weer A-S, Seghers A, et al. Core auditory processing deficits in primary progressive aphasia. Brain. 2016;139:1817–29.

45. Folstein MF, Folstein SE, McHugh PR. Mini-mental state. A practical method for grading the cognitive state of patients for the clinician. J Psychiatr Res. 1975;12:189–98.

46. Hughes CP, Berg L, Danziger WL, Coben LA, Martin RL. A new clinical scale for the staging of dementia. Br J Psychiatry. 1982;140:566–72.

47. Nelissen N, Vandenbulcke M, Fannes K, Verbruggen A, Peeters R, Dupont P, et al. Abeta amyloid deposition in the language system and how the brain responds. Brain. 2007;130:2055–69.

48. Adamczuk K, Schaeverbeke J, Nelissen N, Neyens V, Vandenbulcke M, Goffin K, et al. Amyloid imaging in cognitively normal older adults: comparison between [18F]-flutemetamol and [11C]-Pittsburgh compound B. Eur J Nucl Med Mol Imaging. 2016;43:142–51.

49. Adamczuk K, De Weer AS, Nelissen N, Dupont P, Sunaert S, Bettens K, et al. Functional changes in the language network in response to increased amyloid β deposition in cognitively intact older adults. Cereb Cortex. 2014; 26:358–73.

50. Mariën P, Mampaey E, Vervaet A, Saerens J, De Deyn PP. Normative data for the Boston naming test in native Dutch-speaking Belgian elderly. Brain Lang. 1998;65:447–67.

51. Graetz P, De Bleser R, Willmes K. Akense Afasietest, Nederlandse versie. Lisse: Swets & Zeitlinger; 1992.

52. Crawford JR, Howell DC. Comparing an individual's test score against norms derived from small samples. Clin Neuropsychol. 1998;12:482–6.

53. Kay J, Lesser R, Coltheart M. Psycholinguistic assessments of language processing in aphasia (PALPA): an introduction. Aphasiology; 1996;10:159–180.

54. Howard D, Patterson KE, Thames Valley Test Company. The pyramids and palm trees test. Bury St Edmunds: Thames Valley Test Company Ltd.; 1992;16.

55. Riddoch MJ, Humphreys GW. BORB : Birmingham object recognition battery. Psychol Press. Hove: Lawrence Erlbaum; 1993;388.

56. Bastiaanse R, Maas E. Werkwoorden en Zinnentest, vol. 95. Lisse: Swets & Zeitlinger; 2000.

57. Feiken J, Jonkers R. DIAS : Diagnostisch Instrument voor Apraxie van de Spraak. Houten: Bohn Stafleu van Loghum; 2012;

58. Müller-Gärtner HW, Links JM, Prince JL, Bryan RN, McVeigh E, Leal JP, et al. Measurement of radiotracer concentration in brain gray matter using

59. positron emission tomography: MRI-based correction for partial volume effects. J Cereb Blood Flow Metab. 1992;12:571–83.

59. Ashburner J, Friston KJ. Voxel-based morphometry—the methods. NeuroImage. 2000;11:805–21.

60. Gillebert CR, Schaeverbeke J, Bastin C, Neyens V, Bruffaerts R, De Weer A-S, et al. 3D shape perception in posterior cortical atrophy: a visual neuroscience perspective. J Neurosci. 2015;35:12673–92.

61. Schaeverbeke J, Evenepoel C, Bruffaerts R, Van Laere K, Bormans G, Dries E, et al. Cholinergic depletion and basal forebrain volume in primary progressive aphasia. NeuroImage Clin. 2017;13:271–9.

62. Barnes J, Ridgway GR, Bartlett J, Henley SMD, Lehmann M, Hobbs N, et al. Head size, age and gender adjustment in MRI studies: a necessary nuisance? NeuroImage. 2010;53:1244–55.

63. Adamczuk K, De Weer AS, Nelissen N, Chen K, Sleegers K, Bettens K, et al. Polymorphism of brain derived neurotrophic factor influences beta amyloid load in cognitively intact apolipoprotein E e4 carriers. NeuroImage Clin. 2013;2:512–20.

64. Crawford JR, Garthwaite PH. Comparing patients' predicted test scores from a regression equation with their obtained scores: a significance test and point estimate of abnormality with accompanying confidence limits. Neuropsychology. 2006;20:259–71.

65. Griffiths D, Stirling WD, Weldon KL. Understanding data : principles & practice of statistics. Brisbane: Wiley;1998.

66. Keuleers E, Brysbaert M, New B. SUBTLEX-NL: a new measure for Dutch word frequency based on film subtitles. Behav Res Methods. 2010;42:643–50.

67. Armstrong BC, Tokowicz N, Plaut DC. eDom: norming software and relative meaning frequencies for 544 English homonyms. Behav Res Methods. 2012; 44:1015–27.

68. De Deyne S, Navarro DJ, Storms G. Better explanations of lexical and semantic cognition using networks derived from continued rather than single-word associations. Behav Res Methods. 2013;45:480–98.

69. Code C, Tree J, Ball M. The influence of psycholinguistic variables on articulatory errors in naming in progressive motor speech degeneration. Clin Linguist Phon Taylor & Francis. 2011;25:1074–80.

70. Poline JB, Worsley KJ, Evans a C, Friston KJ. Combining spatial extent and peak intensity to test for activations in functional imaging. NeuroImage. 1997;5:83–96.

71. Dunn LM. Peabody picture vocabulary test. London: Pearson. 2006;

72. Jefferies E, Lambon Ralph MA. Semantic impairment in stroke aphasia versus semantic dementia: a case-series comparison. Brain. 2006;129:2132–47.

73. Badre D, Poldrack RA, Paré-Blagoev EJ, Insler RZ, Wagner AD. Dissociable controlled retrieval and generalized selection mechanisms in ventrolateral prefrontal cortex. Neuron Cell Press. 2005;47:907–18.

74. Binney RJ, Embleton KV, Jefferies E, Parker GJM, Lambon Ralph MA. The ventral and inferolateral aspects of the anterior temporal lobe are crucial in semantic memory: evidence from a novel direct comparison of distortion-corrected fMRI, rTMS, and semantic dementia. Cereb Cortex. 2010;20:2728–38.

75. Hodges JR, Patterson K. Semantic dementia: a unique clinicopathological syndrome. Lancet Neurol. 2007;6:1004–14.

76. Rogers TT, Lambon Ralph MA, Garrard P, Bozeat S, McClelland JL, Hodges JR, et al. Structure and deterioration of semantic memory: a neuropsychological and computational investigation. Psychol Rev. 2004;111:205–35.

77. Gorno-Tempini ML, Brambati SM, Ginex V, Ogar J, Dronkers NF, Marcone A, et al. The logopenic/phonological variant of primary progressive aphasia. Neurology. 2008;71:1227–34.

78. Wagner AD, Paré-Blagoev EJ, Clark J, Poldrack RA. Recovering meaning: left prefrontal cortex guides controlled semantic retrieval. Neuron. 2001;31:329–38.

79. Grindrod CM, Garnett EO, Malyutina S, den Ouden DB. Effects of representational distance between meanings on the neural correlates of semantic ambiguity. Brain Lang. 2014;139:23–35.

80. Ali N, Green DW, Kherif F, Devlin JT, Price CJ. The role of the left head of caudate in suppressing irrelevant words. J Cogn Neurosci. 2010;22:2369–86.

81. Copland D. The basal ganglia and semantic engagement: potential insights from semantic priming in individuals with subcortical vascular lesions, Parkinson's disease, and cortical lesions. J Int Neuropsychol Soc. 2003;9:1041–52.

82. Noonan KA, Jefferies E, Corbett F, Lambon Ralph MA. Elucidating the nature of deregulated semantic cognition in semantic aphasia: evidence for the roles of prefrontal and temporo-parietal cortices. J Cogn Neurosci. 2010;22:1597–613.

83. Alario F-X, Chainay H, Lehericy S, Cohen L. The role of the supplementary motor area (SMA) in word production. Brain Res. 2006;1076:129–43.

84. Whitwell JL, Duffy JR, Strand EA, Xia R, Mandrekar J, Machulda MM, et al. Distinct regional anatomic and functional correlates of neurodegenerative apraxia of speech and aphasia: an MRI and FDG-PET study. Brain Lang. 2013;125:245–52.

85. Catani M, Mesulam MM, Jakobsen E, Malik F, Martersteck A, Wieneke C, et al. A novel frontal pathway underlies verbal fluency in primary progressive aphasia. Brain. 2013;136:2619–28.

86. Mandelli ML, Caverzasi E, Binney RJ, Henry ML, Lobach I, Block N, et al. Frontal white matter tracts sustaining speech production in primary progressive aphasia. J Neurosci. 2014;34:9754–67.

87. Botha H, Duffy JR, Whitwell JL, Strand EA, Machulda MM, Schwarz CG, et al. Clinical and imaging features of primary progressive aphasia and apraxia of speech. Cortex. 2015;69:220–36.

88. Whitwell JL, Duffy JR, Machulda MM, Clark HM, Strand EA, Senjem ML, et al. Tracking the development of agrammatic aphasia: a tensor-based morphometry study. Cortex. 2017;90:138–48.

89. Amici S, Ogar J, Brambati SM, Miller BL, Neuhaus J, Dronkers NL, et al. Performance in specific language tasks correlates with regional volume changes in progressive aphasia. Cogn Behav Neurol. 2007;20:203–11.

90. Wilson SM, Dronkers NF, Ogar JM, Jang J, Growdon ME, Agosta F, et al. Neural correlates of syntactic processing in the nonfluent variant of primary progressive aphasia. J Neurosci. 2010;30:16845–54.

91. Dickson DW. Neuropathologic differentiation of progressive supranuclear palsy and corticobasal degeneration. J Neurol. 1999;246(Suppl):II6–15.

92. Dickson DW, Bergeron C, Chin SS, Duyckaerts C, Horoupian D, Ikeda K, et al. Office of Rare Diseases neuropathologic criteria for corticobasal degeneration. J Neuropathol Exp Neurol. 2002;61:935–46.

93. Ishiki A, Harada R, Okamura N, Tomita N, Rowe CC, Villemagne VL, et al. Tau imaging with [18F]THK-5351 in progressive supranuclear palsy. Eur J Neurol. 2017;24:130–6.

94. Kikuchi A, Okamura N, Hasegawa T, Harada R, Watanuki S, Funaki Y, et al. In vivo visualization of tau deposits in corticobasal syndrome by [18F]-THK5351 PET. Neurology. 2016;87:2309–16.

95. Ling H, Kovacs GG, Vonsattel JPG, Davey K, Mok KY, Hardy J, et al. Astrogliopathy predominates the earliest stage of corticobasal degeneration pathology. Brain. 2016;139:3237–52.

96. Pike KE, Ellis KA, Villemagne VL, Good N, Chételat G, Ames D, et al. Cognition and beta-amyloid in preclinical Alzheimer's disease: data from the AIBL study. Neuropsychologia. 2011;49:2384–90.

97. Josephs KA, Dickson DW, Murray ME, Senjem ML, Parisi JE, Petersen RC, et al. Quantitative neurofibrillary tangle density and brain volumetric MRI analyses in Alzheimer's disease presenting as logopenic progressive aphasia. Brain Lang. 2013;127:127–34.

98. Brown JA, Hua AY, Trujillo A, Attygalle S, Binney RJ, Spina S, et al. Advancing functional dysconnectivity and atrophy in progressive supranuclear palsy. NeuroImage Clin. 2017;16:564–74.

Alzheimer disease pathology and the cerebrospinal fluid proteome

Loïc Dayon[1][*] [iD], Antonio Núñez Galindo[1], Jérôme Wojcik[2], Ornella Cominetti[1], John Corthésy[1], Aikaterini Oikonomidi[3], Hugues Henry[4], Martin Kussmann[1,6], Eugenia Migliavacca[1], India Severin[1], Gene L. Bowman[1] and Julius Popp[3,5]

Abstract

Background: Altered proteome profiles have been reported in both postmortem brain tissues and body fluids of subjects with Alzheimer disease (AD), but their broad relationships with AD pathology, amyloid pathology, and tau-related neurodegeneration have not yet been fully explored. Using a robust automated MS-based proteomic biomarker discovery workflow, we measured cerebrospinal fluid (CSF) proteomes to explore their association with well-established markers of core AD pathology.

Methods: Cross-sectional analysis was performed on CSF collected from 120 older community-dwelling adults with normal ($n = 48$) or impaired cognition ($n = 72$). LC-MS quantified hundreds of proteins in the CSF. CSF concentrations of β-amyloid 1–42 (Aβ$_{1-42}$), tau, and tau phosphorylated at threonine 181 (P-tau181) were determined with immunoassays. First, we explored proteins relevant to biomarker-defined AD. Then, correlation analysis of CSF proteins with CSF markers of amyloid pathology, neuronal injury, and tau hyperphosphorylation (i.e., Aβ$_{1-42}$, tau, P-tau181) was performed using Pearson's correlation coefficient and Bonferroni correction for multiple comparisons.

Results: We quantified 790 proteins in CSF samples with MS. Four CSF proteins showed an association with CSF Aβ$_{1-42}$ levels (p value ≤ 0.05 with correlation coefficient (R) ≥ 0.38). We identified 50 additional CSF proteins associated with CSF tau and 46 proteins associated with CSF P-tau181 (p value ≤ 0.05 with $R \geq 0.37$). The majority of those proteins that showed such associations were brain-enriched proteins. Gene Ontology annotation revealed an enrichment for synaptic proteins and proteins originating from reelin-producing cells and the myelin sheath.

Conclusions: We used an MS-based proteomic workflow to profile the CSF proteome in relation to cerebral AD pathology. We report strong evidence of previously reported CSF proteins and several novel CSF proteins specifically associated with amyloid pathology or neuronal injury and tau hyperphosphorylation.

Keywords: Alzheimer disease, Amyloid, Biomarker, Cerebrospinal fluid, CSF, Mass spectrometry, Proteomics, Tau, Tandem mass tag

Background

Proteome alterations have been identified in a multitude of pathologies, such as cancer, metabolic disorders, and brain diseases [1]. Several circulating protein markers of neurodegenerative diseases, such as Parkinson's disease or Alzheimer disease (AD), have been reported [2], but the ones with consistent findings or of current clinical utility are very few [3]. AD is the most common form of

dementia, and there is still an urgent need for the definition of early detection markers as well as for a better understanding of its pathogenesis. In the latter perspective, cerebrospinal fluid (CSF) represents a key biofluid to decipher altered protein levels and pathways in diseases of the central nervous system (CNS) using large-scale proteomic technologies, such as MS-based platforms.

Because of the proximity of CSF to the brain and the presence of proteins in CSF specific to the brain [4, 5], the CSF proteome can reflect the biochemical and metabolic changes in the CNS. In particular, despite the definitive

---

* Correspondence: loic.dayon@rd.nestle.com
[1]Nestlé Institute of Health Sciences, Lausanne, Switzerland
Full list of author information is available at the end of the article

confirmation of the diagnosis of AD being possible today only at brain autopsy, specific CSF peptides and proteins (i.e., β-amyloid 1–42 [Aβ$_{1-42}$], total tau, and hyperphosphorylated tau [P-tau]) linked to the main hallmarks of AD pathology, such as amyloid plaques and neurofibrillary tangles, can complement clinical examination for the diagnosis of AD [6, 7].

There is now strong evidence that suggests the development of AD pathology begins years to decades prior to the onset of the first clinical signs. Thus, on one hand, elderly persons with normal cognition may already have cerebral AD pathology and be at the preclinical stage of the disease [8]; on the other hand, subjects with cognitive deficits may present with cognitive impairment suggesting AD but not primarily or only partially related to AD pathology. New research criteria consider AD as a biological *continuum* across the clinical spectrum from asymptomatic stage to advanced dementia and emphasize the utility of biomarkers of AD pathology for an accurate diagnosis, in particular at the preclinical and prodromal disease stages [8–10]. In this respect, endophenotype approaches have been proposed as innovative ways to better address AD stages using proxy measures such as the concentrations of the aforementioned CSF markers of core AD pathology [11].

Several studies have characterized the CSF proteome with MS but mainly using sample pools and/or a limited number of samples [12–14]. Because of technical constraints such as limited sample throughput [15], studies in larger clinical cohorts using MS-based proteomics are indeed limited [16–21]. In recent years, our group [22] and other groups [23, 24] have demonstrated that MS-based proteomics enables protein biomarker discovery in large numbers of human clinical samples, providing increased statistical power and result robustness [21, 22, 25]. Although most of these studies were performed with plasma or serum samples [26], the analysis of the CSF proteome and its alteration using MS-based proteomics in larger cohorts has been mostly unexplored.

Our aim in this study was to investigate the CSF proteome in relation to the core elements of CSF-defined AD pathology in older adults (*n* = 120) with normal and impaired cognition using MS-based shotgun proteomics (Fig. 1). We evaluated whether the CSF proteome could relate to AD pathology, defined as the combined presence of both amyloid pathology and tau pathology. We then explored more deeply the relationships of the quantified proteins in CSF with well-established biomarkers of amyloid pathology, neuronal injury, and tau hyperphosphorylation

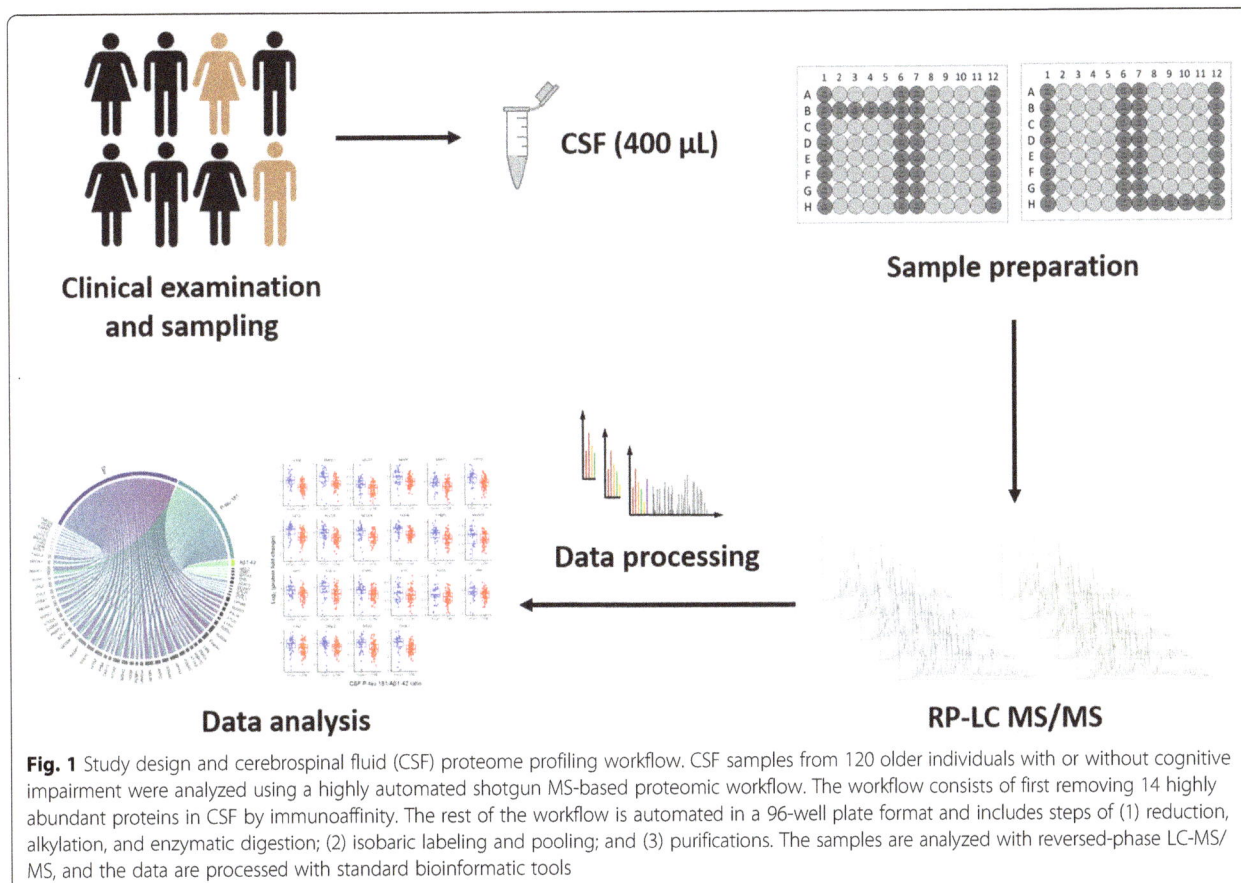

Fig. 1 Study design and cerebrospinal fluid (CSF) proteome profiling workflow. CSF samples from 120 older individuals with or without cognitive impairment were analyzed using a highly automated shotgun MS-based proteomic workflow. The workflow consists of first removing 14 highly abundant proteins in CSF by immunoaffinity. The rest of the workflow is automated in a 96-well plate format and includes steps of (1) reduction, alkylation, and enzymatic digestion; (2) isobaric labeling and pooling; and (3) purifications. The samples are analyzed with reversed-phase LC-MS/MS, and the data are processed with standard bioinformatic tools

(i.e., $A\beta_{1-42}$, tau, and tau phosphorylated at threonine 181 [P-tau181], respectively).

Methods

Study design

One hundred twenty community-dwelling participants were included in this study, of whom 48 were cognitively healthy volunteers and 72 had mild cognitive impairment (MCI) ($n = 63$) or mild dementia of AD type ($n = 9$) [27]. Diagnosis of MCI or dementia was based on neuropsychological and clinical evaluation and made by a consensus conference of psychiatrists and/or neurologists as well as neuropsychologists prior to inclusion in the study. The participants with cognitive impairment were recruited from among outpatients who were referred to the Memory Clinics, Departments of Psychiatry, and Department of Clinical Neurosciences, University Hospitals of Lausanne, Switzerland. They had no major psychiatric disorders or substance abuse or severe or unstable physical illness that might contribute to cognitive impairment, had a Clinical Dementia Rating (CDR) [28] score > 0, and met the clinical diagnostic criteria for MCI [29] or AD mild dementia according to the recommendations of the National Institute on Aging-Alzheimer's Association [30]. In the current study, nine subjects met criteria for probable AD dementia. Because there is a clinical *continuum* between MCI and mild dementia, and because the participants with cognitive impairment were patients from memory clinics recruited in the same way regardless of MCI or mild dementia classification, these subjects were grouped and labeled as cognitively impaired with CDR > 0 (Table 1). The control

subjects were recruited through journal announcements or word of mouth and had no history, symptoms, or signs of relevant psychiatric or neurologic disease and no cognitive impairment (CDR = 0). All participants underwent a comprehensive clinical and neuropsychological evaluation, structural brain imaging, and venous and lumbar punctures [27]. Magnetic resonance imaging (MRI) and computed tomographic scans were used to exclude cerebral pathologies possibly interfering with cognitive performance.

Neuropsychological tests were used to assess cognitive performance in the domains of memory [31], language, and visuoconstructive functions. The Mini Mental State Examination [32] was used to assess participants' global cognitive performance. Depression and anxiety were assessed using the Hospital Anxiety and Depression Scale [33]. The psychosocial and functional assessments included activities of daily living and instrumental activities of daily living, the Neuropsychiatric Inventory Questionnaire, and the Informant Questionnaire on Cognitive Decline in the Elderly [34], and these were completed by family members of the participants. All tests and scales are validated and widely used in the field.

CSF sample collection

Lumbar punctures were performed between 8:30 a.m. and 9:30 a.m. after overnight fasting. A standardized technique with a 22-gauge "atraumatic" spinal needle and a sitting or lying position was applied [35]. A volume of 10–12 ml of CSF was collected in polypropylene tubes. Routine cell count and protein quantification were performed. The remaining CSF was frozen in aliquots

Table 1 Demographics and clinical characteristics

	P-tau181/$A\beta_{1-42}$ ≤ 0.0779 (n = 78)	P-tau181/$A\beta_{1-42}$ > 0.0779 (n = 42)	CDR = 0 (n = 48)	CDR > 0 (n = 72)
Age, yr, mean (SD)	68.4 (8.3)	74.1 (5.6)[a]	66.0 (7.4)	73.3 (6.9)[a]
Gender, n (%) of males	25 (32.05%)	18 (42.86%)	17 (35.42%)	26 (36.11%)
Education, yr, mean (SD)	12.5 (2.7)	12.1 (2.4)	13.2 (2.3)	11.8 (2.7)[a]
CDR, score (% of subjects, number of subjects)	0 (60.2%, 47) or 0.5 (37.2%, 29) or 1 (2.6%, 2)	0 (2.4%, 1) or 0.5 (80.9%, 34) or 1 (16.7%, 7)	0 (100%, 48)	0.5 (87.5%, 63) or 1 (12.5%, 9)
MMSE score, mean (SD)	27.8 (2.3)	25.2 (3.7)[a]	28.5 (1.4)	25.9 (3.5)[a]
APOE ε4 carriers, n (%)	13 (16.67%)	24 (57.14%)[a]	11 (22.92%)	26 (36.11%)[a]
CSF $A\beta_{1-42}$ (pg/ml), mean (SD)	979.9 (196.4)	601.2 (190.0)[a]	957.4 (194.0)	774.0 (281.5)[a]
CSF tau (pg/ml), mean (SD)	235.1 (104.2)	624.2 (322.4)[a]	221.5 (82.9)	471.1 (316.6)[a]
CSF P-tau181 (pg/ml), mean (SD)	46.7 (13.4)	90.3 (44.8)[a]	45.9 (13.3)	72.7 (40.9)[a]
CSF P-tau181/$A\beta_{1-42}$, mean (SD)	0.05 (0.01)	0.16 (0.10)[a]	0.049 (0.015)	0.114 (0.097)[a]
CSF albumin index[b], mean (SD)	5.9 (2.4)	6.4 (2.3)	5.3 (1.9)	6.6 (2.5)[a]

Abbreviations: $A\beta_{1-42}$ β-Amyloid 1–42, APOE Apolipoprotein E, CDR Clinical Dementia Rating, CSF Cerebrospinal fluid, MMSE Mini Mental State Examination, P-tau181 Tau phosphorylated at threonine 181
[a]Statistically different ($p \leq 0.05$) from P-tau181/$A\beta_{1-42}$ ≤ 0.0779, and CDR = 0, respectively, using t tests for continuous variables and binomial proportion tests for categorical variables. [b]CSF albumin index = [CSF albumin]/[serum albumin] × 100

(500 μl) no later than 1 hour after collection and stored at − 80 °C without thawing until experiment and assay.

MS-based proteomics

CSF samples were prepared using a highly automated shotgun proteomic workflow as previously described [36] and isobaric tags [37] for relative quantification of proteins. Reversed-phase LC-MS/MS was performed with a hybrid linear ion trap-Orbitrap Elite and an UltiMate 3000 RSLCnano System (Thermo Scientific, Waltham, MA, USA) as recently described [38]. Protein identification was performed against the human UniProtKB/Swiss-Prot database (08/12/2014 release). All details are provided in Additional file 1: Supplementary Methods.

CSF β-amyloid 1–42, tau, tau phosphorylated at threonine 181, and *APOE* genotyping

The measurements were performed using commercially available enzyme-linked immunosorbent assay kits and Taq-Man assays as described in Additional file 1: Supplementary Methods.

Definition of CSF biomarker profile of Alzheimer pathology

A pathological AD CSF biomarker profile was defined as CSF P-tau181/Aβ$_{1-42}$ ratio > 0.0779 (i.e., "high" ratio for positive CSF profile of AD pathology), based on clinical study site data [39] and in line with previous work (i.e., 0.08) [40]. The cutoff optimized the Youden index [41] of the ROC curve for the prediction of CDR categories (CDR = 0 versus CDR > 0) as previously reported [27], where the cutoff for CSF P-tau181/Aβ$_{1-42}$ ratio was further confirmed to be a highly significant predictor of cognitive decline.

Proteomic data management

Six CSF samples were removed because of aberrant values, leaving CSF proteomic data available for 114 subjects (exclusion of those 6 subjects did not induce bias on the overall population characteristics) (*see* Additional file 1: Table S1)). In total, 790 CSF proteins were quantified.

For exploration of CSF proteins relevant to AD pathology (*see below*), proteins with > 5% missingness were excluded, leaving 541 CSF proteins. The remaining missing data (5% or less per protein) were imputed by randomly drawing a value between the observed range of biomarker values. Log$_2$ of the protein ratio fold changes were scaled to mean zero and SD of 1 prior to statistical analyses. Calculation and statistics were performed with the R version 3.3.2 statistical software (http://www.r-project.org/).

Exploratory analysis of CSF proteins relevant to Alzheimer pathology

In a first exploratory analysis, 541 CSF proteins were tested (one by one) in a logistic regression model as follows:

Positive CSF profile of AD ~ CSF protein biomarkers
+age + gender
+years of education
+presence of *APOE* ε4 allele

where positive CSF profile of AD is defined by categorizing the CSF P-tau181/Aβ$_{1-42}$ ratio into two groups: P-tau181/Aβ$_{1-42}$ > 0.0779 for AD CSF biomarker profile (or "high") and P-tau181/Aβ$_{1-42}$ ≤ 0.0779 for non-AD CSF biomarker profile (or "low"). *p* Values were corrected for multiple testing using the Benjamini-Hochberg procedure. Box plots were produced for the significant hits presenting false discovery rate (FDR) ≤ 5%.

Selection of CSF proteins relevant to Alzheimer pathology

Least absolute shrinkage and selection operator (LASSO) logistic regression [42] selected biomarkers that best predict CSF biomarker profile of AD pathology. A reference model was initially generated, testing variables that are likely to be available to clinicians and known risk factors for AD to provide a benchmark for comparison with the model that included CSF proteins. These inputs included age, gender, years of education, and presence of the apolipoprotein E (*APOE*) ε4 allele, such as:

Positive CSF profile of AD
~ age + gender + years of education
+presence of *APOE* ε4 allele

In addition to all variables used to make the reference models, CSF protein measurements (i.e., 541 CSF proteins) and CSF albumin index were then included in building so-called best models:

Positive CSF profile of AD
~ CSF protein biomarkers
+CSF albumin index + age
+gender + years of education
+presence of *APOE* ε4 allele

A tenfold cross-validation process was performed for each LASSO analysis using the glmnet package [43], which allows estimating the confidence interval of the misclassification error for each value of the regularization parameter λ. The LASSO analyses were repeated 100 times (1000 times for the reference models). The model that minimized the upper limit of the cross-validated misclassification error confidence interval across the 100 runs with less than 20 features (when possible) was selected. The results were formally tested for significance against the reference model using accuracy with a McNemar test. The group differences for the CSF proteins selected in the best models were graphically illustrated in box plots and assessed using t test statistics. In addition, Kruskal-Wallis test statistics produced comparable results (*see* Additional file 1: Tables S2 and S3). Because the tests were applied only to the proteins selected with LASSO, p values obtained from these analyses were not corrected for multiple testing.

Statistical Pearson's correlation and bioinformatic analysis

Correlation analysis was performed on protein fold changes of all 790 quantified proteins using Pearson's correlation coefficient and Bonferroni correction for multiple comparisons. In addition, Spearman's correlation analyses produced comparable results (*see* Additional file 1: Tables S4–S6). Several bioinformatics tools and resources were used for analysis and protein annotation (i.e., Database for Annotation, Visualization and Integrated Discovery [DAVID] 6.8 [44], UniProt tissue annotation database [45], Gene Ontology database [46], Kyoto Encyclopedia of Genes and Genomes [KEGG] database [47], tissue atlas [48], and Venny [http://bioinfogp.cnb.csic.es/tools/venny/]).

Results

Demographic and clinical characteristics of the study population

Demographics and clinical characteristics of the patient cohort are detailed in Table 1. The cognitively impaired subjects (CDR > 0) were older and less educated and had a higher prevalence of *APOE* ε4 genotype than the cognitively intact group (CDR = 0). In cognitive impairment, CSF $A\beta_{1-42}$ was lower, whereas CSF tau, CSF P-tau181, and CSF P-tau181/$A\beta_{1-42}$ were all higher. MS-based proteomic analyses were performed in the CSF of the 120 individuals (Fig. 1). In total, we measured 790 proteins in CSF. Of those, 541 proteins presented < 5% missing values in 114 subjects (*see* the Methods section above).

The following classification analyses of the CSF P-tau181/$A\beta_{1-42}$ ratios were aimed at separating 39 patients with high-expression AD CSF biomarker profiles (i.e., P-tau181/$A\beta_{1-42}$ > 0.0779) from 75 low-expression profile subjects in the complete analysis set, regardless of the clinical diagnosis. Then, the analyses were performed on the subset of cognitively impaired patients, where 38 and 28 subjects had high and low expression of AD CSF biomarker profiles, respectively.

Identification of Alzheimer pathology with CSF proteins

First, we explored whether the CSF proteome presents specific alterations in AD, endophenotypically defined a priori as a CSF P-tau181/$A\beta_{1-42}$ ratio > 0.0779 (*see* the Methods section above). In the whole sample, group comparisons (i.e., "high" when P-tau181/$A\beta_{1-42}$ > 0.0779 and "low" when P-tau181/$A\beta_{1-42}$ ≤ 0.0779) revealed 22 CSF proteins with significant differences between AD versus non-AD CSF biomarker profiles after correction for multiple testing using the Benjamini-Hochberg procedure at FDR ≤ 5% (Fig. 2a and Additional file 1: Table S7). Similarly, in the subset of cognitively impaired subjects (*see* the Methods section above), group comparisons provided ten CSF proteins with significant differences (Fig. 2b and Additional file 1: Table S8). All of these 10 proteins were already present among the 22 proteins (Fig. 2) previously identified in the whole sample.

As a second exploratory approach and ability assessment of the CSF proteome to identify AD, we used LASSO logistic regression to build mathematical models able to classify AD pathology, again defined a priori as a CSF P-tau181/$A\beta_{1-42}$ ratio > 0.0779 (*see* the Methods section above). In the whole sample, the benchmark reference model for classification of CSF P-tau181/$A\beta_{1-42}$ included age and presence of the *APOE* ε4 allele. Its prediction accuracy was 78.3% (as compared with the accuracy of a majority class prediction of 65.8%). CSF protein biomarkers were indeed able to improve the classification of AD CSF biomarker profile with respect to the reference model. The best model accuracy was 100% (McNemar p value 3.35×10^{-7}). It included 26 CSF proteins (from the 541 provided as input) in addition of age and presence of the *APOE* ε4 allele. Only seven selected CSF proteins displayed significant group comparison differences, i.e., 14-3-3 protein ζ/δ (1433Z) ($p = 1.69 \times 10^{-3}$), SPARC-related modular calcium-binding protein 1 (SMOC1) ($p = 5.26 \times 10^{-5}$), KICSTOR complex protein SZT2 (SZT2) ($p = 5.47 \times 10^{-4}$), fatty acid-binding protein, heart (FABPH) ($p = 8.70 \times 10^{-4}$), chitinase-3-like protein 1 (CH3L1) ($p = 1.23 \times 10^{-3}$), neuromodulin (NEUM) ($p = 3.40 \times 10^{-3}$), and keratin, type I cytoskeletal 10 ($p = 0.025$) (Additional file 1: Figure S1a). Many of these CSF proteins were correlated with each other (Additional file 1: Figure S2). Six of the seven proteins (i.e., 1433Z, SMOC1, SZT2, FABPH, CH3L1, and NEUM) were reported in the exploratory group comparisons (Fig. 2a).

In the subset of cognitively impaired subjects (*see* the Methods section above), the benchmark reference model to classify AD CSF biomarker profile included age, gender, years of education, and presence of *APOE* ε4 allele, with a prediction accuracy of 77.8% (majority class prediction of 57.6%). In cognitive impairment, inclusion of

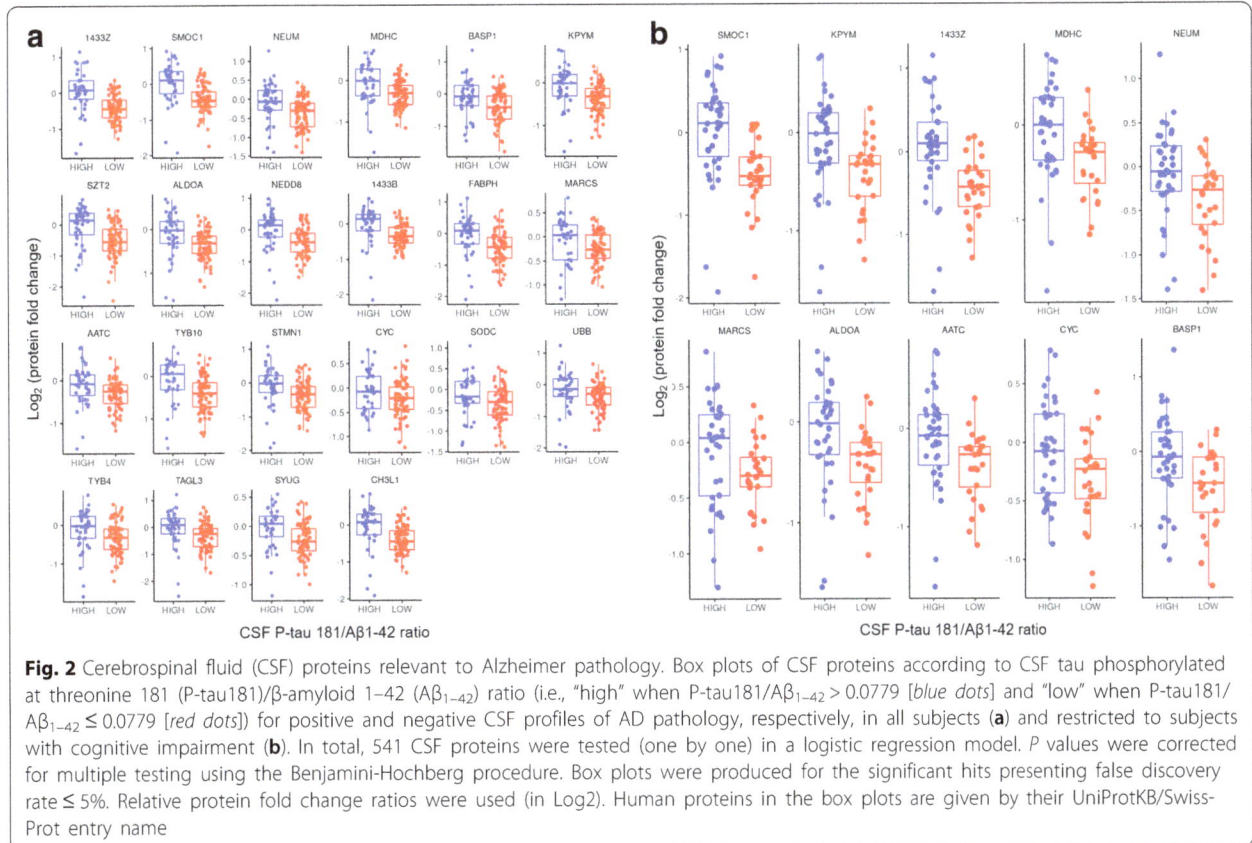

Fig. 2 Cerebrospinal fluid (CSF) proteins relevant to Alzheimer pathology. Box plots of CSF proteins according to CSF tau phosphorylated at threonine 181 (P-tau181)/β-amyloid 1–42 (Aβ$_{1-42}$) ratio (i.e., "high" when P-tau181/Aβ$_{1-42}$ > 0.0779 [*blue dots*] and "low" when P-tau181/Aβ$_{1-42}$ ≤ 0.0779 [*red dots*]) for positive and negative CSF profiles of AD pathology, respectively, in all subjects (**a**) and restricted to subjects with cognitive impairment (**b**). In total, 541 CSF proteins were tested (one by one) in a logistic regression model. *P* values were corrected for multiple testing using the Benjamini-Hochberg procedure. Box plots were produced for the significant hits presenting false discovery rate ≤ 5%. Relative protein fold change ratios were used (in Log2). Human proteins in the box plots are given by their UniProtKB/Swiss-Prot entry name

CSF protein biomarkers again improved significantly the prediction accuracy to 100% (McNemar *p* value of 0.0003). In total, 18 CSF proteins (from the 541 provided as input) were included in this best model in addition to gender and presence of the *APOE* ε4 allele. Among those proteins, four displayed significant differences between the groups: 1433Z ($p = 4.04 \times 10^{-5}$), SMOC1 ($p = 5.49 \times 10^{-5}$), γ-synuclein ($p = 1.19 \times 10^{-3}$), and macrophage colony-stimulating factor 1 receptor ($p = 0.013$) (Additional file 1: Figure S1b). Again, several correlations were observed between the CSF proteins retained in the model (Additional file 1: Figure S3), suggesting that models with fewer variables may still provide high classification performance. Two of the four proteins (i.e., 1433Z and SMOC1) were reported in the exploratory group comparisons (Fig. 2b). The perfect performance to classify the participants with AD pathology indicated that the reported models were very possibly overfitting the data.

Associations of CSF proteins with β-amyloid 1–42, tau, and tau phosphorylated at threonine 181

Next, we separately and more specifically studied the associations of all 790 quantified CSF proteins (no minimal missing value criteria applied) with CSF markers of core AD pathology (i.e., Aβ$_{1-42}$, tau, and P-tau181). Four proteins—cannabinoid receptor 1 (CNR1, correlation coefficient [R] = 0.3929), neuroendocrine convertase 2 (NEC2, R = 0.3818), neuronal pentraxin-2 (NPTX2, R = 0.3868), and somatostatin (SMS, R = 0.4188)—showed an association with CSF Aβ$_{1-42}$, which was significant (*p* value ≤0.05) after Bonferroni correction for multiple testing (Fig. 3a). We found 50 CSF proteins correlated with CSF tau (Fig. 3b) and 46 associated with CSF P-tau181 (Fig. 3c) in a significant manner after Bonferroni correction, of which 41 were in common (Fig. 3d). The five strongest correlations with CSF tau were CSF neurogranin (NEUG), sodium/potassium-transporting ATPase subunit α-2 (AT1A2), brain acid soluble protein 1 (BASP1), 1433Z, and NEUM. The five strongest correlations with CSF P-tau181 were CSF AT1A2, disintegrin and metalloproteinase domain-containing protein 10 (ADA10), N^G,N^G-dimethylarginine dimethylaminohydrolase 1 (DDAH1), NEUG, and SMOC1. In particular, CSF NEUG and NEUM [49], two synaptic proteins, were positively correlated with CSF tau (R = 0.6721 and 0.5287, respectively) and P-tau181 (R = 0.5074 and 0.4741, respectively) (Additional file 1: Figure S4). All the observed associations are summarized in the chord diagram of Additional file 1: Figure S5. With the exception of ectonucleotide

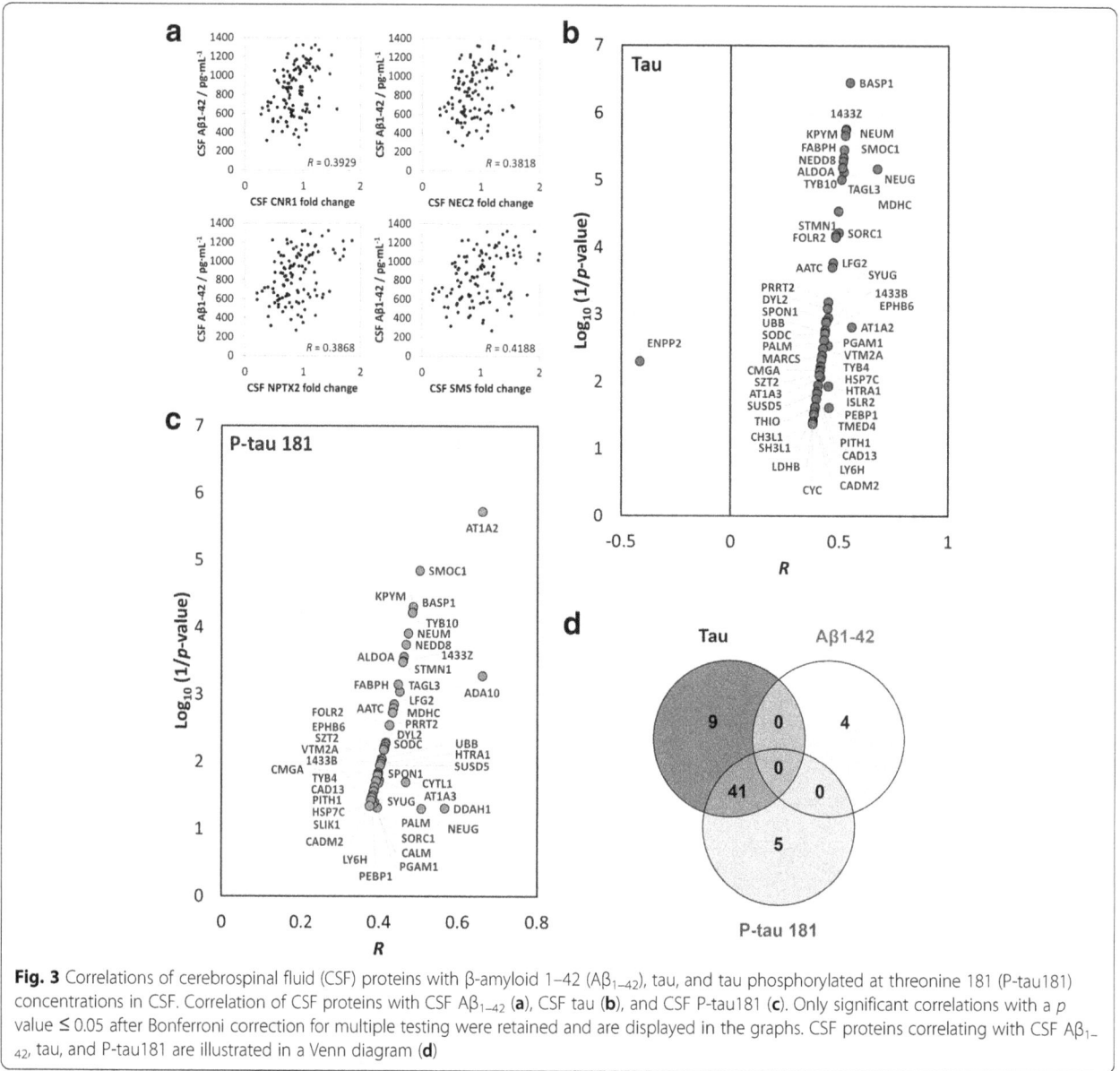

Fig. 3 Correlations of cerebrospinal fluid (CSF) proteins with β-amyloid 1–42 (Aβ$_{1-42}$), tau, and tau phosphorylated at threonine 181 (P-tau181) concentrations in CSF. Correlation of CSF proteins with CSF Aβ$_{1-42}$ (**a**), CSF tau (**b**), and CSF P-tau181 (**c**). Only significant correlations with a p value ≤ 0.05 after Bonferroni correction for multiple testing were retained and are displayed in the graphs. CSF proteins correlating with CSF Aβ$_{1-42}$, tau, and P-tau181 are illustrated in a Venn diagram (**d**)

pyrophosphatase/phosphodiesterase family member 2, which negatively correlated with tau, all reported correlations were positive.

Annotations of CSF proteins correlating with β-amyloid 1–42, tau, and tau phosphorylated at threonine 181

Of the 59 proteins displaying correlations in those analyses (Fig. 3d), most are expressed in the brain, in particular in the fetal brain cortex and Cajal-Retzius cells (Fig. 4a). Moreover, and based on the tissue-based map of the human proteome [48], seven proteins (i.e., SLIT and NTRK-like protein 1, NEUM, NEUG, cell adhesion molecule 2, lymphocyte antigen 6H [LY6H], transgelin-3 [TAGL3], and protein lifeguard) are brain-enriched (i.e., having at least fivefold higher mRNA levels in the brain

as compared with all other tissues) and a total of 22 proteins have elevated gene expression in the brain (i.e., in addition to the seven above, AT1A2, immunoglobulin superfamily containing leucine-rich repeat protein 2 [ISLR2], sodium/potassium-transporting ATPase subunit α-3 [AT1A3], BASP1, CH3L1, CNR1, ephrin type-B receptor 6 [EPHB6], NPTX2, paralemmin-1, NEC2, proline-rich transmembrane protein 2, SMOC1, VPS10 domain-containing receptor SorCS1, SMS, and V-set and transmembrane domain-containing protein 2A).

In Fig. 4b, we identified the myelin sheath as an enriched cellular component. Of the 59 CSF proteins correlating with Aβ$_{1-42}$, tau, and/or P-tau181, 9 proteins pertain to the myelin sheath: TAGL3, malate dehydrogenase, cytoplasmic (MDHC), heat shock cognate 71 kDa protein

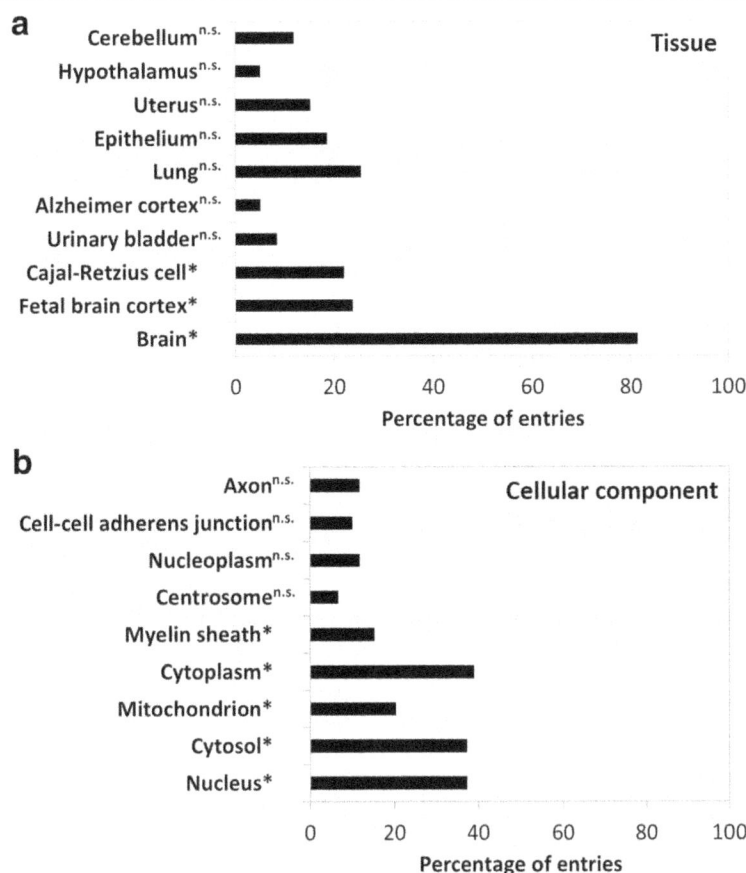

Fig. 4 Annotations of cerebrospinal fluid (CSF) proteins correlating with β-amyloid 1–42 ($A\beta_{1-42}$), tau, and/or tau phosphorylated at threonine 181 (P-tau181) concentrations in CSF. Tissue annotation using the UniProt tissue annotation database (**a**) and Gene Ontology (GO) (cellular component category) annotation (**b**) obtained with DAVID software for the 59 CSF proteins correlating with CSF $A\beta_{1-42}$, tau, and/or P-tau181. Significant enrichment (Benjamini-Hochberg procedure) is indicated with an asterisk. The background used for the enrichment analysis was the 790 detected proteins in CSF. *n.s.* Nonsignificant

(HSP7C), AT1A2, phosphoglycerate mutase 1 (PGAM1), superoxide dismutase [Cu-Zn] (SODC), AT1A3, pyruvate kinase PKM (KPYM), and L-lactate dehydrogenase B chain (LDHB). Those nine proteins were associated with tau and/or P-tau181. Pathway enrichment analysis using the KEGG database did not yield any significant results (data not shown).

Discussion

In the present study, we used MS-based shotgun proteomics to measure the CSF proteomes of 120 older adults and investigate broad CSF protein relationships with core AD pathology. Overall, human CSF proteome coverage was composed of 790 proteins. Four CSF proteins were associated with CSF $A\beta_{1-42}$ levels, 50 proteins with CSF tau, and 46 proteins with CSF P-tau181 levels. The CSF proteins related to $A\beta_{1-42}$ were different from those associated with tau or P-tau181.

To explore the relevance of the CSF proteome to AD pathology, we applied an approach that was unbiased by the clinical diagnosis and defined endophenotypically the disease as the presence of "core" AD pathology (i.e., the combined presence of cerebral amyloid and tau pathology). Unbiased classification based on markers of cerebral amyloid and tau pathology and neuronal injury has been proposed for use across the clinical stages [7]. We first used two exploratory approaches to evaluate and select CSF proteins that were able to stratify subjects according to levels of CSF P-tau181/$A\beta_{1-42}$. Using LASSO logistic regression, we observed that CSF proteins could significantly increase the classification accuracy of non-AD versus AD CSF biomarker profiles as compared with models based only on clinical parameters and the presence of the *APOE* ε4 allele. Nonetheless, those statistical models relying on CSF proteins might be overfitted and should be interpreted with caution; class imbalance also affected their strict performance.

Overall, with both exploratory analyses, we identified specific CSF proteome alterations that are related to AD pathology and may provide novel mechanistic insights. Assessing the whole sample and the subgroup of subjects with cognitive impairment, we could decipher the strong contribution of some CSF proteins, such as SMOC1 and 1433Z (Fig. 2 and Additional file 1: Figure S1). On the basis of this performance, we specifically investigated associations of CSF proteins with individual most validated biomarkers of amyloid pathology, neuronal injury, and tau hyperphosphorylation (i.e., $A\beta_{1-42}$, tau, and P-tau181, respectively) to elaborate further on the involved mechanisms. Most of the correlations of CSF proteins were with CSF tau and P-tau181 (Fig. 3d), suggesting the CSF proteome alterations to be more representative of tau pathology than amyloid pathology. Four CSF proteins not related to tau and P-tau181 were associated with CSF $A\beta_{1-42}$ levels, overall indicating distinct proteome alterations related to either amyloid pathology or tau-related neurodegeneration. The majority of these proteins were brain-enriched proteins, including synaptic proteins, and proteins involved in reelin-producing cells and the myelin sheath. Comparison of the proteins found with different levels in AD versus non-AD CSF biomarker profiles and in the models able to classify CSF-defined AD pathology with those associated with CSF $A\beta_{1-42}$, tau, and P-tau181 in Venn diagrams (Additional file 1: Figures S6 and S7, respectively) revealed mixed overlaps. Interestingly, the 22 proteins with different levels in AD versus non-AD CSF biomarker profiles (Fig. 2a) were all associated with CSF tau; a large majority were associated with CSF P-tau181; but none were associated with CSF $A\beta_{1-42}$ (Additional file 1: Figure S6). Nevertheless, beyond those 22 proteins, 37 proteins, still representing the majority of CSF proteins associated with CSF $A\beta_{1-42}$, tau, and P-tau181, were not evidenced as having a relationship to AD, suggesting they might represent more general makers of amyloid pathology, neuronal injury, and tau hyperphosphorylation.

The CSF proteins CNR1, NEC2, NPTX2, and SMS were associated with CSF $A\beta_{1-42}$ in our study (Fig. 3a). CNR1 and the endocannabinoid system were previously identified as potential targets for treatment of neurological disorders and AD in particular [50, 51]. In line with our results, higher NPTX2, a proinflammatory protein involved in synaptic plasticity, was previously associated with higher CSF $A\beta_{1-42}$ in the Alzheimer's Disease Neuroimaging Initiative study [52]. NEC2, also known as prohormone convertase 2, is essential to the processing of pro-islet amyloid polypeptide [53]. Its role in the processing of hormones and in particular of neuropeptide precursors in the human cortex has been established, but the link with SMS deficiency in AD, for instance, was not confirmed [54]. Relevant to our observations, neuropeptide SMS is known to be decreased in

the CSF of patients with AD [55] and to regulate $A\beta_{1-42}$ via proteolytic degradation [56]. Together, these findings indicate amyloid-related changes in the CSF proteome that may be particularly relevant for early cerebral AD pathology as well as for disease-modifying interventions targeting amyloid and starting at preclinical disease stages.

We found that CSF $A\beta_{1-42}$, tau, and P-tau181 were mainly associated with CSF proteins enriched in brain tissue (Fig. 4a), and this despite the important proportion (about 80%) of proteins in CSF originating from blood [4]. In particular, some are expressed in the fetal brain cortex. We observed positive correlations between CSF tau and/or P-tau181 with 13 CSF proteins (i.e., calmodulin, fructose-bisphosphate aldolase A [ALDOA], DDAH1, HSP7C, KPYM, LDHB, MDHC, PGAM1, phosphatidylethanolamine-binding protein 1 [PEBP1], stathmin, TAGL3, thioredoxin, and 1433Z) known also to be present in reelin-producing Cajal-Retzius cells. In early AD, a massive decline of the number of Cajal-Retzius cells was previously described [57], suggesting a link between their loss, reduction of reelin, impairment of synaptic plasticity, amyloid plaque deposition, and neurofibrillary tangle formation [58]. Interestingly, we also revealed the involvement of nine CSF proteins (i.e., AT1A2, AT1A3, HSP7C, KPYM, LDHB, MDHC, PGAM1, SODC, and TAGL3), again positively correlating with CSF tau and/or P-tau181, being specifically part of the myelin sheath. Although amyloid plaques and neurofibrillary tangles likely induce neuronal and synaptic loss, myelin alteration may also participate in the development of AD dementia. Myelin content changes in the white matter measured with MRI have been linked to CSF AD biomarkers (i.e., lower concentrations of $A\beta_{1-42}$ and higher concentrations of tau and P-tau181), but mainly in association with amyloid pathology [59]. Our results, including associations of AT1A2 and KPYM with both tau and P-tau181, may suggest an underestimated connection between tau-related neurodegeneration and (de)myelination. These specific alterations provide new insights into the disease pathology and deserve further exploration.

Several single relationships between CSF proteins and $A\beta_{1-42}$, tau, and/or P-tau181 levels in our study (Fig. 3) have previously been reported. A first example is the synaptic protein NEUG, which was previously proposed as a novel candidate CSF biomarker for AD and prodromal AD; high CSF NEUG was shown to predict future cognitive decline and to be more specific for AD than tau [60]. In addition, CSF NEUG was reported to be increased in AD and positively correlated with CSF tau [61] and P-tau [49]. In line with our observations, positive associations were identified with NEUM for both tau and P-tau in CSF [49]. BASP1, like NEUM, is a presynaptic membrane protein participating in axon guidance, neurodegeneration, and synaptic plasticity [62] and was found to be significantly downregulated in AD versus control brain samples [63]. Our findings of significant association of CSF BASP1 with both CSF tau and P-tau warrant further investigations. Mutations in the *ADAM10* gene, which encodes the major α-secretase responsible for cleaving APP, have previously been identified in families with late-onset AD [64]. In our study, protein ADA10, which is encoded by *ADAM10*, was only significantly associated with CSF P-tau181. To the best of our knowledge, such an association between those CSF proteins has not been observed before [65].

Further and broader cross-validation of our findings can be made by comparing them with those of a recent study investigating CSF proteins associated with CSF AD biomarkers in 58 cognitively healthy men using an aptamer-based technology (i.e., SOMAscan; SomaLogic, Boulder, CO, USA) [66]. Of the 59 CSF proteins associated with CSF biomarkers of core AD pathology that we report, 28 were also measured with the SOMAscan in that prior study; of those, 22 proteins (i.e., 78.6% overlap) were correlated with CSF Aβ$_{1-42}$, tau, and/or P-tau [66], confirming part of our observations in an independent cohort and using a different technology. Those proteins are ALDOA, dynein light chain 2, cytoplasmic, polyubiquitin B, ISLR2, EPHB6, MDHC, SH3 domain-binding glutamic acid-rich-like protein, PEBP1, NPTX2, chromogranin A, cytochrome c, SMS, 1433Z, LDHB, SMOC1, 14–3-3 protein β/α, spondin-1, FABPH, transmembrane emp24 domain-containing protein 4, PGAM1, cytokine-like protein 1, and HSP7C.

Altogether, our shotgun MS-based proteomic approach [22] was confirmed to provide relevant findings and to be complementary to alternative proteomic technologies. In this perspective, the identification of novel and strongly significant associations of CSF proteins with CSF biomarkers of AD core pathology in our study is of specific interest. In particular, proteins AT1A2 and KPYM implicated in energy production, as well as 1433Z, DDAH1, and SMOC1, showing some of the strongest associations with tau and/or P-tau181 in addition to NEUG and NEUM, could appear relevant. Our results in a relatively large group of subjects including both participants with cognitive impairment and healthy volunteers are therefore encouraging. Sample fractionation would have allowed deeper proteome coverage but with a throughput incompatible with the analysis of 120 clinical samples in a reasonable time frame. The proteins we have identified would deserve additional research.

Conclusions

Using an MS-based proteomic workflow, we have quantified a number of CSF proteins in 120 older adults with normal cognition and with cognitive impairment. We report strong evidence of known and new CSF proteins related to amyloid pathology, neuronal injury, and tau hyperphosphorylation. Although we confirmed several previous findings of CSF proteins related to AD pathology, our work reveals a large number of additional CSF proteome alterations involving in particular reelin-producing cells and the myelin sheath.

Abbreviations

1433B: 14-3-3 protein β/α; 2LFG2: Protein lifeguard; AD: Alzheimer disease; ADA10: Disintegrin and metalloproteinase domain-containing protein 10; ALDOA: Fructose-bisphosphate aldolase A; *APOE*: Apolipoprotein E; AT1A2: Sodium/potassium-transporting ATPase subunit α-2; AT1A3: Sodium/potassium-transporting ATPase subunit α-3; AUC: Area under the curve; BASP1: Brain acid soluble protein 1; CADM2: Cell adhesion molecule 2; CALM: Calmodulin; CDR: Clinical Dementia Rating; CH3L1: Chitinase-3-like protein 1; CMGA: Chromogranin-A; CNR1: Cannabinoid receptor 1; CNS: Central nervous system; CSF: Cerebrospinal fluid; DDAH1: N^G,N^G-dimethylarginine dimethylaminohydrolase 1; CSF1R: Macrophage colony-stimulating factor 1 receptor; CYC: Cytochrome c; CYTL1: Cytokine-like protein 1; DYL2: Dynein light chain 2, cytoplasmic; ENPP2: Ectonucleotide pyrophosphatase/phosphodiesterase family member 2; EPHB6: Ephrin type- B receptor 6; FABPH: Fatty acid-binding protein, heart; FDR: False discovery rate; HSP7C: Heat shock cognate 71 kDa protein; ISLR2: Immunoglobulin superfamily containing leucine-rich repeat protein 2; K1C10: Keratin, type I cytoskeletal 10; KPYM: Pyruvate kinase PKM; LASSO: Least absolute shrinkage and selection operator regression; LC: Liquid chromatography; LDHB: L-lactate dehydrogenase B chain; MCI: Mild cognitive impairment; MDHC: Malate dehydrogenase, cytoplasmic; MMSE: Mini Mental State Examination; MS: Mass spectrometry; MS/MS: Tandem mass spectrometry; MRI: Magnetic resonance imaging; NEC2: Neuroendocrine convertase 2; NEUG: Neurogranin; NEUM: Neuromodulin; NPTX2: Neuronal pentraxin-2; PALM: Paralemmin-1; PEBP1: Phosphatidylethanolamine-binding protein 1; PGAM1: Phosphoglycerate mutase 1; PRRT2: Proline-rich transmembrane protein 2; P-tau: Hyperphosphorylated tau; P-tau181: Tau phosphorylated at threonine 181; RP: Reversed-phase; SLIK1: SLIT and NTRK-like protein 1; SMOC1: SPARC-related modular calcium-binding protein 1; SMS: Somatostatin; SODC: Superoxide dismutase [Cu-Zn]; SORC1: VPS10 domain-containing receptor SorCS1; SPON1: Spondin-1; STMN1: Stathmin; SYUG: γ-Synuclein; SZT2: KICSTOR complex protein SZT2; TAGL3: Lymphocyte antigen 6H (LY6H), transgelin-3; Aβ$_{1-42}$: β-Amyloid 1--42; 1433Z: 14-3-3 protein ζ/δ

Acknowledgements
We thank Barbara Moullet and Domilė Tautvydaitė for their assistance with and contributions to data acquisition.

Funding
This study was supported by grants from the Swiss National Research Foundation (to JP) (SNF 320030_141179) and funding from the Nestlé Institute of Health Sciences.

Authors' contributions

LD was responsible for study conception and design, acquisition of data, supervision of data acquisition, analysis of data, interpretation of the analysis, and writing of the manuscript. ANG was responsible for acquisition of data and critical revision of the manuscript. JW was responsible for study conception and design, the statistical analysis plan, statistical analysis, drafting of the statistical analysis section, and critical revision of the manuscript. OC was responsible for statistical analysis and critical revision of the manuscript. JC was responsible for acquisition of data and critical revision of the manuscript. AO was responsible for acquisition of data and critical revision of the manuscript. HH was responsible for supervision of data acquisition and critical revision of the manuscript. MK was responsible for supervision of data acquisition and critical revision of the manuscript. EM was responsible for the statistical analysis plan and critical revision of the manuscript. IS was responsible for interpretation of the analysis and critical revision of the manuscript. GLB was responsible for study conception and design, the statistical analysis plan, critical revision of the manuscript, and overall study supervision. JP was responsible for study conception and design, interpretation of the analysis, critical revision of the manuscript, and overall study supervision. All authors read and approved the final version of the manuscript.

Competing interests

LD, ANG, OC, JC, MK, EM, and IS are employees of Nestlé Institute of Health Sciences. JW is an employee and shareholder of Precision for Medicine and received consultation honoraria from Nestlé Institute of Health Sciences. AO and HH report no competing interests. GLB is an employee of Nestlé Institute of Health Sciences, an unpaid scientific advisor of the H2020 EU-funded project PROPAG-AGEING whose aim is to identify new molecular signatures for early diagnosis of neurodegenerative diseases, and receives research support related to cognitive decline from the National Institute on Aging of the National Institutes of Health. JP received consultation honoraria from Nestlé Institute of Health Sciences.

Author details

[1]Nestlé Institute of Health Sciences, Lausanne, Switzerland. [2]Precision for Medicine, Geneva, Switzerland. [3]Old Age Psychiatry, Department of Psychiatry, CHUV, Lausanne, Switzerland. [4]Department of Laboratories, CHUV, Lausanne, Switzerland. [5]Geriatric Psychiatry, Department of Mental Health and Psychiatry, HUG, Geneva, Switzerland. [6]Present address: Liggins Institute, University of Auckland, Auckland, New Zealand.

References

1. Aebersold R, Bader GD, Edwards AM, Van Eyk JE, Kussmann M, Qin J, Omenn GS. The biology/disease-driven Human Proteome Project (B/D-HPP): enabling protein research for the life sciences community. J Proteome Res. 2013;12:23–7.
2. Shi M, Caudle WM, Zhang J. Biomarker discovery in neurodegenerative diseases: a proteomic approach. Neurobiol Dis. 2009;35:157–64.
3. Agrawal M, Biswas A. Molecular diagnostics of neurodegenerative disorders. Front Mol Biosci. 2015;2:54.
4. Begcevic I, Brinc D, Drabovich AP, Batruch I, Diamandis EP. Identification of brain-enriched proteins in the cerebrospinal fluid proteome by LC-MS/MS profiling and mining of the human protein atlas. Clin Proteomics. 2016;13:11.
5. Fang Q, Strand A, Law W, Faca VM, Fitzgibbon MP, Hamel N, et al. Brain-specific proteins decline in the cerebrospinal fluid of humans with Huntington disease. Mol Cell Proteomics. 2009;8:451–66.
6. Galasko DR, Shaw LM. Alzheimer disease: CSF biomarkers for Alzheimer disease-approaching consensus. Nat Rev Neurol. 2017;13:131–2.
7. Jack CR Jr, Bennett DA, Blennow K, Carrillo MC, Feldman HH, Frisoni GB, et al. A/T/N: an unbiased descriptive classification scheme for Alzheimer disease biomarkers. Neurology. 2016;87:539–47.
8. Sperling RA, Aisen PS, Beckett LA, Bennett DA, Craft S, Fagan AM, et al. Toward defining the preclinical stages of Alzheimer's disease: recommendations from the National Institute on Aging-Alzheimer's Association workgroups on diagnostic guidelines for Alzheimer's disease. Alzheimers Dement. 2011;7:280–92.
9. Albert MS, DeKosky ST, Dickson D, Dubois B, Feldman HH, Fox NC, et al. The diagnosis of mild cognitive impairment due to Alzheimer's disease: recommendations from the National Institute on Aging-Alzheimer's Association workgroups on diagnostic guidelines for Alzheimer's disease. Alzheimers Dement. 2011;7:270–9.
10. Dubois B, Feldman HH, Jacova C, Hampel H, Molinuevo JL, Blennow K, et al. Advancing research diagnostic criteria for Alzheimer's disease: the IWG-2 criteria. Lancet Neurol. 2014;13:614–29.
11. Baird AL, Westwood S, Lovestone S. Blood-based proteomic biomarkers of Alzheimer's disease pathology. Front Neurol. 2015;6:236.
12. Guldbrandsen A, Vethe H, Farag Y, Oveland E, Garberg H, Berle M, et al. In-depth characterization of the cerebrospinal fluid (CSF) proteome displayed through the CSF proteome resource (CSF-PR). Mol Cell Proteomics. 2014;13:3152–63.
13. Schutzer SE, Liu T, Natelson BH, Angel TE, Schepmoes AA, Purvine SO, et al. Establishing the proteome of normal human cerebrospinal fluid. PLoS One. 2010;5:e10980.
14. Zhang Y, Guo Z, Zou L, Yang Y, Zhang L, Ji N, et al. A comprehensive map and functional annotation of the normal human cerebrospinal fluid proteome. J Proteome. 2015;119:90–9.
15. Dayon L, Kussmann M. Proteomics of human plasma: a critical comparison of analytical workflows in terms of effort, throughput and outcome. EuPA Open Proteom. 2013;1:8–16.
16. Cole RN, Ruczinski I, Schulze K, Christian P, Herbrich S, Wu L, et al. The plasma proteome identifies expected and novel proteins correlated with micronutrient status in undernourished Nepalese children. J Nutr. 2013;143:1540–8.
17. García-Bailo B, Brenner DR, Nielsen D, Lee HJ, Domanski D, Kuzyk M, et al. Dietary patterns and ethnicity are associated with distinct plasma proteomic groups. Am J Clin Nutr. 2012;95:352–61.
18. Johansson Å, Enroth S, Palmblad M, Deelder AM, Bergquist J, Gyllensten U. Identification of genetic variants influencing the human plasma proteome. Proc Natl Acad Sci U S A. 2013;110:4673–8.
19. Lee SE, Stewart CP, Schulze KJ, Cole RN, Wu LSF, Yager JD, et al. The plasma proteome is associated with anthropometric status of undernourished Nepalese school-aged children. J Nutr. 2017;147:304–13.
20. Lee SE, West KP Jr, Cole RN, Schulze KJ, Christian P, Wu LSF, et al. Plasma proteome biomarkers of inflammation in school aged children in Nepal. PLoS One. 2015;10:e0144279.
21. Oller Moreno S, Cominetti O, Núñez Galindo A, Irincheeva I, Corthésy J, Astrup A, et al. The differential plasma proteome of obese and overweight individuals undergoing a nutritional weight loss and maintenance intervention. Proteomics Clin Appl. 2018;12:1600150.
22. Cominetti O, Núñez Galindo A, Corthésy J, Oller Moreno S, Irincheeva I, Valsesia A, et al. Proteomic biomarker discovery in 1000 human plasma samples with mass spectrometry. J Proteome Res. 2016;15:389–99.
23. Geyer PE, Wewer Albrechtsen NJ, Tyanova S, Grassl N, Iepsen EW, Lundgren J, et al. Proteomics reveals the effects of sustained weight loss on the human plasma proteome. Mol Syst Biol. 2016;12:901.
24. Liu Y, Buil A, Collins BC, Gillet LCJ, Blum LC, Cheng LY, et al. Quantitative variability of 342 plasma proteins in a human twin population. Mol Syst Biol. 2015;11:786.

25. Dayon L, Núñez Galindo A, Cominetti O, Corthésy J, Kussmann M. A highly automated shotgun proteomic workflow: clinical scale and robustness for biomarker discovery in blood. Methods Mol Biol. 2017;1619:433–49.

26. Geyer PE, Holdt LM, Teupser D, Mann M. Revisiting biomarker discovery by plasma proteomics. Mol Syst Biol. 2017;13:942.

27. Popp J, Oikonomidi A, Tautvydaitė D, Dayon L, Bacher M, Migliavacca E, et al. Markers of neuroinflammation associated with Alzheimer's disease pathology in older adults. Brain Behav Immun. 2017;62:203–11.

28. Morris JC. The Clinical Dementia Rating (CDR): current version and scoring rules. Neurology. 1993;43:2412–4.

29. Winblad B, Palmer K, Kivipelto M, Jelic V, Fratiglioni L, Wahlund LO, et al. Mild cognitive impairment - beyond controversies, towards a consensus: report of the international working group on mild cognitive impairment. J Intern Med. 2004;256:240–6.

30. McKhann GM, Knopman DS, Chertkow H, Hyman BT, Jack CR Jr, Kawas CH, et al. The diagnosis of dementia due to Alzheimer's disease: recommendations from the National Institute on Aging-Alzheimer's Association workgroups on diagnostic guidelines for Alzheimer's disease. Alzheimers Dement. 2011;7:263–9.

31. Buschke H, Sliwinski MJ, Kuslansky G, Lipton RB. Diagnosis of early dementia by the double memory test: encoding specificity improves diagnostic sensitivity and specificity. Neurology. 1997;48:989–97.

32. Folstein MF, Folstein SE, McHugh PR. "Mini-mental state": a practical method for grading the cognitive state of patients for the clinician. J Psychiatr Res. 1975;12:189–98.

33. Zigmond AS, Snaith RP. The Hospital Anxiety and Depression Scale. Acta Psychiatr Scand. 1983;67:361–70.

34. Jorm AF, Jacomb PA. The Informant Questionnaire on Cognitive Decline in the Elderly (IQCODE): socio-demographic correlates, reliability, validity and some norms. Psychol Med. 1989;19:1015–22.

35. Popp J, Riad M, Freymann K, Jessen F. Diagnostic lumbar puncture performed in the outpatient setting of a memory clinic: frequency and risk factors of post-lumbar puncture headache. Nervenarzt. 2007;78:547–51.

36. Núñez Galindo A, Kussmann M, Dayon L. Proteomics of cerebrospinal fluid: throughput and robustness using a scalable automated analysis pipeline for biomarker discovery. Anal Chem. 2015;87:10755–61.

37. Dayon L, Sanchez JC. Relative protein quantification by MS/MS using the tandem mass tag technology. Methods Mol Biol. 2012;893:115–27.

38. Dayon L, Núñez Galindo A, Corthésy J, Cominetti O, Kussmann M. Comprehensive and scalable highly automated MS-based proteomic workflow for clinical biomarker discovery in human plasma. J Proteome Res. 2014;13:3837–45.

39. Tautvydaitė D, Antonietti JP, Henry H, von Gunten A, Popp J. Relations between personality changes and cerebrospinal fluid biomarkers of Alzheimer's disease pathology. J Psychiatr Res. 2017;90:12–20.

40. Duits FH, Teunissen CE, Bouwman FH, Visser PJ, Mattsson N, Zetterberg H, et al. The cerebrospinal fluid "Alzheimer profile": easily said, but what does it mean? Alzheimers Dement. 2014;10:713–23.

41. Youden WJ. Index for rating diagnostic tests. Cancer. 1950;3:32–5.

42. Tibshirani R. Regression shrinkage and selection via the lasso: a retrospective. J R Stat Soc Ser B Stat Methodol. 2011;73:273–82.

43. Friedman J, Hastie T, Tibshirani R. Regularization paths for generalized linear models via coordinate descent. J Stat Softw. 2010;33:1–22.

44. Huang DW, Sherman BT, Lempicki RA. Systematic and integrative analysis of large gene lists using DAVID bioinformatics resources. Nat Protoc. 2009;4:44–57.

45. Bateman A, Martin MJ, O'Donovan C, Magrane M, Alpi E, Antunes R, et al. UniProt: the universal protein knowledgebase. Nucleic Acids Res. 2017;45:D158–69.

46. Carbon S, Dietze H, Lewis SE, Mungall CJ, Munoz-Torres MC, Basu S, et al. Expansion of the gene ontology knowledgebase and resources. Nucleic Acids Res. 2017;45:D331–8.

47. Kanehisa M, Furumichi M, Tanabe M, Sato Y, Morishima K. KEGG: new perspectives on genomes, pathways, diseases and drugs. Nucleic Acids Res. 2017;45:D353–61.

48. Uhlén M, Fagerberg L, Hallström BM, Lindskog C, Oksvold P, Mardinoglu A, et al. Tissue-based map of the human proteome. Science. 2015;347:1260419.

49. Remnestål J, Just D, Mitsios N, Fredolini C, Mulder J, Schwenk JM, et al. CSF profiling of the human brain enriched proteome reveals associations of neuromodulin and neurogranin to Alzheimer's disease. Proteomics Clin Appl. 2016;10:1242–53.

50. Scotter EL, Abood ME, Glass M. The endocannabinoid system as a target for the treatment of neurodegenerative disease. Br J Pharmacol. 2010;160:480–98.

51. Stumm C, Hiebel C, Hanstein R, Purrio M, Nagel H, Conrad A, et al. Cannabinoid receptor 1 deficiency in a mouse model of Alzheimer's disease leads to enhanced cognitive impairment despite of a reduction in amyloid deposition. Neurobiol Aging. 2013;34:2574–84.

52. Swanson A, Willette AA. Neuronal pentraxin 2 predicts medial temporal atrophy and memory decline across the Alzheimer's disease spectrum. Brain Behav Immun. 2016;58:201–8.

53. Wang J, Xu J, Finnerty J, Furuta M, Steiner DF, Verchere CB. The prohormone convertase enzyme 2 (PC2) is essential for processing pro-islet amyloid polypeptide at the NH_2-terminal cleavage site. Diabetes. 2001;50:534–9.

54. Winsky-Sommerer R, Grouselle D, Rougeot C, Laurent V, David JP, Delacourte A, et al. The proprotein convertase PC2 is involved in the maturation of prosomatostatin to somatostatin-14 but not in the somatostatin deficit in Alzheimer's disease. Neuroscience. 2003;122:437–47.

55. Nilsson CL, Brinkmalm A, Minthon L, Blennow K, Ekman R. Processing of neuropeptide Y, galanin, and somatostatin in the cerebrospinal fluid of patients with Alzheimer's disease and frontotemporal dementia. Peptides. 2001;22:2105–12.

56. Saito T, Iwata N, Tsubuki S, Takaki Y, Takano J, Huang SM, et al. Somatostatin regulates brain amyloid β peptide $A\beta_{42}$ through modulation of proteolytic degradation. Nat Med. 2005;11:434–9.

57. Baloyannis SJ. Morphological and morphometric alterations of Cajal-Retzius cells in early cases of Alzheimer's disease: a Golgi and electron microscope study. Int J Neurosci. 2005;115:965–80.

58. Kocherhans S, Madhusudan A, Doehner J, Breu KS, Nitsch RM, Fritschy JM, Knuesel I. Reduced reelin expression accelerates amyloid-β plaque formation and tau pathology in transgenic Alzheimer's disease mice. J Neurosci. 2010;30:9228–40.

59. Dean DC III, Hurley SA, Kecskemeti SR, O'Grady JP, Canda C, Davenport-Sis NJ, et al. Association of amyloid pathology with myelin alteration in preclinical Alzheimer disease. JAMA Neurol. 2017;74:41–9.

60. Blennow K. A review of fluid biomarkers for Alzheimer's disease: moving from CSF to blood. Neurol Ther. 2017;6:15–24.

61. De Vos A, Jacobs D, Struyfs H, Fransen E, Andersson K, Portelius E, et al. C-terminal neurogranin is increased in cerebrospinal fluid but unchanged in plasma in Alzheimer's disease. Alzheimers Dement. 2015;11:1461–9.

62. Forsova OS, Zakharov VV. High-order oligomers of intrinsically disordered brain proteins BASP1 and GAP-43 preserve the structural disorder. FEBS J. 2016;283:1550–69.

63. Musunuri S, Wetterhall M, Ingelsson M, Lannfelt L, Artemenko K, Bergquist J, et al. Quantification of the brain proteome in Alzheimer's disease using multiplexed mass spectrometry. J Proteome Res. 2014;13:2056–68.

64. Kim J, Suh J, Romano D, Truong MH, Mullin K, Hooli B, et al. Potential late-onset Alzheimer's disease-associated mutations in the ADAM10 gene attenuate α-secretase activity. Hum Mol Genet. 2009;18:3987–96.

65. Yuan XZ, Sun S, Tan CC, Yu JT, Tan L. The role of ADAM10 in Alzheimer's disease. J Alzheimers Dis. 2017;58:303–22.

66. Westwood S, Liu B, Baird AL, Anand S, Nevado-Holgado AJ, Newby D, et al. The influence of insulin resistance on cerebrospinal fluid and plasma biomarkers of Alzheimer's pathology. Alzheimers Res Ther. 2017;9:31.

Permissions

List of Contributors

Venexia M. Walker, Neil M. Davies and Richard M. Martin
Bristol Medical School: Population Health Sciences, University of Bristol, Bristol, UK
MRC Integrative Epidemiology Unit, University of Bristol, Bristol, UK

Patrick G. Kehoe
Dementia Research Group, University of Bristol, Bristol, UK
Bristol Medical School: Translational Health Sciences, University of Bristol, Bristol, UK

Clayton J. Vesperman, Lena L. Law, Jennifer M. Oh and Sanjay Asthana
Geriatric Research Education and Clinical Center, William S. Middleton Memorial Veterans Hospital, Madison, WI 53705, USA
Wisconsin Alzheimer's Disease Research Center, University of Wisconsin School of Medicine and Public Health, Madison, WI 53792, USA

Vincent Pozorski
Geriatric Research Education and Clinical Center, William S. Middleton Memorial Veterans Hospital, Madison, WI 53705, USA
Department of Neurology, University of Wisconsin School of Medicine and Public Health, Madison, WI 53705, USA

Cynthia M. Carlsson, Barbara B. Bendlin and Sterling C. Johnson
Geriatric Research Education and Clinical Center, William S. Middleton Memorial Veterans Hospital, Madison, WI 53705, USA
Wisconsin Alzheimer's Disease Research Center, University of Wisconsin School of Medicine and Public Health, Madison, WI 53792, USA
Wisconsin Alzheimer's Institute,University of Wisconsin School of Medicine and Public Health, Madison, WI 53705, USA

Ozioma C. Okonkwo
Geriatric Research Education and Clinical Center, William S. Middleton Memorial Veterans Hospital, Madison, WI 53705, USA
Wisconsin Alzheimer's Disease Research Center, University of Wisconsin School of Medicine and Public Health, Madison, WI 53792, USA

Wisconsin Alzheimer's Institute,University of Wisconsin School of Medicine and Public Health, Madison, WI 53705, USA
Department of Medicine and Alzheimer's Disease Research Center, University of Wisconsin School of Medicine and Public Health, Madison, WI 53792, USA

Catherine L. Gallagher
Geriatric Research Education and Clinical Center, William S. Middleton Memorial Veterans Hospital, Madison, WI 53705, USA
Wisconsin Alzheimer's Disease Research Center, University of Wisconsin School of Medicine and Public Health, Madison, WI 53792, USA
Department of Neurology, University of Wisconsin School of Medicine and Public Health, Madison, WI 53705, USA

Yue Ma
Wisconsin Alzheimer's Disease Research Center, University of Wisconsin School of Medicine and Public Health, Madison, WI 53792, USA

Mark A. Sager
Wisconsin Alzheimer's Disease Research Center, University of Wisconsin School of Medicine and Public Health, Madison, WI 53792, USA
Wisconsin Alzheimer's Institute,University of Wisconsin School of Medicine and Public Health, Madison, WI 53705, USA

Bruce P. Hermann
Wisconsin Alzheimer's Disease Research Center, University of Wisconsin School of Medicine and Public Health, Madison, WI 53792, USA
Wisconsin Alzheimer's Institute,University of Wisconsin School of Medicine and Public Health, Madison, WI 53705, USA
Department of Neurology, University of Wisconsin School of Medicine and Public Health, Madison, WI 53705, USA

Ryan J. Dougherty
Wisconsin Alzheimer's Disease Research Center, University of Wisconsin School of Medicine and Public Health, Madison, WI 53792, USA
Department of Kinesiology, University of Wisconsin School of Education, Madison, WI 53792, USA

Howard A. Rowley
Wisconsin Alzheimer's Disease Research Center, University of Wisconsin School of Medicine and Public Health, Madison, WI 53792, USA
Department of Radiology, University of Wisconsin School of Medicine and Public Health, Madison, WI 53705, USA

Dane B. Cook
Department of Kinesiology, University of Wisconsin School of Education, Madison, WI 53792, USA
Research Service, William S. Middleton Memorial Veterans Hospital, Madison, WI 53705, USA

Elizabeth Boots
Department of Psychology, University of Illinois-Chicago, Chicago, IL 60607, USA
Rush Alzheimer's Disease Center, Rush University Medical Center, Chicago, IL 60612, USA

Monica Shin, Joseph Therriault, Kok Pin Ng, Andrea L. Benedet and Serge Gauthier
Translational Neuroimaging Laboratory, The McGill University Research Centre for Studies in Aging, 6825 LaSalle Boulevard, Verdun, QC H4H 1R3,Canada

Tharick A. Pascoal, Min Su Kang and Sulantha Mathotaarachchi
Translational Neuroimaging Laboratory, The McGill University Research Centre for Studies in Aging, 6825 LaSalle Boulevard, Verdun, QC H4H 1R3,Canada
Montreal Neurological Institute, 3801 University Street, Montreal, QC H3A 2B4, Canada

Pedro Rosa-Neto
Translational Neuroimaging Laboratory, The McGill University Research Centre for Studies in Aging, 6825 LaSalle Boulevard, Verdun, QC H4H 1R3,Canada
Montreal Neurological Institute, 3801 University Street, Montreal, QC H3A 2B4, Canada. 4Douglas Hospital, McGill University, 6875 La Salle Blvd—FBC room 3149, Montreal, QC H4H 1R3, Canada

Mira Chamoun, Daniel Chartrand, Robert Hopewell, Reda Bouhachi, Hung-Hsin Hsiao, Jean-Paul Soucy and Gassan Massarweh
Montreal Neurological Institute, 3801 University Street, Montreal, QC H3A 2B4, Canada

Idriss Bennacef
Translational Biomarkers, Merck and Co., Inc., 770 Sumneytown Pike, West Point, PA 19486, USA

Shraddha Sapkota and Joel Ramirez
Hurvitz Brain Sciences Research Program, Sunnybrook Research Institute, Sunnybrook Health Sciences Centre, 2075 Bayview Avenue, M6-192, Toronto,ON M4N 3M5, Canada

Donald T. Stuss
Hurvitz Brain Sciences Research Program, Sunnybrook Research Institute, Sunnybrook Health Sciences Centre, 2075 Bayview Avenue, M6-192, Toronto,ON M4N 3M5, Canada
Departments of Medicine, University of Toronto, 190 Elizabeth Street, R. Fraser Elliot Building, 3-805, Toronto, ON M5G 2C4,Canada
Department of Psychology, University of Toronto, 100 St. George Street, 4th Floor, Sidney Smith Hall, Toronto, ON M5S 3G3, Canada
Rotman Research Institute of Baycrest Centre, 3560 Bathurst Street, Toronto, ON M6H 4A6, Canada

Mario Masellis and Sandra E. Black
Department of Medicine (Neurology), University of Toronto, 190 Elizabeth Street, R. Fraser Elliot Building, 3-805, Toronto, ON M5G 2C4,Canada

Umesh Gangishetti, Kelly D. Watts and Alexander Kollhoff
Department of Neurology, Emory University, 615 Michael Street, 505F, Atlanta, GA 30322, USA

J. Christina Howell and William T. Hu
Department of Neurology, Emory University, 615 Michael Street, 505F, Atlanta, GA 30322, USA
Department of Alzheimer's Disease Research Center, Emory University, Atlanta, GA, USA

Richard J. Perrin
Knight Alzheimer's Disease Research Center, Washington University, St. Louis, MO, USA.
Department of Pathology, Washington University, St. Louis, MO, USA

Anne M. Fagan and John C. Morris
Knight Alzheimer's Disease Research Center, Washington University, St. Louis, MO, USA
Department of Neurology, Washington University, St. Louis, MO, USA

Natalia Louneva
Department of Pathology, Washington University, St. Louis, MO, USA

John Q. Trojanowski
Penn Memory Center, University of Pennsylvania, Philadelphia, PA, USA
Center for Neurodegenerative Disease Research, University of Pennsylvania, Philadelphia, PA, USA.
Department of Pathology and Laboratory Medicine, University of Pennsylvania, Philadelphia, PA, USA

Steven E. Arnold
Penn Memory Center, University of Pennsylvania, Philadelphia, PA, USA
Center for Neurodegenerative Disease Research, University of Pennsylvania, Philadelphia, PA, USA.
Present Address: Massachusetts General Hospital, Boston, MA, USA

David A. Wolk
Penn Memory Center, University of Pennsylvania, Philadelphia, PA, USA
Department of Neurology, University of Pennsylvania, Philadelphia, PA, USA

Murray Grossman
Center for Neurodegenerative Disease Research, University of Pennsylvania, Philadelphia, PA, USA
Penn FTD Center, University of Pennsylvania, Philadelphia, PA, USA
Department of Neurology, University of Pennsylvania, Philadelphia, PA, USA

Leslie M. Shaw
Department of Pathology and Laboratory Medicine, University of Pennsylvania, Philadelphia, PA, USA

Marieke P. Hoevenaar-Blom, Willem A. van Gool and Jan-Willem van Dalen
Department of Neurology, Academic Medical Center (AMC), Meibergdreef 9, 1105, AZ, Amsterdam, the Netherlands

Tessa van Middelaar and Edo Richard
Department of Neurology, Academic Medical Center (AMC), Meibergdreef 9, 1105, AZ, Amsterdam, the Netherlands
Department of Neurology, Donders Institute for Brain, Cognition and Behaviour, Radboud University Medical Center, Nijmegen, the Netherlands

Eric P. Moll van Charante
Department of General Practice, Amsterdam Public Health Research Institute, Academic Medical Center (AMC), Amsterdam, the Netherlands

Kay Deckers and Sebastian Köhler
Department of Psychiatry and Neuropsychology, Alzheimer Center Limburg, Maastricht University, Maastricht, the Netherlands

Jana Crum and Jeffrey Wilson
Arizona State University, Tempe, AZ, USA

Marwan Sabbagh
Department of Neurology, Barrow Neurological Institute, Phoenix, AZ, USA
Cleveland Clinic Lou Ruvo Center for Brain Health, 888 W. Bonneville Ave, Las Vegas, NV 89106, USA

Yu An, Xiaona Zhang, Ying Wang, Yushan Wang, Lingwei Tao and Rong Xiao
School of Public Health, Capital Medical University, No.10 Xitoutiao, You An Men Wai, Beijing 100069, China

Lingli Feng
School of Public Health, Capital Medical University, No.10 Xitoutiao, You An Men Wai, Beijing 100069, China
Peking university First Hospital, Beijing, China

Yanhui Lu
School of Public Health, Capital Medical University, No.10 Xitoutiao, You An Men Wai, Beijing 100069, China
Linyi Mental Health Center, Linyi, Shandong, China

Zhongsheng Qin
Jincheng People's Hospital, Jincheng, Shanxi, China

Gloria Benson and Claudia Schwarz
NeuroCure Clinical Research Center, Department of Neurology, Charité –Universitätsmedizin Berlin, Freie Universität Berlin, Humboldt-Universität zu Berlin, Berlin Institute of Health, Berlin, Germany

Theresa Köbe
NeuroCure Clinical Research Center, Department of Neurology, Charité –Universitätsmedizin Berlin, Freie Universität Berlin, Humboldt-Universität zu Berlin, Berlin Institute of Health, Berlin, Germany.
Department of Psychiatry, McGill University, Montreal, Quebec, Canada

Douglas Mental Health University Institute, Studies on Prevention of Alzheimer's Disease Centre, Montreal, Quebec, Canada

Miranka Wirth
NeuroCure Clinical Research Center, Department of Neurology, Charité –Universitätsmedizin Berlin, Freie Universität Berlin, Humboldt-Universität zu Berlin, Berlin Institute of Health, Berlin, Germany
Center for Stroke Research Berlin, Charité – Universitätsmedizin Berlin, Freie Universität Berlin, Humboldt-Universität zu Berlin, Berlin Institute of Health, Berlin, Germany

Andrea Hildebrandt
Department of Psychology, University Medicine Greifswald, Greifswald, Germany
Department of Psychology, Humboldt-Universität zu Berlin, Berlin, Germany

Werner Sommer
Department of Psychology, Humboldt-Universität zu Berlin, Berlin, Germany

Catharina Lange
Department of Nuclear Medicine, Charité – Universitätsmedizin Berlin, Freie Universität Berlin, Humboldt-Universität zu Berlin, Berlin Institute of Health, Berlin,Germany

Agnes Flöel
Department of Neurology, University Medicine Greifswald, Greifswald, Germany

Elles Konijnenberg, Mara ten Kate, Jori Tomassen, Linda Wesselman, Matteo Demuru, Femke H. Bouwman and Philip Scheltens
Alzheimer Center, Department of Neurology, VU University Medical Center, Neuroscience Amsterdam, PO Box 7057, 1007 MB Amsterdam, The Netherlands

Anouk den Braber
Alzheimer Center, Department of Neurology, VU University Medical Center, Neuroscience Amsterdam, PO Box 7057, 1007 MB Amsterdam, The Netherlands
Department of Biological Psychology, VU University, Neuroscience Amsterdam, Amsterdam, The Netherlands

Pieter Jelle Visser
Alzheimer Center, Department of Neurology, VU University Medical Center, Neuroscience Amsterdam, PO Box 7057, 1007 MB Amsterdam, The Netherlands
Department of Psychiatry and Neuropsychology, School for Mental Health and Neuroscience, Alzheimer Center Limburg, Maastricht University, Maastricht, The Netherlands

Stephen F. Carter, Chinenye Amadi, Karl Herholz and Neil Pendleton
Wolfson Molecular Imaging Centre, Division of Neuroscience and Experimental Psychology, University of Manchester, Manchester, UK

Dorret I. Boomsma
Department of Biological Psychology, VU University, Neuroscience Amsterdam, Amsterdam, The Netherlands

Hoang-Ton Nguyen, Annette C. Moll, Frank D. Verbraak and Jacoba A. van de Kreeke
Department of Ophthalmology, VU University Medical Center, Neuroscience Amsterdam, Amsterdam, The Netherlands

Maqsood Yaqub, Adriaan A. Lammertsma and Bart N. M. van Berckel
Department of Radiology and Nuclear Medicine, VU University Medical Center, Neuroscience Amsterdam, Amsterdam, The Netherlands

Frederik Barkhof
Department of Radiology and Nuclear Medicine, VU University Medical Center, Neuroscience Amsterdam, Amsterdam, The Netherlands
Institutes of Neurology and Healthcare Engineering, UCL, London, UK

Charlotte E. Teunissen
Neurochemistry Laboratory, Department of Clinical Chemistry, VU University Medical Center, Neuroscience Amsterdam, Amsterdam, The Netherlands

Arjan Hillebrand
Department of Clinical Neurophysiology, VU University Medical Center, Neuroscience Amsterdam, Amsterdam, The Netherlands

Erik H. Serné
Department of Internal Medicine, VU University Medical Center, Neuroscience Amsterdam, Amsterdam, The Netherlands

Rainer Hinz
Wolfson Molecular Imaging Centre, Division of Informatics, Imaging and Data Sciences, Faculty of Medicine, Biology and Health, University of Manchester, Manchester, UK

Ananya Chakraborty, Ruud D. Fontijn and Helga E. de Vries
Department of Molecular Cell Biology and Immunology, Amsterdam Neuroscience, VU University Medical Center, De Boelelaan 1108, 1007 MB Amsterdam, The Netherlands

Madhurima Chatterjee, Harry Twaalfhoven, Marta Del Campo Milan and Charlotte E. Teunissen
Department of Clinical Chemistry, VU University Medical Center, Amsterdam, The Netherlands

Philip Scheltens
Alzheimer Centre and Department of Neurology, Amsterdam Neuroscience, VU University Medical Center, Amsterdam, The Netherlands

Wiesje M. van Der Flier
Alzheimer Centre and Department of Neurology, Amsterdam Neuroscience, VU University Medical Center, Amsterdam, The Netherlands
Department of Epidemiology and Biostatistics, Amsterdam Neuroscience, VU University Medical Centrer, Amsterdam, The Netherlands

Lara Paracchini, Luca Beltrame and Sergio Marchini
Department of Oncology, Istituto di Ricerche Farmacologiche Mario Negri IRCCS, Via La Masa 19, 20156 Milan, Italy

Lucia Boeri
Dipartimento di Chimica, Materialie Ingegneria Chimica "G. Natta", Politecnico di Milano, Piazza Leonardo da Vinci 32, 20133 Milan, Italy

Federica Fusco, Diego Albani and Gianluigi Forloni
Department of Neuroscience, Istituto di Ricerche Farmacologiche Mario Negri IRCCS, Via La Masa 19, 20156 Milan, Italy

Paolo Caffarra
Department of Neuroscience, Istituto di Neurologia, Università di Parma, Via Gramsci 14, 43100 Parma, Italy

Dahyun Yi and Min Soo Byun
Institute of Human Behavioral Medicine, Medical Research Center Seoul National University, Seoul, Republic of Korea

Dong Young Lee
Institute of Human Behavioral Medicine, Medical Research Center Seoul National University, Seoul, Republic of Korea
Department of Neuropsychiatry, Seoul National University Hospital, Seoul, Republic of Korea
Department of Psychiatry, Seoul National University College of Medicine, 101 Daehak-ro, Jongno-gu, Seoul 03080, Republic of Korea

Younghwa Lee, Jun Ho Lee and Kang Ko
Department of Neuropsychiatry, Seoul National University Hospital, Seoul, Republic of Korea

Bo Kyung Sohn
Department of Psychiatry, Sanggye Paik Hospital, Inje University College of Medicine, Seoul, Republic of Korea

Young Min Choe
Department of Neuropsychiatry, University of Ulsan College of Medicine, Ulsan University Hospital, Ulsan, Republic of Korea

Hyo Jung Choi
Department of Neuropsychiatry, SMG-SNU Boramae Medical Center, Seoul, Republic of Korea

Hyewon Baek
Department of Neuropsychiatry, Kyunggi Provincial Hospital for the Elderly, Yongin, Republic of Korea

Chul-Ho Sohn
Department of Radiology, Seoul National University College of Medicine and Seoul National University Hospital, Seoul, Republic of Korea

Yu Kyeong Kim
Department of Nuclear Medicine, SMG-SNU Boramae Medical Center, Seoul, Republic of Korea

Simon Hsu, Joanne B. Norton, Adia Louden, Carlos Cruchaga and Celeste M. Karch
Department of Psychiatry, Washington University School of Medicine, 425 S. Euclid Ave, Campus Box 8134, St. Louis, MO 63110, USA

Brian A. Gordon and Russ Hornbeck
Department of Radiology, Washington University School of Medicine, St. Louis, MO, USA

Tammie L. S. Benzinger
Department of Radiology, Washington University School of Medicine, St. Louis, MO, USA
Mallinckrodt Institute of Radiology, Washington University School of Medicine, St. Louis, MO 63110,USA

Denise Levitch, Ellen Ziegemeier, Gregory S. Day, Eric McDade, John C. Morris, Anne M. Fagan and Randall J. Bateman
Department of Neurology, Washington University School of Medicine, St. Louis, MO, USA

Robert Laforce Jr.
Clinique Interdisciplinaire de Mémoire du CHU de Québec, Département des Sciences Neurologiques, Faculté de Médecine, Université Laval, Québec City, Québec, Canada

Jasmeer Chhatwal
Massachusetts General Hospital/ Martinos Center for Biomedical Imaging, 149 13th Street, Gerontology Research Room 2669, Charlestown, MA 02129, USA

Alison M. Goate
Department of Neuroscience, Mount Sinai School of Medicine, New York, NY, USA

Mara ten Kate and Philip Scheltens
Alzheimer Center and Department of Neurology, VU University Medical Center, PO Box 7057, 1007 MB Amsterdam, the Netherlands

Pieter Jelle Visser
Alzheimer Center and Department of Neurology, VU University Medical Center, PO Box 7057, 1007 MB Amsterdam, the Netherlands
Alzheimer Centrum Limburg, Department of Psychiatry and Neuropsychology, Maastricht University, Maastricht, the Netherlands

Alberto Redolfi, Enrico Peira and Silvia Bianchetti
Laboratory of Epidemiology and Neuroimaging, IRCCS San Giovanni di Dio Fatebenefratelli, Brescia, Italy

Giovanni Frisoni
Laboratory of Epidemiology and Neuroimaging, IRCCS San Giovanni di Dio Fatebenefratelli, Brescia, Italy
University of Geneva, Geneva, Switzerland

Isabelle Bos, Stephanie J. Vos and Frans R. J. Verhey
Alzheimer Centrum Limburg, Department of Psychiatry and Neuropsychology, Maastricht University, Maastricht, the Netherlands

Rik Vandenberghe, Silvy Gabel, Jolien Schaeverbeke
University Hospital Leuven, Leuven, Belgium
Laboratory for Cognitive Neurology, Department of Neurosciences, KU Leuven, Leuven, Belgium

Olivier Blin
AP-HM, CHU Timone, CIC CPCET, Service de Pharmacologie Clinique et Pharmacovigilance, Marseille, France

Jill C. Richardson
Neurosciences Therapeutic Area Unit, GlaxoSmithKline R&D, Stevenage, UK

Regis Bordet
U1171 Inserm, CHU Lille, Degenerative and Vascular Cognitive Disorders, University of Lille, Lille, France

Anders Wallin and Carl Eckerstrom
Sahlgrenska Academy, Institute of Neuroscience and Physiology, Section for Psychiatry and Neurochemistry, University of Gothenburg, Gothenburg, Sweden

José Luis Molinuevo
Barcelona βeta Brain Research Center, Pasqual Maragall Foundation, Barcelona, Spain

Sebastiaan Engelborghs
Reference Center for Biological Markers of Dementia (BIODEM), Institute Born-Bunge, University of Antwerp, Antwerp, Belgium

Department of Neurology and Memory Clinic, Hospital Network Antwerp (ZNA) Middelheim and Hoge Beuken, Antwerp, Belgium

Johannes Streffer
Reference Center for Biological Markers of Dementia (BIODEM), Institute Born-Bunge, University of Antwerp, Antwerp, Belgium
UCB Biopharma SPRL, Braine-l'Alleud, Belgium

Christine Van Broeckhoven
Neurodegenerative Brain Diseases, Center for Molecular Neurology, VIB, Antwerp, Belgium. Laboratory of Neurogenetics, Institute Born-Bunge, University of Antwerp, Antwerp, Belgium

Pablo Martinez-Lage
Department of Neurology, Center for Research and Advanced Therapies, CITA-Alzheimer Foundation, San Sebastian, Spain

Julius Popp
Department of Psychiatry, University Hospital of Lausanne, Lausanne, Switzerland
Geriatric Psychiatry, Department of Mental Health and Psychiatry, Geneva University Hospitals, Geneva, Switzerland

Magdalini Tsolaki
Memory and Dementia Center, 3rd Department of Neurology, "G Papanicolau" General Hospital, Aristotle University of Thessaloniki, Thessaloniki, Greece

Alison L. Baird and Simon Lovestone
University of Oxford, Oxford, UK

Cristina Legido-Quigley
King's College London, London, UK

Valerija Dobricic
Lübeck Interdisciplinary Platform for Genome Analytics, University of Lübeck, Lubeck, Germany

Lars Bertram
Lübeck Interdisciplinary Platform for Genome Analytics, University of Lübeck, Lubeck, Germany. School of Public Health, Imperial College London, London, UK
Department of Psychology, University of Oslo, Oslo,Norway

Henrik Zetterberg
Department of Psychiatry and Neurochemistry, University of Gothenburg, Mölndal, Sweden. Department of Molecular Neuroscience, UCL Institute of Neurology, Queen Square, London, UK
UK Dementia Research Institute at UCL, London, UK
Clinical Neurochemistry Laboratory, Sahlgrenska University Hospital, Mölndal, Sweden

Gerald P. Novak
Janssen Pharmaceutical Research and Development, Titusville, NJ, USA

Jerome Revillard
MAAT, Archamps, France

Mark F. Gordon
Teva Pharmaceuticals, Inc., Malvern, PA, USA
Boehringer Ingelheim Pharmaceuticals, Inc., Ridgefield, CT, USA

Zhiyong Xie
Worldwide Research and Development, Pfizer Inc, Cambridge, MA, USA

Viktor Wottschel
Department of Radiology and Nuclear Medicine, VUMC, Amsterdam, the Netherlands

Frederik Barkhof
Department of Radiology and Nuclear Medicine, VUMC, Amsterdam, the Netherlands
Institutes of Neurology and Healthcare Engineering, UCL, London, UK

Karen Meersmans and Antonietta Gabriella Liuzzi
Laboratory for Cognitive Neurology, Department of Neurosciences, KU Leuven, Herestraat 49, 3000 Leuven, Belgium

Jolien Schaeverbeke, Silvy Gabel, Charlotte Evenepoel and Patrick Dupont
Laboratory for Cognitive Neurology, Department of Neurosciences, KU Leuven, Herestraat 49, 3000 Leuven, Belgium
Alzheimer Research Centre KU Leuven, Leuven Research Institute for Neuroscience and Disease, KU Leuven, Herestraat 49, 3000 Leuven, Belgium

Rose Bruffaerts and Rik Vandenberghe
Laboratory for Cognitive Neurology, Department of Neurosciences, KU Leuven, Herestraat 49, 3000 Leuven, Belgium
Alzheimer Research Centre KU Leuven, Leuven Research Institute for Neuroscience and Disease, KU Leuven, Herestraat 49, 3000 Leuven, Belgium.
Neurology Department, University Hospitals Leuven, Herestraat 49 - box 7003, 3000 Leuven, Belgium

Koen Van Laere
Alzheimer Research Centre KU Leuven, Leuven Research Institute for Neuroscience and Disease, KU Leuven, Herestraat 49, 3000 Leuven, Belgium.
Nuclear Medicine and Molecular Imaging, University Hospitals Leuven, Herestraat 49, 3000 Leuven, Belgium

Eva Dries and Karen Van Bouwel
Neurology Department, University Hospitals Leuven, Herestraat 49 - box 7003, 3000 Leuven, Belgium.

Anne Sieben
Neurodegenerative Brain Diseases Group, Center for Molecular Neurology, VIB, Universiteitsplein 1, 2610 Antwerp, Belgium
Institute Born-Bunge,Neuropathology and Laboratory of Neurochemistry and Behavior, University of Antwerp, Universiteitsplein 1, 2610 Antwerp, Belgium
Neurology Department, University Hospitals Ghent, Corneel Heymanslaan 10, 9000 Ghent, Belgium

Yolande Pijnenburg
Old Age Psychiatry Department, GGZinGeest, Van Hilligaertstraat 21, 1072 JX Amsterdam, The Netherlands
Alzheimer Center and Department of Neurology, VU University Medical Center, De Boelelaan 1117, 1081 HV Amsterdam, The Netherlands

Ronald Peeters
Radiology Department, University Hospitals Leuven, Herestraat 49, Leuven 30000, Belgium

Guy Bormans and Michel Koole
Laboratory of Radiopharmaceutical Research, KU Leuven, Herestraat 49, 3000 Leuven,Belgium
Nuclear Medicine and Molecular Imaging, University Hospitals Leuven, Herestraat 49, 3000 Leuven, Belgium

Loïc Dayon, Antonio Núñez Galindo, Ornella Cominetti, John Corthésy, Eugenia Migliavacca and India Severin
Nestlé Institute of Health Sciences, Lausanne, Switzerland

Martin Kussmann
Nestlé Institute of Health Sciences, Lausanne, Switzerland
Present address: Liggins Institute, University of Auckland, Auckland, New Zealand

Jérôme Wojcik
Precision for Medicine, Geneva, Switzerland

Aikaterini Oikonomidi
Old Age Psychiatry, Department of Psychiatry, CHUV, Lausanne, Switzerland

Gene L. Bowman and Julius Popp
Old Age Psychiatry, Department of Psychiatry, CHUV, Lausanne, Switzerland
Geriatric Psychiatry, Department of Mental Health and Psychiatry, HUG, Geneva, Switzerland

Hugues Henry
Department of Laboratories, CHUV,Lausanne, Switzerland

Index

A

Alzheimer Disease, 1, 17-18, 20, 32, 44-45, 54-55, 65, 71, 87, 99-100, 110, 118, 137, 148-149, 169, 187-188, 190, 199-201

Amyloid, 16, 19-20, 22, 24, 30, 32, 41, 45-49, 53-55, 66, 68-70, 87, 100-102, 104-107, 109-111, 114-115, 117-119, 122, 135-142, 144, 147-150, 153-172, 174, 178, 182-183, 185-193, 195-199, 201

Amyloid Pathology, 54-55, 101-102, 107, 109-110, 118, 140, 148, 158-159, 162, 164-169, 188, 190-191, 198-199, 201

Apoe, 18, 24, 35, 38, 42-43, 45, 47-49, 66-70, 102, 104-105, 107, 110-112, 118-122, 139, 142, 144, 147-149, 158-169, 192-195, 197, 199

Apoe Genotyping, 48, 120, 122, 160, 166, 193

Autopsy, 53, 66-70, 118, 152, 191

Autosomal Dominant, 99, 119, 150, 153, 156-157

B

Braak Stages, 66, 68-69, 71

C

Cardiorespiratory Fitness, 12-13, 15-18

Cell-based Assays, 150, 156

Cerebral Amyloid Deposition, 139

Cerebral Glucose Imaging, 141

Cerebral Glucose Metabolism, 139-140, 144, 146-147

Cerebral Vascular Dysfunction, 113

Cerebrospinal Fluid, 36, 44, 46-47, 53-55, 101-102, 105, 110-113, 115, 117-119, 136-137, 151, 159, 167, 169, 172, 174, 186, 188, 190-192, 195-197, 199-201

Cerebrovascular Pathology, 89-90, 96, 98-99

Cognitive Control Networks, 89-90, 98-99

Cognitive Function, 13, 15, 17-18, 63-64, 66, 72-73, 75, 84, 87-88, 98-99, 103, 111, 148

Cognitive Impairment, 17, 19-20, 24-27, 29-31, 33-36, 40-41, 43-48, 51-55, 66-67, 71-73, 84, 86-88, 95, 99-101, 103, 107, 110, 118, 158-159, 163-169, 191-192, 194-195, 198-201

Cognitive Pattern, 72

Cognitive Reserve, 33, 35-36, 39-40, 43-45, 89, 93, 97, 99-100

Crf Attenuates, 12, 15

D

Dementia, 1-5, 7-11, 13, 17, 19-21, 30-61, 63-67, 70-74, 77-79, 87-89, 99-103, 105, 107, 110-115, 117-118, 120, 122, 136-137, 140-141, 147-149, 156-164, 167-169, 174, 176, 180, 190-192, 201

Donepezil, 1-3, 5, 7, 9, 11

E

Exome Sequencing, 119-123, 137, 151-152

F

False Discovery Rate (FDR), 49, 75

Fatty Acid Binding Protein, 46-47, 50-51, 53, 55

Flair, 12-13, 18, 89, 92, 100, 104, 110, 114, 160-161

Frontotemporal Dementia, 33-34, 36, 43-44, 47, 54, 137, 171, 201

Ftld, 54-55, 171, 185-186

Functional Connectivity, 44, 89-90, 92-98, 100, 106, 168

G

Galantamine, 1-3, 5, 7, 9, 11

Genomic Dna, 112, 136, 141, 151

I

Interleukin-10, 46

L

Libra Index, 56-61, 63-64

M

Magnetoencephalography, 101, 106, 110, 112

Mass Spectrometry, 55, 112, 190, 199-201

Memantine, 1-3, 5, 9-11

Mild Cognitive Impairment, 17, 19, 24-27, 29-31, 33, 36, 43-48, 51-52, 54, 66-67, 71, 73, 87-88, 95, 100, 118, 158-159, 163-168, 192, 199-201

Modifiable Dementia, 56-57, 63

Monozygotic Twins, 101, 108

Mri, 12-14, 17, 21, 30-32, 44-45, 89-90, 92, 100, 103-104, 106-107, 110-112, 114, 118, 139-141, 147, 149, 151, 157-162, 164-169, 171-172, 177-178, 184-186, 188-189, 192, 198-199

N

Neurofibrillary Tangles, 19-20, 25-26, 28-29, 31-32, 66, 101, 114, 147, 150, 159, 198

Neurofilament Light Chain, 46-47, 50-52, 54

Neuropsychological Testing, 103, 107, 159, 177

Non-beta-amyloid, 46, 53

O

Oxysterol, 72-73, 87

P

Pathogenicity Algorithm, 150-152

Positron Emission Tomography (PET), 19, 101, 139, 141, 171

Post Mortem, 66, 71

Prediva Trial, 56, 63-64

Principal Component Analysis (PCA), 72, 74

Psen1, 119, 135-136, 150-157, 169

Psen2, 119, 135, 150-157

R

R615h, 119-123, 135-136

Randomised Controlled Trial, 56-57, 64

Rivastigmine, 1-3, 5, 7, 9, 11

S

Seizure-related Gene 6 (SEZ6), 119, 138

Senile Plaques, 66, 114

Single-word Comprehension Deficits, 170-171, 178, 180, 183-185

Support Vector Machine, 158-159, 165-167, 169

Synergistic Interaction, 32, 139-140, 144

T

Tandem Mass Tag, 190, 201

Tau Cerebrospinal Fluid, 46

Tau Positron Emission Tomography, 19

Threonine 181, 47, 54, 151, 190, 192, 195-197, 199

U

Ultrasound Carotid Artery, 104

V

Vascular Dementia, 5, 8, 34, 43-44, 113-115, 117-118

Vascular Endothelial Growth Factor, 113-115, 117-118

Ventricular Atrophy, 34

Ventricular Size, 33-43

W

White Matter Hyperintensities, 12-15, 17-18, 36, 40, 43, 45, 99-100, 114, 161

White Matter Lesions (WML), 89, 96

www.ingramcontent.com/pod-product-compliance
Lightning Source LLC
Chambersburg PA
CBHW082037190326
41458CB00010B/3394